# Our Shrinking Globe: Implications for Child Safety

*Editor*

AVINASH K. SHETTY

# PEDIATRIC CLINICS OF NORTH AMERICA

www.pediatric.theclinics.com

*Consulting Editor*
BONITA F. STANTON

February 2016 • Volume 63 • Number 1

**ELSEVIER**

1600 John F. Kennedy Boulevard • Suite 1800 • Philadelphia, Pennsylvania, 19103-2899

http://www.theclinics.com

**THE PEDIATRIC CLINICS OF NORTH AMERICA Volume 63, Number 1**
**February 2016 ISSN 0031-3955, ISBN-13: 978-0-323-41708-2**

Editor: Kerry Holland
Developmental Editor: Casey Jackson

*The Pediatric Clinics of North America* (ISSN 0031-3955) is published bimonthly by Elsevier Inc., 360 Park Avenue South, New York, NY 10010-1710. Months of issue are February, April, June, August, October, and December. Periodicals postage paid at New York, NY and additional mailing offices. Subscription prices are $200.00 per year (US individuals), $556.00 per year (US institutions), $270.00 per year (Canadian individuals), $740.00 per year (Canadian institutions), $325.00 per year (international individuals), $740.00 per year (international institutions), $100.00 per year (US students and residents), and $165.00 per year (international and Canadian residents and students). To receive students/resident rare, orders must be accompanied by name of affiliated institution, date of term, and the signature of program/residency coordinator on institution letterhead. Orders will be billed at individual rate until proof of status is received. Foreign air speed delivery is included in all *Clinics* subscription prices. All prices are subject to change without notice. **POSTMASTER:** Send address changes to *The Pediatric Clinics of North America*, Elsevier Health Sciences Division, Subscription Customer Service, 3251 Riverport Lane, Maryland Heights, MO 63043. **Customer Service: 1-800-654-2452 (US and Canada). From outside of the US and Canada: 1-314-447-8871. Fax: 1-314-447-8029. For print support, E-mail: JournalsCustomerService-usa@elsevier.com. For online support, E-mail: JournalsOnlineSupport-usa@elsevier.com.**

*Reprints.* For copies of 100 or more, of articles in this publication, please contact the Commercial Reprints Department, Elsevier Inc., 360 Park Avenue South, New York, NY 10010-1710. Tel.: 212-633-3874; Fax: 212-633-3820; E-mail: reprints@elsevier.com.

*The Pediatric Clinics of North America* is also published in Spanish by McGraw-Hill Inter-americana Editores S.A., Mexico City, Mexico; in Portuguese by Riechmann and Affonso Editores, Rua Comandante Coelho 1085, CEP 21250, Rio de Janeiro, Brazil; and in Greek by Althayia SA, Athens, Greece.

*The Pediatric Clinics of North America* is covered in *MEDLINE/PubMed (Index Medicus), Excerpta Medica, Current Contents, Current Contents/Clinical Medicine, Science Citation Index, ASCA, ISI/BIOMED,* and *BIOSIS.*

Printed in the United States of America.

## PROGRAM OBJECTIVE

The goal of the *Pediatric Clinics of North America* is to keep practicing physicians and residents up to date with current clinical practice in pediatrics by providing timely articles reviewing the state-of-the-art in patient care.

## TARGET AUDIENCE

All practicing pediatricians, physicians and healthcare professionals who provide patient care to pediatric patients.

## LEARNING OBJECTIVES

Upon completion of this activity, participants will be able to:

1. Review prevention and control of childhood illness through global delivery of vaccines and special care of vulnerable populations.
2. Discuss the ethical, environmental, and safety issues in pediatric global health.
3. Recognize how globalization and new age technology are impacting global maternal, newborn, and child health.

## ACCREDITATION

The Elsevier Office of Continuing Medical Education (EOCME) is accredited by the Accreditation Council for Continuing Medical Education (ACCME) to provide continuing medical education for physicians.

The EOCME designates this enduring material for a maximum of 15 *AMA PRA Category 1 Credit*(s)™. Physicians should claim only the credit commensurate with the extent of their participation in the activity.

All other health care professionals requesting continuing education credit for this enduring material will be issued a certificate of participation.

## DISCLOSURE OF CONFLICTS OF INTEREST

The EOCME assesses conflict of interest with its instructors, faculty, planners, and other individuals who are in a position to control the content of CME activities. All relevant conflicts of interest that are identified are thoroughly vetted by EOCME for fair balance, scientific objectivity, and patient care recommendations. EOCME is committed to providing its learners with CME activities that promote improvements or quality in healthcare and not a specific proprietary business or a commercial interest.

**The planning committee, staff, authors and editors listed below have identified no financial relationships or relationships to products or devices they or their spouse/life partner have with commercial interest related to the content of this CME activity:**
Lisa Adams, MD; Andrew Adesman, MD; Olakunle Alonge, MBBS, MPH, PhD; Alexandra Bailin; Jennifer Beard, PhD, MA, MPH; Malcolm Bryant, MBBS, MPH; Jaya Chandna, MSc; Mohammod J. Chisti, MBBS, MMed, PhD; Ricky Choi, MD, MPH; Holly B. Fontenot, PhD, RN; Anjali Fortna; Caitlin Hansen, MD; Kerry Holland; Adnan A. Hyder, MD, MPH, PhD; Cara Jacobson; Uzma R. Khan, MBBS, MSc; Indu Kumari; Tim Lahey, MD, MMSc; Philip J. Landrigan, MD, MSc, FAAP; Daniel T. Leung, MD, MSc; Julie M. Linton, MD; Sharon E. Mace, MD, FAAP, FACEP; Melanie A. Marty, PhD; Fernando Mendoza, MD, MPH; Ruth Milanaik, DO; Mark D. Miller, MD, MPH; Elijah Paintsil, MD; Andrew T. Pavia, MD; Atif Rahman, MB BS, PhD; Avinash K. Shetty, MD, FAAP, FIDSA; Bonita F. Stanton, MD; Megan Suermann; Gautham K. Suresh, MD, DM, MS, FAAP; Nadja van Ginneken, MRCGP, PhD; Jannah Wigle, MSc; Lawrence S. Wissow, MD, MPH.

**The planning committee, staff, authors and editors listed below have identified financial relationships or relationships to products or devices they or their spouse/life partner have with commercial interest related to the content of this CME activity:**
**Gregory D. Zimet, PhD** is a consultant/advisor for, with research support from, Merck & Co., Inc.

## UNAPPROVED/OFF-LABEL USE DISCLOSURE

The EOCME requires CME faculty to disclose to the participants:

1. When products or procedures being discussed are off-label, unlabelled, experimental, and/or investigational (not US Food and Drug Administration [FDA] approved); and
2. Any limitations on the information presented, such as data that are preliminary or that represent ongoing research, interim analyses, and/or unsupported opinions. Faculty may discuss information about pharmaceutical agents that is outside of FDA-approved labelling. This information is intended solely for CME and is not intended to promote off-label use of these medications. If you have any questions, contact the medical affairs department of the manufacturer for the most recent prescribing information.

**TO ENROLL**
To enroll in the *Pediatric Clinics of North America* Continuing Medical Education program, call customer service at 1-800-654-2452 or sign up online at http://www.theclinics.com/home/cme. The CME program is available to subscribers for an additional annual fee of USD 290.

**METHOD OF PARTICIPATION**
In order to claim credit, participants must complete the following:
1. Complete enrolment as indicated above.
2. Read the activity.
3. Complete the CME Test and Evaluation. Participants must achieve a score of 70% on the test. All CME Tests and Evaluations must be completed online.

**CME INQUIRIES/SPECIAL NEEDS**
For all CME inquiries or special needs, please contact elsevierCME@elsevier.com.

# Contributors

## CONSULTING EDITOR

**BONITA F. STANTON, MD**
Vice Dean for Research and Professor of Pediatrics, School of Medicine, Wayne State University, Detroit, Michigan

## EDITOR

**AVINASH K. SHETTY, MD, FAAP, FIDSA**
Professor of Pediatrics, Chief, Pediatric Infectious Diseases; Director, Pediatric HIV Program, Associate Dean for Global Health, Director, Global Health Education, Wake Forest School of Medicine, Attending Physician, Brenner Children's Hospital, Winston-Salem, North Carolina

## AUTHORS

**LISA ADAMS, MD**
Associate Dean for Global Health, Associate Professor of Medicine, Associate Professor of Community and Family Medicine, Section of Infectious Diseases and International Health, Geisel School of Medicine at Dartmouth, Hanover, New Hampshire

**ANDREW ADESMAN, MD**
Division of Developmental and Behavioral Pediatrics, Cohen Children's Medical Center of New York, Northwell Health, Lake Success, New York

**OLAKUNLE ALONGE, MBBS, MPH, PhD**
International Injury Research Unit, Department of International Health, Johns Hopkins University Bloomberg School of Public Health, Baltimore, Maryland

**ALEXANDRA BAILIN**
Division of Developmental and Behavioral Pediatrics, Cohen Children's Medical Center of New York, Northwell Health, Lake Success, New York

**JENNIFER BEARD, PhD, MA, MPH**
Assistant Professor, Department of Global Health, Center for Global Health and Development, Boston University School of Public Health, Boston, Massachusetts

**MALCOLM BRYANT, MBBS, MPH**
Clinical Associate Professor, Department of Global Health, Center for Global Health and Development, Boston University School of Public Health, Boston, Massachusetts

**JAYA CHANDNA, MSc**
Department of Psychological Sciences, Institute of Psychology, Health and Society, University of Liverpool, Liverpool, United Kingdom

**MOHAMMOD J. CHISTI, MBBS, MMed, PhD**
Centre for Nutrition and Food Security, ICU and Respiratory Wards, Dhaka Hospital, International Centre for Diarrhoeal Disease Research, Dhaka, Bangladesh

**RICKY CHOI, MD, MPH**
Pediatrics, Asian Health Services Community Health Center, Oakland, California

**HOLLY B. FONTENOT, PhD, RN**
W.F. Connell School of Nursing, Boston College, Chestnut Hill, Massachusetts

**CAITLIN HANSEN, MD**
Associate Research Scientist, Department of Pediatrics, Yale University School of Medicine, New Haven, Connecticut

**ADNAN A. HYDER, MD, MPH, PhD**
International Injury Research Unit, Department of International Health, Johns Hopkins University Bloomberg School of Public Health, Baltimore, Maryland

**CARA JACOBSON**
Division of Developmental and Behavioral Pediatrics, Cohen Children's Medical Center of New York, Northwell Health, Lake Success, New York

**UZMA R. KHAN, MBBS, MSc**
Department of Emergency Medicine, Aga Khan University, Karachi, Pakistan

**TIM LAHEY, MD, MMSc**
Director of Education, The Dartmouth Institute for Health Policy and Clinical Practice; Associate Professor of Medicine, Geisel School of Medicine at Dartmouth, Hanover, New Hampshire; Staff Physician, Section of Infectious Diseases and International Health; Chair, Clinical Ethics Committee, Dartmouth-Hitchcock Medical Center, Lebanon, New Hampshire

**PHILIP J. LANDRIGAN, MD, MSc, FAAP**
Dean for Global Health, Arnhold Institute for Global Health, Professor of Preventive Medicine and Pediatrics, Icahn School of Medicine at Mount Sinai, New York, New York

**DANIEL T. LEUNG, MD, MSc**
Division of Infectious Diseases, Department of Medicine; Division of Microbiology and Immunology, Department of Pathology, University of Utah School of Medicine, Salt Lake City, Utah

**JULIE M. LINTON, MD**
Assistant Professor of Pediatrics, Department of Pediatrics, Wake Forest School of Medicine, Winston-Salem, North Carolina

**SHARON E. MACE, MD, FAAP, FACEP**
Professor of Medicine, Department of Emergency Medicine, Cleveland Clinic Lerner College of Medicine, Case Western Reserve University, Cleveland Clinic; Director of Research and Director of Observation Unit, Emergency Services Institute, Cleveland Clinic, Cleveland, Ohio

**MELANIE A. MARTY, PhD**
Acting Deputy Director, Office of Environmental Health Hazard Assessment, California Environmental Protection Agency, Sacramento, California

**FERNANDO MENDOZA, MD, MPH**
Professor of Pediatrics, Division of General Pediatrics, Lucile Packard Children Hospital; Associate Dean of Minority Advising and Programs, Stanford, California

**RUTH MILANAIK, DO**
Division of Developmental and Behavioral Pediatrics, Cohen Children's Medical Center of New York, Northwell Health, Lake Success, New York

**MARK D. MILLER, MD, MPH**
Director, Children's Environmental Health Program, Office of Environmental Health Hazard Assessment, California EPA, Oakland, California; Assistant Clinical Professor and Director, Western States Pediatric Environmental Health Specialty Unit, University of California, San Francisco, California

**ELIJAH PAINTSIL, MD**
Associate Professor of Pediatrics, Departments of Pediatrics, Pharmacology, and Public Health, Yale University School of Medicine, New Haven, Connecticut

**ANDREW T. PAVIA, MD**
Department of Pediatrics, University of Utah School of Medicine, Salt Lake City, Utah

**ATIF RAHMAN, MB BS, PhD**
Department of Psychological Sciences, Institute of Psychology, Health and Society, University of Liverpool, Liverpool, United Kingdom

**AVINASH K. SHETTY, MD, FAAP, FIDSA**
Professor of Pediatrics, Chief, Pediatric Infectious Diseases; Director, Pediatric HIV Program, Associate Dean for Global Health, Director, Global Health Education, Wake Forest School of Medicine, Attending Physician, Brenner Children's Hospital, Winston-Salem, North Carolina

**GAUTHAM K. SURESH, MD, DM, MS, FAAP**
Chief Medical Officer and Service Chief, The Newborn Center, Texas Children's Hospital, Professor of Pediatrics, Baylor College of Medicine, Houston, Texas

**NADJA VAN GINNEKEN, MRCGP, PhD**
Department of Health Services Research, Institute of Psychology, Health and Society, University of Liverpool, Liverpool, United Kingdom

**JANNAH WIGLE, MSc**
Division of Social and Behavioural Health Sciences, Dalla Lana School of Public Health, University of Toronto, Toronto, Ontario, Canada

**LAWRENCE S. WISSOW, MD, MPH**
Center for Mental Health in Pediatric Primary Care, Department of Health, Behavior, and Society, Johns Hopkins School of Public Health, Baltimore, Maryland

**GREGORY D. ZIMET, PhD**
Department of Pediatrics, Indiana University School of Medicine, Indianapolis, Indiana

# Contents

> Considerable progress has been made towards reducing under-5 childhood mortality in the Millennium Development Goals era. Reduction in newborn mortality has lagged behind maternal and child mortality. Effective implementation of innovative, evidence-based, and cost-effective interventions can reduce maternal and newborn mortality. Interventions aimed at the most vulnerable group results in maximal impact on mortality. Intervention coverage and scale-up remains low, inequitable and uneven in low-income countries due to numerous health-systems bottle-necks. Innovative service delivery strategies, increased integration and linkages across the maternal, newborn, child health continuum of care are vital to accelerate progress towards ending preventable maternal and newborn deaths.

> Children have rights, as enumerated in the Declaration of the Rights of the Child, and need protection from violence, exploitation, and abuse. Global threats to child safety exist. These threats include lack of basic needs (food, clean water, sanitation), maltreatment, abandonment, child labor, child marriage, female genital mutilation, child trafficking, disasters, and armed conflicts/wars. Recent disasters and armed conflicts have led to a record number of displaced people especially children and their families. Strategies and specific programs can be developed and implemented for eliminating threats to the safety of children.

> "Infectious diseases of poverty" (IDoP) describes infectious diseases that are more prevalent among poor and vulnerable populations, namely human immunodeficiency virus (HIV) infection, tuberculosis (TB), malaria, and neglected tropical diseases (NTDs). In 2013, 190,000 children died of HIV-related causes and there were 550,000 cases and 80,000 TB deaths in children. Children under age 5 account for 78% of malaria deaths

annually. NTDs remain a public health challenge in low- and middle-income countries. This article provides an overview of the major IDoP that affect children. Clinicians must be familiar with the epidemiology and clinical manifestations to ensure prompt diagnosis and treatment.

Pneumonia and diarrhea are the 2 leading infectious causes of death in children younger than 5 years worldwide, most of which occur in low- and middle-income countries (LMICs) in sub-Saharan Africa and Southern Asia. The past decade has seen large reductions in global childhood mortality, partly due to expansion of nonspecific public health interventions and vaccines against *Streptococcus pneumoniae, Haemophilus influenzae*, and rotavirus in LMICs. Further progress in this field depends on the international community's commitment to fund and implement programs using currently available vaccines and development of new vaccines against pathogens common to children in LMICs.

Worldwide, cervical cancer is the fourth most common cancer among women. Human papillomavirus (HPV) vaccination, if broadly implemented, has the potential to significantly reduce global rates of morbidity and mortality associated with cervical and other HPV-related cancers. More than 100 countries around the world have licensed HPV vaccines. As of February, 2015, there were an estimated 80 national HPV immunization programs and 37 pilot programs. This article discusses global implementation of HPV vaccination programs and issues such as vaccine financing and different approaches to HPV vaccine delivery.

Children's mental health problems are among global health advocates' highest priorities. Nearly three-quarters of adult disorders have their onset or origins during childhood, becoming progressively harder to treat over time. Integrating mental health with primary care and other more widely available health services has the potential to increase treatment access during childhood, but requires re-design of currently-available evidence-based practices to fit the context of primary care and place a greater emphasis on promoting positive mental health. While some of this re-design has yet to be accomplished, several components are currently well-defined and show promise of effectiveness and practicality.

Demographics indicate that pediatricians increasingly care for children in immigrant families in routine practice. Although these children may be at risk for health disparities relating to socioeconomic disadvantage and cultural or linguistic challenges, immigrant families have unique strengths and potential for resilience. Adaptive and acculturation processes concerning health and well-being can be mediated by cultural media. Pediatricians have a professional responsibility to address the medical, mental health, and social needs of immigrant families. Advocacy and research at the practice level and beyond can further explore the unique needs of this population and evidence-based strategies for health promotion.

In Sub-Saharan Africa, 15.1 million children have been orphaned because of human immunodeficiency virus (HIV). They face significant vulnerabilities, including stigma and discrimination, trauma and stress, illness, food insecurity, poverty, and difficulty accessing education. Millions of additional children who have living parents are vulnerable because their parents or other relatives are infected. This article reviews the current situation of orphans and vulnerable children, explores the underlying determinants of vulnerability and resilience, describes the response by the global community, and highlights the challenges as the HIV pandemic progresses through its fourth decade.

Children are especially vulnerable to environmental pollution, a major cause of disease, death, and disability in countries at every level of development. This article reviews threats to children, including air and water pollution, toxic industrial chemicals, pesticides, heavy metals, and hazardous wastes. Global climate change is expected to exacerbate many of these issues. Examples of innovative nongovernmental organizations and governmental programs that address the impacts of environmental hazards on children are included. International travel, adoption, migration, and movement of goods and pollutants worldwide make these conditions concerns for all pediatricians.

Unintentional injuries are a leading cause of deaths for children of all ages. Globally, they accounted for 15.4% of 2.6 million deaths recorded among children aged 1 to 14 years in 2013. The 12 highest burden countries in the world by absolute death count and mortality are low- and middle-income countries (LMIC) except for Russia and Equatorial Guinea. These countries accounted for 58% of the 406,442 unintentional injury deaths among 1 to 14 year olds in 2013. Globalization drives inequalities in the distribution of economic gains, risks, and opportunities for preventing child unintentional injuries between high-income countries and LMIC.

# PEDIATRIC CLINICS OF NORTH AMERICA

# Foreword

# Our Shrinking Globe: Implications for Child Safety

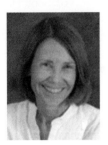

Bonita F. Stanton, MD
*Consulting Editor*

There are so many reasons why every pediatrician and child health care provider in the United States needs to know about global pediatric health issues.

There are practical reasons.

Virtually all pediatric practices will have contact with immigrant children. Approximately 14 million children living in the United States were born in another country. Roughly the same number was born in the United States to foreign-born parents. About one in four children live with at least one foreign-born parent.[1]

Virtually every pediatric practice will take care of children who have travelled abroad. Over 30 million Americans travel abroad each year; about one-tenth of adults are travelling with children[2]. Over the last half-century, the number travelling by air has been increasing—and is expected to continue to increase—by 5% to 10% per year.[3] Geographic boundaries have become virtually meaningless in terms of the spread of disease and are increasingly porous in terms of containment of violence.

More importantly, there are moral reasons.

It matters that every American pediatrician know about pediatric global health issues because children everywhere depend on adults. As child health providers, we are all morally and professionally obligated to advocate for the child—everywhere. Nowhere in any of our oaths did we promise to care only for children living in, born in, or naturalized in our country.

We care for them because they are children. We also care for them because we are preparing them to be tomorrow's adults. As child health care providers, we now know that the kind of adults they become will reflect the kind of childhood they enjoyed—or endured. We want tomorrow's adults to be propelled by love, excitement, creativity, and vision—not shackled by hatred, despair, and anger.

Pediatr Clin N Am 63 (2016) xv–xvi
http://dx.doi.org/10.1016/j.pcl.2015.10.002
0031-3955/16/$ – see front matter © 2016 Published by Elsevier Inc.

**pediatric.theclinics.com**

It is because we care for children that we must increase our understanding of childhood disease states and health status around the world.

Bonita F. Stanton, MD
School of Medicine
Wayne State University
1261 Scott Hall
540 East Canfield, Suite 1261
Detroit, MI 48201, USA

E-mail address:
bstanton@med.wayne.edu

**REFERENCES**

1. Available at: http://www.census.gov/newsroom/pdf/cspan_fb_slides.pdf.
2. Available at: http://perceptivetravel.com/blog/2010/12/21/american-tourist-statistics/.
3. Tatem AJ, Rogers DJ, Hay SI. Global transport networks and infectious disease spread. Adv Parasitol 2006;62:293–343.

# Preface

# Keeping Children Healthy and Safe Worldwide in the Era of Sustainable Development

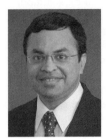

Avinash K. Shetty, MD, FAAP, FIDSA
*Editor*

Despite the shrinking world around us due to increased international trade, investment, spread of technology, and cultural exchange, global unevenness and inequalities persist across countries, regions, and communities that significantly impact the health of children. In September 2015, the United Nations member states formally adopted the new Sustainable Development Goals (SDGs), consisting of 17 goals and 169 targets toward achieving an integrated global goal of population health, economic prosperity, and social and environmental sustainability by 2030. Women and children remain the key to sustainable development. In the SDG era, children must be provided with an equal opportunity to live healthy lives and have access to education, good nutrition, and safe physical environment, regardless of their country of origin or obstacles they encounter. The current issue of *Pediatric Clinics of North America* entitled "Our Shrinking Globe: Implications for Child Safety" is devoted to address the myriad complex global health problems affecting children worldwide that seriously compromise their health, safety, and survival.

Despite substantial gains made in under-5 child survival, preventable maternal deaths and neonatal deaths continue to occur in low-income countries (LIC). Infectious diseases (eg, HIV, tuberculosis, malaria, and neglected tropical diseases) disproportionately affect children living in poverty. Combating poverty is the key to preventing and controlling infectious diseases in LIC. There is an urgent need to address the needs of orphans and vulnerable children due to HIV/AIDS in sub-Saharan Africa. Besides discovery of lifesaving interventions (eg, development of new and improved vaccines), we also need to do a better job at bridging the knowledge-implementation gap and increase the effectiveness of proven interventions. For example, despite the availability of effective vaccines to prevent pneumococcal pneumonia, rotavirus gastroenteritis, and human papilloma virus-related diseases (eg, cervical cancer), use of these

Pediatr Clin N Am 63 (2016) xvii–xviii
http://dx.doi.org/10.1016/j.pcl.2015.10.001
0031-3955/16/$ – see front matter © 2016 Published by Elsevier Inc.

**pediatric.theclinics.com**

vaccines remains suboptimal in LIC. Emerging and re-emerging infectious diseases (such as the 2014–2015 Ebola outbreak in West Africa) underscore the need for strengthening the existing fragile health systems in LIC, address complex ethical issues, and maintain effective community engagement, governance, and outbreak preparedness response and management.

Children are vulnerable for environmental health hazards (eg, contaminated water, poor sanitation, air pollution, toxic chemicals, and climate change) and unintentional injuries, which can result in mortality, morbidity, and disability. Other unique threats to child and adolescent safety include sex trafficking, sexual exploitation, violence and abuse, especially during wars, conflicts, and natural disasters. The explosion of new-age technology poses a considerable risk to children and adolescents. Pediatricians can play a vital role in promoting child health and development by providing services to the disadvantaged, socially isolated, and impoverished children and families in their local communities. Improving access, equity, and quality of care for immigrant and newly arrived refugee children in the United States remains a challenge. There is also an unmet need for mental health services for children and adolescents in the United States and worldwide.

As pediatricians, we must recognize that the health of children is a fundamental human right and strongly advocate for marginalized, low-income families. To protect children from toxic stress and reduce health inequalities, we must actively engage our patients and develop collaborative partnerships between various disciplines and across research, education, and service. Pediatricians engaged in global health service and research programs need to be aware of diverse sociocultural and ethical issues.

I am most grateful to all the authors for writing the state-of-the-art articles that will inspire pediatricians to remain strong advocates for promoting child health worldwide. I also want to thank Dr Bonita Stanton, consulting editor for this issue, and Casey Jackson and Kerry Holland at Elsevier for their continued support, cooperation, and advice in the preparation of this issue.

Avinash K. Shetty, MD, FAAP, FIDSA
Wake Forest School of Medicine
Department of Pediatrics
Brenner Children's Hospital
Medical Center Boulevard
Meads Hall, 3rd Floor
Winston-Salem, NC 27157, USA

E-mail address:
ashetty@wakehealth.edu

# Global Maternal, Newborn, and Child Health

## Successes, Challenges, and Opportunities

Avinash K. Shetty, MD*

## KEYWORDS

- Maternal health • Newborn health • Child health • Millennium Development Goals
- Sustainable development • Reproductive health

## KEY POINTS

- Considerable progress has occurred in the Millennium Development Goals era with substantial reductions in the mortality of children younger than 5 years.
- Reduction in newborn mortality has consistently lagged behind maternal and child mortality, and progress is uneven between countries and regions.
- Reduction of maternal, newborn, and child mortality is achievable through effective implementation of many innovative, high-impact, cost-effective, evidence-based interventions.
- Rapid scale-up of effective interventions, innovative service delivery strategies, and smart integration and linkages across the continuum of care is vital to accelerate progress toward improving maternal, newborn, and child survival.
- The goal of ending preventable maternal, newborn, and child deaths worldwide is achievable with the convergence of reproductive, maternal, newborn, child, and adolescent health with multi-stakeholder partnerships, multi-sectoral collaboration, and strong political leadership.

## INTRODUCTION

In recent years, increased attention has been focused on global reproductive, maternal, newborn, and child health (RMNCH).[1-7] The Millennium Development Goals (MDGs) were established in the year 2000 by leaders of 189 nations to achieve a set of targets by 2015 compared with the 1990 baseline level.[8] (**Box 1**). Health-related MDG4

Disclosure Statement: The author has nothing to disclose.
Pediatric HIV Program, Pediatric Infectious Diseases, Global Health Education, Wake Forest School of Medicine, Brenner Children's Hospital, Medical Center Boulevard, Winston-Salem, NC 27157, USA
* Department of Pediatrics, Wake Forest School of Medicine, Meads Hall, 3rd Floor, Medical Center Boulevard, Winston-Salem, NC 27157-1042.
E-mail address: ashetty@wakehealth.edu

Pediatr Clin N Am 63 (2016) 1–18
http://dx.doi.org/10.1016/j.pcl.2015.08.001
0031-3955/16/$ – see front matter © 2016 Elsevier Inc. All rights reserved.

**pediatric.theclinics.com**

was aimed at reducing child mortality by two-thirds, whereas MDG5 was aimed at reducing maternal mortality by three-quarters and achieving universal access to reproductive health by the year 2015; but other MDGs also impact the health of women and children.[8] Although considerable progress has occurred in the MDG era with substantial reductions in child mortality for those younger than 5 years, MDG4 targets will not be met in 2015.[9,10] In addition, decline in newborn mortality has consistently lagged behind the maternal mortality rate and the mortality rate of children younger than 5 years. Reduction of maternal, newborn, and child mortality is achievable through effective implementation of many innovative, evidence-based, cost-effective interventions.[11–18] Targeted interventions aimed at the most vulnerable group results in maximal impact on mortality.[4] However, maternal, newborn, and child health (MNCH) intervention coverage and scale-up remains low, inequitable, and uneven between low- and middle-income countries (LMIC) and regions because of numerous health-system bottlenecks, such as workforce, financing, and service delivery.[19,20]

The MDGs that end in September 2015 will be followed by a new set of goals: the Sustainable Development Goals (SDGs). Leaders representing the MNCH global community have recommended inclusion of new goals and targets for ending preventable newborn deaths and stillbirths as well as preventable maternal and child deaths in the post-2015 agenda.[21–23] More intensified and coordinated efforts will be needed by governments, multilateral organizations, and other stakeholders, including nongovernmental organizations, civil society, private sector, and policy makers from high-income countries (HIC), to accelerate progress and achieve sustainable, high-quality services to improve MNCH in the post-2015 era.[21–23]

## CURRENT SCOPE OF THE PROBLEM
### Maternal Health and Global Mortality Trends

Maternal health is defined as the health of women during pregnancy, childbirth, and post partum (first 42 days after delivery). In 2010, the maternal mortality ratio (MMR) in LMIC was estimated at 240 per 100,000 live births compared with 16 per 100,000 live births in HIC.[24] Between 1990 and 2013, maternal mortality rates declined by 45%; in 1990, an estimated 523,000 maternal deaths occurred compared with 289,000 deaths in 2013.[24] Although progress has been made, this decline in maternal

---

**Box 1**
**MDGs**

Goal 1: Eradicate extreme poverty and hunger

Goal 2: Achieve universal primary education

Goal 3: Promote gender equality and empower women

Goal 4: Reduce child mortality

Goal 5: Improve maternal health

Goal 6: Combat human immunodeficiency virus/AIDS, malaria, and other diseases

Goal 7: Ensure environmental sustainability

Goal 8: Develop a global partnership for development

*From* United Nations. Millennium Development Goals. New York: United Nations; 2014. Available at: http://www.un.org/millenniumgoals/. Accessed July 25 2015.

mortality rates fails to meet the MDG target of a 75% reduction between 1990 and 2015.[19,21] The MMR can vary markedly from country to country. For example, South Sudan has an MMR of 956.8 (685.1–1262.8), whereas Iceland has an MMR of 2.4 (1.6–3.6) in 2013.[25] Besides the risk of dying during pregnancy, labor, and post partum, women in LMIC also experience severe acute or chronic morbidities and disabilities with impaired quality of life.[26,27]

Most of the maternal deaths are largely preventable and occur in sub-Saharan Africa and Southern Asia; approximately 50% of maternal deaths occur in India, Nigeria, Pakistan, Afghanistan, Ethiopia, and the Democratic Republic of Congo.[8,24,25] Although the causes of death may vary from region to region, severe hemorrhage, pregnancy-induced hypertensive disorders, and sepsis account for more than half of preventable maternal deaths globally[28] (**Box 2**). The highest risk of maternal mortality occurs during the intrapartum or postpartum period.[25] Other important causes of maternal mortality include unsafe abortion and obstructed labor. Indirect and late causes of maternal mortality include infectious diseases of poverty, such as human immunodeficiency virus (HIV), malaria, and tuberculosis, and other preexisting conditions, such as diabetes, obesity, anemia, sickle cell disease, and chronic kidney disease.[28]

### Child and Newborn Global Mortality Trends

Child health is defined as the health of children younger than 5 years (perinatal <7 days old, neonate <29 days old, child <5 years of age). Between 1990 and 2013, mortality rates of children younger than 5 years declined by approximately 50%; in 1990, an estimated 12.7 million deaths occurred in children younger than 5 years compared with approximately 6.3 million deaths in 2013.[9,10] From 2000 to 2012, remarkable declines in child deaths have been noted in 22 high-burden countries in sub-Saharan Africa and South Asia, with annual rates of reduction in the mortality rates of children younger than 5 years of 4.4% or higher.[29]

---

**Box 2**
**Leading causes of maternal and younger-than-5 deaths worldwide**

*Maternal*

- Hemorrhage (27%)

- Pregnancy-induced hypertensive disorders (14%)

- Sepsis (11%)

- Unsafe abortions (8%)

- Other direct causes (12%)

- Other indirect causes (28%)

*Younger-than-5 deaths*

- Preterm birth complications (15.4%)

- Pneumonia (14.9%)

- Intrapartum complications (10.5%)

*Data from* Say L, Chou D, Gemmill A, et al. Global causes of maternal health: a WHO systematic analysis. Lancet Glob Health 2014;2:e323–33; and Liu L, Oza S, Hogan D, et al. Global, regional, and national causes of child mortality in 2000-13, with projections to inform post-2015 priorities: an updated systematic analysis. Lancet 2015;385:430–40.

Of the 6.3 million deaths of children younger than 5 years in 2013, 51.8% (3.257 million) were caused by infectious disease.[30] Pneumonia, diarrhea, and malaria are major causes of preventable deaths of children younger than 5 years beyond the neonatal period.[30] Pneumonia and diarrhea accounted for 15% and 9% of the estimated 6.3 million deaths of children younger than 5 years in 2013 globally.[9,30,31] It is estimated that childhood undernutrition (stunting, wasting, and micronutrient deficiencies) contributes to nearly 50% of child deaths (3.1 million deaths) annually.[15,21]

From 1990 to 2013, the annual rate of reduction (ARR) in maternal mortality was 3.5% and reduction in the mortality of children younger than 5 years was 3.6%; in contrast, ARR in neonatal mortality (deaths in the first 28 days of life) has lagged behind (2.2%).[3,9,24] In 2013, neonatal deaths accounted for 44% (2.761 million) of the 6.3 million deaths of children younger than 5 years.[30] There is variation in neonatal mortality rates across countries[32] (**Table 1**). The 5 highest-burden countries account for more than 50% of neonatal deaths.[32]

Preterm birth complications, intrapartum complications (birth asphyxia), and infections (sepsis, meningitis, pneumonia) remain primary causes of neonatal mortality[32] (see **Box 2**). In sub-Saharan Africa and South Asia, more than 80% of the neonatal deaths occurred in low-birthweight babies (typically preterm infants).[22] Data from 2000 to 2012 indicate slow progress (<20% reduction) toward prevention of deaths due to prematurity.[22,32] Approximately 2.6 million stillbirths (defined by the World Health Organization [WHO] as fetal death at a weight $\geq$1000 g and/or $\geq$28 weeks' gestation) occur annually; of these, 1.2 million deaths occur during the intrapartum period, usually due to poor care.[33–35]

### Factors Affecting Maternal, Newborn, and Child Health

In LMIC, women are at an increased health risk during pregnancy and childbirth. There are many social, economic, cultural, or behavioral factors that affect maternal and child health.[12,36,37] Key determinants, such as maternal education, poverty and

**Table 1**
**The 10 countries with the highest burden of neonatal and maternal deaths**

| Country | Neonatal Deaths, 2012 (No.) | Maternal Deaths, 2013 (No.) |
|---|---|---|
| India | 779,000 | 50,000 |
| Nigeria | 267,000 | 40,000 |
| Pakistan | 202,400 | 7900 |
| China | 157,400 | 5900 |
| Democratic Republic of the Congo | 118,100 | 21,000 |
| Ethiopia | 87,800 | 13,000 |
| Bangladesh | 75,900 | 5200 |
| Indonesia | 72,400 | 8800 |
| United Republic of Tanzania | 39,500 | 7900 |
| Kenya | 40,000 | 6300 |

*Data from* UNICEF, WHO, World Bank, UN. UN Inter-agency Group for Child Mortality Estimation. Levels and trends in child mortality: report 2014. New York: United Nations Children's Fund; 2014; and Lawn JE, Blencowe H, Oza S, et al. Every newborn: progress, priorities, and potential beyond survival. Lancet 2014;384:189–205.

poor housing, inequity in intervention coverage, community and social network systems, nutrition, lack of empowerment, financial autonomy, and armed conflict, can adversely affect MNCH outcomes.[19,38–41] About 800,000 neonatal deaths each year are attributable to maternal undernutrition.[15]

In South Asia and sub-Saharan Africa, children living in congested, urban informal settlements (or slums) are at an increased health risk because of air pollution or absence of clean water and sewage systems.[42–45] In both rural areas and urban slums, poor access to quality health care poses a serious threat to maternal and child health and survival.[12,44]

Conflicts, displacement, and natural disasters account for 60% of preventable maternal mortality, 54% of younger-than-5 mortality, and 45% of neonatal mortality.[9,24,46] Other unique health risks for girls and women include gender inequity and social inequalities in health.[47] Stigma and discrimination faced by HIV-infected women remain a hurdle to eliminate mother-to-child HIV transmission and achieve maternal and child health goals in LMIC.[48,49]

## INTERVENTIONS TO REDUCE MATERNAL, NEWBORN, AND CHILD MORTALITY

Many essential, evidence-based, low-cost, and high-impact interventions across the continuum of care can reduce maternal, newborn, and child morbidity and mortality[4,11–18,50] (**Box 3**).

Scale-up of effective high-impact, low-cost interventions during preconception (before and between pregnancy), antenatal, intrapartum, and postnatal periods could avert an estimated 71% of neonatal deaths, 33% of still births, and 54% of maternal deaths annually.[4] Care provided is cost-effective: savings are estimated to be $1298 for each life saved for an annual investment of $5.65 billion ($1.15 per person).[4] Innovative new newborn interventions, such as chlorhexidine cord cleansing and management of small and ill newborn infants, can be nested within other care packages and could save nearly 600,000 newborns per year by 2025 when care is delivered in sub-district and district-level facilities.[4] Chlorhexidine cord cleansing is associated with a 27% reduction in incidence of omphalitis and a 23% reduction in the risk of neonatal mortality.[53,54] Most effective packages of care are cost-effective and can avert 87% of maternal and neonatal deaths.[4]

## GAPS IN COVERAGE, EQUITY, AND QUALITY OF CARE

Substantial progress has been made toward achieving the MDG targets related to health. According to the 2015 WHO "Statistics Report," child undernutrition has declined by four-fifths, child mortality by two-thirds, maternal mortality by three-fifths, and in increasing access to sanitation by three-fifths.[55] Despite these advances, approximately 17,000 children younger than 5 years die each day, primarily from preventable causes.[9] High newborn mortality and stillbirths in Bangladesh, Afghanistan, Nepal, India, Pakistan, Malawi, and Uganda remain a major concern.[56] Uneven progress and significant disparities have been observed across many countries of the South Asian Association for Regional Cooperation.[56] High coverage of key MNCH interventions correlates with lower maternal and child death rates.[19] **Table 2** depicts the current coverage of selected key maternal and newborn interventions in the 75 high-burden countries.[4] Major emphasis for scaling-up essential interventions is focused on the 75 countdown countries where greater than 95% of all maternal and child deaths occur.[57,58]

Despite the existence of interventions to end preventable maternal and newborn deaths, coverage is poor and uneven in many LMIC.[4,19] Gaps in intervention coverage,

---

**Box 3**
**Key interventions to reduce maternal, newborn, and child mortality**

*Preconception and adolescent health interventions*
- Reduce unintended pregnancy
- Sex education
- Universal access to family planning services
- Optimize birth spacing
- Improve nutritional status (micronutrient supplementation)

*Antenatal interventions*
- Antenatal care (at least 4 visits)
- Vaccination (tetanus toxoid)
- Screening, treatment, and prevention of infectious diseases (HIV, syphilis, other sexually transmitted infections, malaria [intermittent preventive therapy], insecticide-treated bed nets)
- Management of chronic noncommunicable diseases (diabetes, hypertension)
- Management of pregnancy-induced disorders
- Diagnosis and management of in utero growth retardation
- Prevention of rhesus D alloimmunization
- Promotion of psychosocial health and support
- Cessation of smoking and substance use during pregnancy
- Nutritional supplementation for mothers before and during pregnancy
  - Folic acid supplementation and fortification
  - Multiple micronutrient supplementation (including iron and balanced energy supplementation)

*Intrapartum interventions*
- Skilled attendant at birth
- Emergency obstetric care
- Antenatal corticosteroids for preterm labor
- Antibiotics for premature rupture of membranes
- Management of preterm labor and post-term pregnancy

*Newborn and neonatal interventions*
- Essential newborn care at time of birth
  - Warming, drying, tactile stimulation, hygiene, and thermal care
  - Neonatal resuscitation for babies who do not breathe at birth
  - Umbilical cord care (including chlorhexidine application) and skin care
  - Newborn immunization
  - Early exclusive breastfeeding
  - Vitamin K administration
- Diagnosis and management of neonatal infection
- Management of birth-related complications
- Interventions for small and ill babies
  - Prevention of hypothermia

    ■ Kangaroo mother care (skin-to-skin care)
  - Management of respiratory distress syndrome
  - Management of infection (pneumonia and sepsis)

○ Management of hyperbilirubinemia
○ Topical emollient and massage therapy

*Child health interventions*

- Detection and management of severe childhood illness
  ○ Pneumonia, diarrhea, malaria

- Management of malnutrition

- Immunization (pneumococcus, *Haemophilus influenzae* type b, rotavirus, measles, and diphtheria and tetanus toxoids and pertussis vaccine)

- Nutritional interventions (vitamin A and zinc supplementation)

- Infant and young child feeding

- HIV prevention and treatment

- Water, sanitation, and hygiene interventions

*Data from* Refs.[4,12,17,51,52]

equity and quality of care around birth, care of small and ill newborn babies, reproductive health, and case management of pneumonia, diarrhea, and malaria in children younger than 5 years exists in many LMIC.[4,19,21] These gaps include weak health systems; lack of access to facilities, basic equipment, medication, and supplies and in some settings; poor birth-attendant skills; insufficient numbers of trained health care providers; lack of financial support; and poor quality of care.[4,20,59,60] Based on a systematic evaluation, frequently cited implementation bottlenecks for effective coverage of newborn health interventions in low-income countries included health workforce, financing, and service delivery.[20]

## INNOVATIVE APPROACHES TO ACCELERATE SCALE-UP

Rapid scale-up of key high-impact MNCH interventions targeting hard-to-reach mothers and newborns in high-burden countries can achieve reductions in excess mortality and reduce inequalities.[61,62] A recent cross-sectional analysis from 81 demographic and health surveys from 35 countries in sub-Saharan Africa suggested that improved coverage of proven life-saving interventions will result in further declines in mortality in children younger than 5 years.[63]

### Outreach Delivery Pathways

Given the severe shortage of health professionals in LMIC,[64] innovative strategies have been developed to improve access and deliver services to the mothers and newborns most in need, such as development of community-based delivery platforms led by community health workers (CHW), community mobilization, leadership and engagement, mobile health technology platforms, child health days, integrated management of childhood illness, and financial incentives, such as conditional cash transfer programs.[4,12,65]

*Community delivery platforms* can result in increased coverage of critical interventions to prevent morbidity and mortality from childhood pneumonia and diarrhea and improve maternal and child nutrition in LMIC.[15,50,66] The deployment of trained CHW (task-shifting approach) to deliver care packages to hard-to-reach populations (eg, rural communities) has been shown to be beneficial in the provision of expanded antenatal care, emergency obstetric care, newborn resuscitation, perinatal and newborn

**Table 2**
**Current coverage of selected key maternal and newborn interventions in the 75 high-burden countries**

| Key Interventions | Coverage (%) |
|---|---|
| Antenatal | |
| Tetanus toxoid immunization | 68 |
| ITPp or ITN | 37 |
| Syphilis screening and therapy | 23 |
| ANC ($\geq$4 visits) | 48 |
| Labor and delivery | |
| Steroids for preterm labor | 41 |
| Antibiotics for PROM | 41 |
| Skilled birth attendance | 61 |
| Facility delivery | 55 |
| Clean birth practices | 49 |
| Immediate newborn care/care of healthy neonate | |
| Neonatal resuscitation | 25 |
| Clean postnatal practices | 11 |
| Exclusive breastfeeding at 1 mo | 62 |
| Care of the small and ill neonate | |
| Simple thermal care of neonate | 11 |
| Oral antibiotics for neonatal infections | 8 |
| Hospital care of neonatal infection | 25 |
| Hospital care of preterm newborns | 25 |

*Abbreviations:* ANC, antenatal care; ITN, insecticide-treated mosquito net; ITPp, intermittent preventive treatment during pregnancy; PROM, premature rupture of membranes.
  *Data from* Refs.[4,52]

care, and administration of antibiotics for neonatal sepsis; the improvement of maternal and child nutrition; the treatment of uncomplicated pneumonia and diarrhea; the treatment and prevention of malaria (eg, insecticide-treated nets and antimalarial prophylaxis); and the management of infectious diseases of poverty, such as HIV/AIDS, tuberculosis, and neglected tropical diseases.[12,50,66–72] Ongoing training, support, and supervision of CHW is crucial to maintain the quality of health services.[12,73] Community mobilization in conjunction with home visits by CHW during the antenatal and postnatal period has been shown to improve newborn survival in Southern Asia.[74] Women's groups practicing participatory learning and action delivered at high population coverage have shown improved maternal and neonatal survival in LMIC.[75,76]

*Mobile health systems and other technology platforms* are increasingly being evaluated to promote MNCH service utilization and delivery and modify patient or provider behaviors to improve child survival and development.[77,78] In Kenya, use of mobile phone text-message reminders to health workers improved compliance to malaria case management practices in the outpatient setting.[79]

The *child health days (CHDs)* strategy is an innovative outreach delivery pathway to improve coverage of a variety of high-impact child health interventions, such as oral rehydration salts and zinc for diarrhea, promote breastfeeding, vitamin A supplementation, ready-to-use supplementary food for children with moderate malnutrition, vaccines to prevent pneumonia and diarrhea, deworming, and delivery of insecticide-treated bed nets to prevent malaria.[80] Another innovative delivery pathway includes administration of seasonal malaria chemoprevention to children at the highest risk of malaria acquisition in high-burden countries in sub-Saharan Africa.[81] The CHDs program is typically implemented 2 to 4 times a year and remains an important strategy to eliminate missed MDG4 opportunities.[80]

The *integrated management of childhood illness (IMCI)* strategy was developed by the WHO and the United Nations Children's Fund (UNICEF) in the mid-1990s to address mortality caused by childhood diseases, such as diarrhea, pneumonia, malaria, and malnutrition.[82] In a cluster-based trial in Bangladesh, the IMCI case management approach demonstrated improved child survival, high breastfeeding rates, and decreased stunting.[83] However, successful implementation of IMCI strategies in various LMIC warrants functioning health systems, improved home and community practices, and strong financial and political support.[84]

*Conditional cash transfer (CCT)* programs may improve uptake of child health interventions and service utilization in poverty-stricken communities in LMIC, but additional research is necessary.[85,86] In Brazil, a large CCT program has demonstrated a 9.3% decrease in overall infant mortality rates (24.3% decrease in postneonatal mortality rates) during a 5-year implementation period.[87]

*Quality health care for women and children* is essential to successfully scale-up MNCH interventions in under-resourced settings.[4] In recent years, increasing emphasis has been focused on the development of quality-improvement systems and tools throughout the continuum of care for MNCH in primary health systems and referral hospitals.[4] Linear, mathematical modeling tools, such as the Lives Saved Tool (LiST), can estimate the gains achieved in maternal, newborn, and child mortality by scaling-up a set of key MNCH interventions.[12,66,88]

## FUTURE DIRECTIONS
### *Advance Newborn and Stillbirth Agenda*

Reduction in newborn deaths has lagged behind maternal and child deaths, with 44% of younger-than-5 mortality currently among newborns.[30] Thus, improved coverage of focused and targeted interventions to reach the world's poorest and the most vulnerable communities remains a high priority to address newborn survival.[18,22] In 2014, the WHO and UNICEF launched the Every Newborn Action Plan (ENAP) to improve the quality of maternal and newborn care at the time of birth, reduce social inequalities, engage communities, and achieve universal coverage to save an estimated 3 million lives each year.[5] Many high-burden countries have incorporated newborn health action plans, and progress has been made.[23] Effective implementation of the ENAP will require political leadership and country ownership, cooperation, and continued support from United Nations (UN) agencies and other stakeholders, functional health systems (trained workforce, adequate commodities), availability of innovative interventions and technologies to address newborn health, financial support, and robust monitoring and evaluations systems to track progress.[4,20,22,23]

### *Advance Global Nutrition Agenda*

Although evidence-based nutritional interventions exist to address maternal and childhood undernutrition, coverage rates for some essential nutritional interventions remain poor in LMIC.[15,21,52] Given the vital linkage between nutrition and health, survival, and child development, RMNCH programs must effectively integrate proven nutritional interventions throughout the continuum of care (preconception, first 1000 days from conception through 2 years of age, childhood, and adolescence).[21,89] The dual burden of undernutrition and overnutrition in LMIC must be effectively addressed in the post-2015 era.

### Advance Reproductive Health and Adolescent Health Agenda

Family planning needs (including safe abortion) are largely unmet for women in LMIC.[90] Other challenges include lack of reproductive freedom or decision making, insufficient birth spacing, child marriage, violence against women and girls, intimate partner violence, female genital cutting, and gender inequalities.[47] Unmet sexual and reproductive health needs can significantly affect the survival, health, and economic well-being of adolescent girls, women, and their children.[91] Addressing the adolescent health and family planning needs of women as well as advocacy and education for both men and women in sub-Saharan Africa and South Asia must remain a high priority in the post-2015 global development agenda.[92,93]

### Scale-up High-Quality, Integrated Care Delivery to Mothers and Children

Rapid scale-up, access to quality services through innovative service delivery strategies, smart integration, and strong linkages across the RMNCH continuum of care at various levels of health systems (eg, community health facility, primary health center, district hospital) are key strategies to accelerate progress toward ending preventable maternal and newborn deaths.[4,12,14,15,21,57,65,66,94,95] For example, integration of HIV/tuberculosis/malaria care programs with RMNCH services has the potential to enhance program effectiveness and sustainability, while addressing multiple needs.[96] Gaps in coverage for key interventions, such as family planning, newborn health, and case management of diarrhea, pneumonia, and malaria, must be urgently addressed.[19]

### Foster Human Rights and Respectful Maternal and Neonatal Care

A fundamental human rights–based RMNCA strategy across the life course has been the recent focus of an international expert meeting in Abu Dhabi, United Arab Emirates (Abu Dhabi Declaration).[97] In 2014, the WHO released a statement endorsing respectful maternity and neonatal care, especially during facility-based childbirth.[7,98]

### Survival and Development Agenda

The post-2015 era of sustainable development holds promise to improve individual and population health with integration of economic, social, and environmental initiatives. The MDGs, which end in September 2015, will be replaced by a new set of goals: the SDGs. The SDGs were developed after enormous consultations involving member-states and consists of 17 goals and 169 targets, agreed on by more than 190 countries.[99] In a recent review of national mortality rates and trends to quantify the UN 2030 SDG, the investigators suggested that it is possible to avoid 40% of the premature deaths of individuals younger than 70 years in each country by 2030 by consolidating certain important MDG targets, such as child health (MDG4), maternal health (MDG5), major infectious diseases (MDG6), noncommunicable diseases, and universal health coverage, into one universally achievable health goal.[100] Currently, approximately 35% of births and approximately 60% of deaths are not registered, indicating the crucial need to strengthen civil registration and vital statistics (CRVS).[101] Funding and building robust CRVS systems will provide an accurate estimate of births and deaths worldwide, better inform the WHO's health statistics or global burden of disease in determining population's health and health systems, and improve health outcomes.[102] Given the significant overlap of important risk factors affecting child survival and early childhood development, an integrated child survival and development strategy must be a top priority in the post-2015 sustainable development agenda.[103]

*Mobilize Resources and Invest in Research to Advance Reproductive, Maternal, Newborn, and Child Health*

Several new global initiatives and programs with broad support have been developed for advancing the health of mothers, newborns, and children worldwide, such as the

---

**Box 4**
**Global initiatives for maternal, newborn, child, and reproductive health**

- Helping Babies Breathe
  American Academy of Pediatrics
  http://www.helpingbabiesbreathe.org

- Every Women Every Child
  http://www.everywomaneverychild.org/

- United Nations Global Strategy for Women's and Children' Health
  http://www.who.int/pmnch/topics/maternal/20100914_gswch_en.pdf

- Every Newborn Action Plan
  http://www.everynewborn.org/every-newborn-action-plan/

- Partnership for Maternal, Newborn, and Child Health
  http://www.who.int/pmnch/en/

- Grand Challenge in Development: Saving Lives at Birth
  http://www.savinglivesatbirth.net

- Ending Preventable Maternal Mortality
  Strategies toward ending preventable maternal mortality (EPMM). Geneva: World Health Organization, 2015.
  http://who.int/reproductivehealth/topics/maternal_perinatal/epmm/en/

- United Nations Commission on Life-Saving Commodities for Women and Children Implementation Plan
  http://www.everywomaneverychild.org/images/UN_Commission_Report_September_2012_Final.pdf

- UNICEF/USAID Committing to Child Survival: A Promise Renewed
  http://www.apromiserenewed.org/

- Global Action Plan for the Prevention of Pneumonia and Diarrhea
  http://www.apps.who.int/iris/bitstream/10665/79200/1/9789241505239_eng.pdf

- Global Vaccine Action Plan 2011 to 2020
  http://www.who.int/immunization/global_vaccine_action_plan/en/

- United Nations Sustainable Energy for All Initiative
  http://www.un.org/wcm/content/site/sustainableenergyforall/home/Initiative

- Global Fund New Funding Model
  http://www.theglobalfund.org/en/fundingmodel

- United Nations Commission on Information and Accountability
  http://www.everywomaneverychild.org/accountability/coia

- Campaign for Reduction of Maternal Mortality in Africa
  http://carmma.org/

- Canada's Leadership in Maternal, Newborn, and Child Health—The Muskoka Initiative (2010–2015)
  http://mnch.international.gc.ca/en/topics/leadership-muskoka_initiative.html

UN Secretary General Ban Ki-moon's Every Woman, Every Child initiative, the Every Newborn Action Plan, and the Partnership for Maternal, Newborn, and Child Health (**Box 4**). Research in RMNCH through innovative collaborations and partnerships remain priorities.[1] Academic institutions must engage in scientific research tailored to the needs of individual programs and policy makers to improve the MNCH Continuum of Care.[1] Unique partnerships and research networks between the US National Institutes of Health and the Bill and Melinda Gates Foundation have resulted in the development of an innovative priority research agenda in MNCH, established research infrastructure, and promoted public health in LMIC.[104] Continued donor funding is needed to accelerate progress toward improving RMNCH outcomes.[2] Global and national commitments at the highest level are needed to rapidly translate research evidence to policy and practice. A broader, more inclusive, coherent strategy; collaboration and cooperation between humanitarian agencies; development; and a RMNCA health community are crucial to achieve a common goal: end preventable maternal, newborn, and child deaths worldwide.[105]

## REFERENCES

1. Crockett M, Avery L, Blanchard J. Program science—a framework for improving global maternal, newborn, and child health. JAMA 2015;169:305–6.
2. Arregoces L, Daly F, Pitt C, et al. Countdown to 2015: changes in official development assistance to reproductive, maternal, newborn, and child health, and assessment of progress between 2003 and 2012. Lancet Glob Health 2015;3: e410–21.
3. Darmstadt GL, Kinney MV, Chopra M, et al. Who has been caring for the baby? Lancet 2014;384:174–88.
4. Bhutta ZA, Das JK, Bahl R, et al. Can available interventions end preventable deaths in mothers, newborn babies, and stillbirths, and at what cost? Lancet 2014;384:347–70.
5. WHO. Every newborn: an action plan to end preventable deaths (ENAP). Geneva (Switzerland): World Health Organization; 2014. Available at: http://www.everynewborn.org/every-newborn-action-plan/. Accessed July 25, 2015.
6. WHO. Strategies toward ending preventable maternal mortality (EPMM). Geneva (Switzerland): World Health Organization; 2015. Available at: http://who.int/reproductivehealth/topics/maternal_perinatal/epmm/en/. Accessed July 25, 2015.
7. Sacks E, Kinney MV. Respectful maternal and newborn care: building a common agenda. Reprod Health 2015;12:46.
8. United Nations. Millennium development goals. New York: United Nations; 2014. Available at: http://www.un.org/milleniumgoals/2014%20MDG%20report/MDG%202014%20English%20web.pdf. Accessed July 25, 2015.
9. UNICEF, WHO, World Bank, UN. UN inter-agency group for child mortality estimation. Levels and trends in child mortality: report 2014. New York: United Nations Children's Fund; 2014. Available at: http://www.childmortality.org. Accessed June 21, 2015.
10. Wang H, Liddell CA, Coates MM, et al. Global, regional, and national levels of neonatal, infant, and under-five mortality during 1990-2013: a systematic analysis for the Global Burden of Disease Study. Lancet 2014;384:957–79.
11. Jones G, Steketee RW, Black RE, et al. How many child deaths can we prevent this year? Lancet 2003;362:65–71.
12. Bhutta ZA, Black RE. Global health: global maternal, newborn, and child health – so near and yet so far. N Engl J Med 2013;369:2226–35.

13. Darmstadt GL, Bhutta ZA, Cousens S, et al. Evidence-based, cost-effective interventions: how many newborn babies can we save? Lancet 2005;365:977–88.
14. Ekman B, Pathmanathan I, Liljestrand J. Integrating health interventions for women, newborn babies, and children: a framework for action. Lancet 2008; 372(9642):990–1000.
15. Bhutta ZA, Das JK, Rizvi A, et al. Evidence-based interventions for improvement of maternal and child nutrition: what can be done and at what cost? Lancet 2013;382:452–77.
16. Bhutta ZA, Ali S, Cousens S, et al. Alma-Ata: rebirth and revision 6: interventions to address maternal, newborn and child survival: what difference can integrated primary health care strategies make? Lancet 2008;372:972–89.
17. The Partnership for Maternal, Newborn & Child Health. A global review of the key interventions related to reproductive, maternal, newborn and child health (RMNCH). Geneva (Switzerland): The Partnership for Maternal, Newborn & Child Health; 2011.
18. Lawn JE, Cousens SN, Darmstadt GL, et al, Lancet Neonatal Survival Series steering Team. 1 year after the Lancet Neonatal Survival Series – was the call for action heard? Lancet 2006;367:1541–7.
19. Requejo J, Bryce J, Barros A, et al. Countdown to 2015 and beyond: fulfilling the health agenda for women and children. Lancet 2015;385:466–76.
20. Dickson KE, Simen-Kapeu A, Kinney MV, et al, Lancet Every Newborn Study Group. Every newborn: health-systems bottlenecks and strategies to accelerate scale-up in countries. Lancet 2014;384:438–54.
21. Requejo JH, Bhutta ZA. The post-2015 agenda: staying the course in maternal and child survival. Arch Dis Child 2015;100(Suppl 1):s76–81.
22. Darmstadt GL, Shiffman J, Lawn JE. Advancing the newborn and stillbirth global agenda: priorities for the next decade. Arch Dis Child 2015;100(Suppl 1):s13–8.
23. Kinney MV, Cocoman O, Dickson KE, et al. Implementation of the every newborn action plan: progress and lessons learned. Semin Perinatol 2015;39:326–37.
24. WHO, UNICEF, UNFPA. The World Bank, United Nations population division. Trends in maternal mortality: 1990-2013. Geneva (Switzerland): World Health Organization; 2014. Available at: http://www.who.int/reproductivehealth/publications/monitoring/maternal-mortality-2013/en/.
25. Kassebaum NJ, Bertozzi-Villa A, Coggesha MS, et al. Global, regional, and national levels and causes of maternal mortality during 1990–2013: a systematic analysis for the Global Burden of Disease Study 2013. Lancet 2014;384: 980–1004.
26. Storeng KT, Murray SF, Akoum MS, et al. Beyond body counts: a qualitative study of lives and loss in Burkina Faso after 'near-miss' obstetric complications. Soc Sci Med 2010;71:1749–56.
27. Koblinsky M, Chowdhury ME, Moran A, et al. Maternal morbidity and disability and their consequences: neglected agenda in maternal health. J Health Popul Nutr 2012;30:124–30.
28. Say L, Chou D, Gemmill A, et al. Global causes of maternal health: a WHO systematic analysis. Lancet Glob Health 2014;2:e323–33.
29. Requejo J, Bryce J, Victoria C, Countdown to 2015 Writing Team. Countdown to 2015 and beyond: fulfilling the health agenda for women and children. Geneva (Switzerland): UNICEF and WHO; 2014. p. 1–229.
30. Liu L, Oza S, Hogan D, et al. Global, regional, and national causes of child mortality in 2000-13, with projections to inform post-2015 priorities: an updated systematic analysis. Lancet 2015;385:430–40.

31. WHO. Global health observatory. Causes of child mortality. Available at: http://www.who.int/gho/child_health/mortality/causes/en/. Accessed August 10, 2015.
32. Lawn JE, Blencowe H, Oza S, et al. Every newborn: progress, priorities, and potential beyond survival. Lancet 2014;384:189–205.
33. Lawn JE, Kinney MV, Black RE, et al. Newborn survival: a multi-country analysis of a decade of change. Health Policy Plan 2012;27(Suppl 3):iii6–28.
34. Lawn JE, Blencowe H, Pattinson R, et al. Stillbirths: where? when? why? How to make the data count? Lancet 2011;377:1448–63.
35. Cousens S, Blencowe H, Stanton C, et al. National, regional, and worldwide estimates of stillbirth rates in 2009 with trends since 1995: a systematic analysis. Lancet 2011;377:1319–30.
36. Commission on Social Determinants of Health. Closing the gap in a generation: health equity through action on the social determinants of health. Final report of the Commission on Social Determinants of Health. Geneva (Switzerland): World Health Organization; 2008.
37. Bhutta ZA. Paediatrics in the tropics. In: Farrar J, Hotez PJ, Junghanss T, et al, editors. Manson's tropical diseases. 23rd edition. Philadelphia: Saunders/Elsevier; 2014. p. 1197–214.
38. Gakidou E, Cowling K, Lozano R, et al. Increased educational attainment and its effect on child mortality in 175 countries between 1970 and 2009: a systematic analysis. Lancet 2010;376:959–74.
39. Barros AJ, Ronsmans C, Axelson H, et al. Equity in maternal, newborn, and child health interventions in countdown to 2015: a retrospective review of survey data from 54 countries. Lancet 2012;379:1225–33.
40. Southall D. Armed conflict women and girls who are pregnant, infants and children; a neglected public health challenge. What can health professionals do? Early Hum Dev 2011;87:735–42.
41. Walker SP, Wachs TD, Gardner JM, et al. Child development: risk factors for adverse outcomes in developing countries. Lancet 2007;369:145–57.
42. Awasthi S, Agarwal S. Determinants of childhood mortality and morbidity in urban slums in India. Indian Pediatr 2003;40:1145–61.
43. Matthews Z, Channon A, Neal S, et al. Examining the "urban advantage" in maternal health care in developing countries. PLoS Med 2010;7:e1000327.
44. Bocquier P, Beguy D, Zulu EM, et al. Do migrant children face greater health hazards in slum settlements? Evidence from Nairobi, Kenya. J Urban Health 2011;88(Suppl 2):S266–81.
45. Corburn J, Hildebrand C. Slum sanitation and the social determinants of women's health in Nairobi, Kenya. J Environ Public Health 2015;2015:209505.
46. Organization for Economic Co-operation and Development (OECD). States of fragility 2015: meeting post-2015 ambitions. OECD Publishing, Paris: Organization for Economic Co-operation and Development. 2015. Available at: http://dx.doi.org/10.1787/9789264227699-en. Accessed September 29, 2015.
47. Yamin AE, Bazile J, Knight L, et al. Tracing shadows: how gendered power relations shape the impacts of maternal death on living children in sub Saharan Africa. Soc Sci Med 2015;135:143–50.
48. Nayar US, Stangl AL, De Zalduondo B, et al. Reducing stigma and discrimination to improve child health and survival in low- and middle-income countries: promising approaches and implications for future research. J Health Commun 2014;19(Suppl 1):142–63.

49. Turan JM, Nyblade L. HIV-related stigma as a barrier to achievement of global PMTCT and maternal health goals: a review of the evidence. AIDS Behav 2013; 17:2528–39.
50. Lassi ZS, Bhutta ZA. Community-based intervention packages for reducing maternal and neonatal morbidity and mortality and improving neonatal outcomes. Cochrane Database Syst Rev 2015;(3):CD007754.
51. Dean SV, Imam AM, Lassi ZS, et al. Importance of intervening in the preconception period to impact pregnancy outcomes. Nestle Nutr Inst Workshop Ser 2013; 74:63–73.
52. Gaffey MF, Das JK, Bhutta ZA. Millennium development goals 4 and 5: past and future progress. Semin Fetal Neonatal Med 2015. [Epub ahead of print].
53. Imdad A, Bautista RMM, Semem KAA, et al. Umbilical cord antiseptics for preventing sepsis and death among newborns. Cochrane Database Syst Rev 2006;(4):CD008635.
54. World Health Organization. WHO recommendations on postnatal care of the mother and newborn. 2013. Available at: http://www.healthynewbornnetwork. org/resource/who-recommendations-postnatal-care-mpther-and-newborn-2013. Accessed August 4, 2015.
55. World Health Organization. WHO's world health statistics 2015. Available at: http://www.who.int/gho/publications/world_health_statistics/2015/en/index.html. Accessed September 29, 2015.
56. Das JK, Rizvi A, Bhatti Z, et al. State of neonatal health care in eight countries of the SAARC region, South Asia: how can we make a difference? Paediatr Int Child Health 2015. 2046905515Y0000000046. [Epub ahead of print].
57. Kerber KJ, de Graft-Johnson JE, Bhutta ZA, et al. Continuum of care for maternal, newborn, and child health: from slogan to service delivery. Lancet 2007;370:1358–69.
58. Partnership for Maternal Newborn and Child Health. Fact sheet: RMNCH continuum of care. 2011. Available at: http://www.who.int/pmnch/about/continuum_of_care/en/. Accessed August 10, 2015.
59. Requejo J, Bryce J, Victoria C, et al. Countdown to 2015 for maternal, newborn and child survival: accountability for maternal, newborn and child survival. Geneva (Switzerland): World Health Organization; 2013. Available at: http://www.countdown2015mnch.org/documents/2013Report/Countdown_2013-Update_noprofiles.pdf.
60. Baker U, Peterson S, Marchant T, et al. Identifying implementation bottlenecks for maternal and newborn health interventions in rural districts of the United Republic of Tanzania. Bull World Health Organ 2015;93(6):380–9.
61. Victora CG, Barros AJ, Axelson H, et al. How changes in coverage affect equity in maternal and child health interventions in 35 countdown to 2015 countries: an analysis of national surveys. Lancet 2012;380:1149–56.
62. United Nations Population Fund (UNFPA). Roadmap to accelerate achievement of maternal and newborn survival and reach MDGs4 and 5(A&B). 2014. Available at: http://www.unfpa.org/resources/roadmap-accelerate-achievement-0f-maternal-and-newborn-survival-and-reach-mdgs-4-and-5ab. Accessed August 12, 2015.
63. Corsi DJ, Subramanian SV. Association between coverage of maternal and child health interventions, and under-5 mortality: a repeated cross-sectional analysis of 35 sub-Saharan countries. Glob Health Action 2014;7:24765.
64. Crisp N, Chen L. Global supply of health professionals. N Engl J Med 2014;370: 950–7.

65. Bhutta ZA, Lassi ZS, Pariyo G, et al. Global experience of community health workers for delivery of health-related millennium development goals: a systematic review, country case studies, and recommendations for integration into national health systems. Geneva (Switzerland): World Health Organization; 2010.

66. Bhutta ZA, Das JK, Walker N, et al. Interventions to address deaths from childhood pneumonia and diarrhoea equitably: what works and at what cost? Lancet 2013;381(9875):1417–29.

67. Bhutta ZA, Soofi S, Cousens S, et al. Improvement of perinatal and newborn care in rural Pakistan through community-based strategies: a cluster-randomised effectiveness trial. Lancet 2011;377:403–12.

68. Lewin S, Munabi-Babigumira S, Glenton C, et al. Lay health workers in primary and community health care for maternal and child health and the management of infectious diseases. Cochrane Database Syst Rev 2010;(3):CD004015.

69. Christopher JB, Le May A, Lewin S, et al. Thirty years after Alma-Ata: a systematic review of the impact of community health workers delivering curative interventions against malaria, pneumonia and diarrhoea on child mortality and morbidity in sub-Saharan Africa. Hum Resour Health 2011;9(1):2770.

70. Gilmore B, McAuliffe E. Effectiveness of community health workers delivering preventive interventions for maternal and child health in low- and middle-income countries: a systematic review. BMC Public Health 2013;13:847.

71. Escott S, Walley J. Listening to those on the frontline: lessons for community-based tuberculosis programmes from a qualitative study in Swaziland. Soc Sci Med 2005;61(8):1701–10.

72. Sodahlon YK, Dorkenoo AM, Morgah K, et al. A success story: Togo is moving toward becoming the first sub-Saharan African nation to eliminate lymphatic filariasis through mass drug administration and countrywide morbidity alleviation. PLoS Negl Trop Dis 2013;7(4):e2080.

73. Tran NT, Portela A, de Bernis L, et al. Developing capacities of community health workers in sexual and reproductive, maternal, newborn, child, and adolescent health: a mapping and review of training resources. PLoS One 2014;9(4):e94948.

74. Gogia S, Sachdev HS. Home visits by community health workers to prevent neonatal deaths in developing countries: a systematic review. Bull World Health Organ 2010;88:658–66.

75. Prost A, Colbourn T, Seward N, et al. Women's groups practicing participatory learning and action to improve maternal and newborn health in low-resource settings: a systematic review and meta-analysis. Lancet 2013;18(381):1736–46.

76. Fottrell E, Azad K, Kuddus A, et al. The effect of increased coverage of participatory women's groups on neonatal mortality in Bangladesh: a cluster randomized trial. JAMA Pediatr 2013;167:816–25.

77. Higgs ES, Goldberg AB, Labrique AB, et al. Understanding the role of mHealth and other media interventions for behavior change to enhance child survival and development in low- and middle-income countries: an evidence overview. J Health Commun 2014;19:164–89.

78. Free C, Phillips G, Watson L, et al. The effectiveness of mobile-health technologies to improve health care service delivery processes: a systematic review and meta-analysis. PLoS Med 2013;10:e1001363.

79. Zurovac D, Sudoi RK, Akhwale WS, et al. The effect of mobile phone text-message reminders on Kenyan health workers' adherence to malaria treatment guidelines: a cluster randomised trial. Lancet 2011;378:795–803.

80. The MDG Health Alliance. No more missed MDG4 opportunities: optimizing existing health platforms for child survival. Available at: http://www.mdghealthenvoy.org/wp-content/uploads/2014/05/Child-Health-Weeks-and-Days1.pdf. Accessed August 20, 2015.
81. Tine RC, Ndour CT, Faye B, et al. Feasibility, safety and effectiveness of combining home based malaria management and seasonal malaria chemoprevention in children less than 10 years in Senegal: a cluster-randomised trial. Trans R Soc Trop Med Hyg 2014;108:13–21.
82. World Health Organization/UNICEF. Handbook: IMCI integrated management of childhood illness. WHO 2005. Available at: http://apps.who.int/iris/bitstream/10665/42939/1/9241546441.pdf. Accessed August 20, 2015.
83. Arifeen SE, Hoque DM, Akter T, et al. Effect of the integrated management of childhood illness strategy on childhood mortality and nutrition in a rural area in Bangladesh: a cluster randomised trial. Lancet 2009;374:393–403.
84. Duke T. Child survival and IMCI: in need of sustained global support. Lancet 2009;374:361–2.
85. Bassani DG, Arora P, Wazny K, et al. Financial incentives and coverage of child health interventions: a systematic review and meta-analysis. BMC Public Health 2013;13(Suppl 3):S30.
86. Rasella D, Aquino R, Santos CA, et al. Effect of a conditional cash transfer programme on childhood mortality: a nationwide analysis of Brazilian municipalities. Lancet 2013;382:57–64.
87. Shei A. Brazil's conditional cash transfer program associated with declines in infant mortality rates. Health Aff (Millwood) 2013;32:1274–81.
88. Walker N, Tam Y, Friberg IK. Overview of the Lives Saved Tool (LiST). BMC Public Health 2013;13(Suppl 3):S1.
89. Christian P, Mullany LC, Hurley KM, et al. Nutrition and maternal, neonatal, and child health. Semin Perinatol 2015;39:361–72.
90. Alkema L, Kantorova V, Menozzi C, et al. National, regional, and global rates and trends in contraceptive prevalence and unmet need for family planning between 1990 and 2015: a systematic and comprehensive analysis. Lancet 2013;381:1642–52.
91. UNICEF. Committing to child survival: a promise renewed. Progress report 2013. New York: UNICEF; 2013. Available at: http://www.unicef.org/lac/Committing_to_Child_Survival_APR_9_Sept_2013.pdf. Accessed Aug 19, 2015.
92. Fabic MS, Choi Y, Bongaarts J. Meeting demand for family planning within a generation: the post-2015 agenda. Lancet 2015;385:1928–31.
93. Lassi ZS, Salam RA, Das JK, et al. An unfinished agenda on adolescent health: opportunities for interventions. Semin Perinatol 2015;39(5):353–60.
94. Starrs AM. Survival convergence: bringing maternal and newborn health together for 2015 and beyond. Lancet 2014;384:211–3.
95. Mason E, McDougall L, Lawn JE, et al. From evidence to action to deliver a healthy start for the next generation. Lancet 2014;384:455–67.
96. Chimbwandira F, Mhango E, Makombe S, et al. Impact of an innovative approach to prevent mother-to-child transmission of HIV – Malawi, July 2011-September 2012. MMWR Morb Mortal Wkly Rep 2013;62:148–51.
97. The Abu Dhabi declaration. 2015. Available at: http://www.everywomaneverychild.org/images/The _Abu_Dhabi_Declaration_Feb_2015_7.pdf. Accessed July 27, 2015.

98. World Health Organization. The prevention and elimination of disrespect and abuse during facility-based childbirth. Geneva (Switzerland): World Health Organization; 2014.

99. Sustainable development platform. Outcome document—open working group on sustainable development goals. 2014. Available at: https://sustainabledevelopment.un.org/focussdgs.html. Accessed August 22, 2015.

100. Norheim OF, Jha P, Admasu K, et al. Avoiding 40% of the premature deaths in each country, 2010–30: review of national mortality trends to help quantify the UN sustainable development goal for health. Lancet 2015;385(9964):239–52.

101. Lancet series on counting births and deaths. 2015. Available at: http://www.thelancet.com/series/counting-births-and-deaths. Accessed September 29, 2015.

102. CRVS systems: a cornerstone of sustainable development. Lancet 2015;385: 1917.

103. Jensen SK, Bouhouch RR, Walson JL, et al. Enhancing the child survival agenda to promote, protect, and support early child development. Semin Perinatol 2015; 39(5):373–86.

104. Koso-Thomas M, McClure EM. Global network for women's and children's health research investigators. Semin Fetal Neonatal Med 2015. [Epub ahead of print]. Available at: http://dx.doi.org/10.1016/j.siny.2015.04.004.

105. Zeid S, Bustreo F, Barakat MT, et al. Women, children, and adolescents: the post-2015 agenda. Lancet 2015;385:1919–20.

# Global Threats to Child Safety

Sharon E. Mace, MD[a,b,]*

## KEYWORDS

- Needs of the child • Vulnerable children • Violence toward children
- Exploitation of children • Abuse of children • Child protection

## KEY POINTS

- Children in a disaster or armed conflict and children outside of family care are especially vulnerable to violence, exploitation, and abuse. Other factors include ethnic, racial, religious, or social minorities; disabled children, gender, age, and socioeconomic status.
- Global threats to child safety exist: lack of basic needs (food, clean water, sanitation, shelter), maltreatment, abandonment, child labor, child marriage, female genital mutilation, child trafficking, disasters, and armed conflicts.
- Children have rights, as enumerated in the Declaration of the Rights of the Child, and need protection from violence, exploitation, and abuse; especially during disasters and armed conflicts/wars.
- Strategies and specific programs can be developed and implemented for eliminating threats to the safety of children.

## INTRODUCTION

A recent United Nations (UN) report estimates there was a record number of refugees last year with 59.5 million people forced from their homes by armed conflicts/wars all over the world.[1] The armed conflict/war in Syria alone has resulted in nearly 3.9 million migrants, with 1.59 million of these refugees in nearby Turkey.[1] A significant portion of these individuals are children. Reports indicate that it is not unusual to see migrant children begging in the streets of Turkey. Of these 59.5 million people, 38.2 million were displaced within their own countries.[2]

There was a 16% increase in displaced people in one year alone from 51.2 million in 2013 to 59.5 million in 2014. Moreover, this trend seems to be escalating and it is likely that the numbers will only increase further this year. The mass refugee exodus from

Disclosure: The author has nothing to disclose.
a Department of Emergency Medicine, Cleveland Clinic Lerner College of Medicine, Case Western Reserve University, Cleveland Clinic, 9500 Euclid Avenue, E-19, Cleveland, OH 44195, USA;
b Observation Unit, Emergency Services Institute, Cleveland Clinic, 9500 Euclid Avenue, E-19, Cleveland, OH 44195, USA
* Emergency Department, Cleveland Clinic, 9500 Euclid Avenue, E-19, Cleveland, OH 44195.
E-mail address: maces@ccf.org

Pediatr Clin N Am 63 (2016) 19–35
http://dx.doi.org/10.1016/j.pcl.2015.09.003
0031-3955/16/$ – see front matter © 2016 Elsevier Inc. All rights reserved.

armed conflicts/war all over the world represents a monumental humanitarian crisis and is the worst refugee crisis in years. According to the BBC (British Broadcasting Corporation) "The number of people living as refugees from war or persecution exceeded 50 million in 2013, for the first time since World War Two, the UN says."[3]

In 2012, worldwide, it was estimated that more than 172 million people were directly affected by armed conflicts. This number (172 million) includes conflict affected residents (CARs) (86.6% of the total at 149 million), internally displaced people (18 million or 10.5%) and refugees (5 million or 2.9%). The actual numbers are likely much higher than this because the figures include only 24 countries for which comparable and validated data were available.[4] Again, most of this population includes families with children and orphans or children without family support.[4]

Migrant, displaced, and orphan children or children without family support are especially vulnerable to violence, exploitation, and abuse. These reports and other current headlines highlight the worldwide problems for child safety. This article deals with several key issues facing global child safety, discusses advocacy, and references some strategies and successful programs for combating the violence toward, exploitation of, and abuse of children worldwide (**Box 1**).

## BACKGROUND

The human body cannot survive without meeting its physiologic needs. Obligatory physiologic needs must be met; otherwise, the human body is unable to function properly and will eventually fail, leading to the demise of the individual. The 3 metabolic requirements for survival are air, water, and food; clothing and shelter bestow protection from the elements.

After meeting the physiologic needs, which are the physical requirements for human survival, safety needs are next. Physical safety may be difficult to attain for many reasons including war, armed conflicts, disasters, family violence, and maltreatment (abuse). Once the individual's physical needs are met, safety needs become the priority. Safety and security needs encompass personal security, financial security, health and well-being, and a safety net to prevent accidents, illnesses, or diseases, with their resultant consequences.

---

**Box 1**
**Types of violence, exploitation, and abuse that children experience**

- Failure to provide adequate basic needs: food, water, shelter (including clothing), health care (including immunizations), and education
- Lack of official recording of births
- Child maltreatment (abuse): physical, sexual, verbal, medical child abuse (Munchausen's by proxy, fabricated, or induced illness)
- Child abandonment
- Child labor
- Child marriage
- Female genital mutilation/cutting
- Trafficking
- Sexual exploitation
- Child soldiers

According to Maslow's hierarchy of need, physiologic needs come first, then safety needs, next is love/belonging, followed by esteem, and, finally, self-actualization.[5] Others group basic human needs into several levels: physiologic needs, followed by safety needs, and then psychological needs. These levels of needs may vary across cultures because of the availability of resources, including during peacetime and war. During times of war, the physiologic and safety needs may become of paramount importance and may merge into a survival mode.[6]

*More than a billion people cannot count on meeting their basic needs for food, sanitation, and clean water. Their children die from simple, preventable diseases. They lack a minimally decent quality of life.*[7]

From an international perspective, what are the challenges faced in meeting the basic physiologic and safety needs of children?

## PHYSIOLOGIC NEEDS: WORLD HUNGER

World hunger is defined as the want or scarcity of food in the world.[4] Food security exists "when all people, at all times, have access to sufficient, safe, nutritious food to maintain a healthy and active life."[8] According to the Food and Agriculture Organization in 2011 to 2013, 12% of the world's population or approximately 842 million people were undernourished; 98% of these reside in the developing world.[8]

It is estimated that 1 in 9 people in the world, or 805 million of the world's 7.3 billion people, are chronically undernourished. Most of the people with hunger, about 791 million, live in developing countries where 1 of 8 people or 13.5% of the population is undernourished; compared with 11 million malnourished people in the developed world.[4] Statistics about world hunger do not include micronutrient deficiencies. Micronutrient deficiency is the deficiency of specific vitamins and minerals, such as vitamin A or D.[4]

Eight Millennium Development Goals (MDGs) were set by world leaders in 2000. The first goal or MDG 1 is to eradicate extreme poverty and hunger. Children are greatly affected by undernutrition. About 45% of all child deaths in 2011, or 3.1 million deaths annually, have been attributed to undernutrition.[5] Undernutrition worsens the effect of any given disease and is an underlying cause of death for most illnesses; it is an underlying cause of death in 52% to 61% of those with pneumonia, malaria, or diarrhea.[4]

"Poverty is the principle cause of hunger."[4] Harmful political and economic systems, conflicts/wars (CARs, which include refugees and internally displaced persons), population growth, poverty, food/agricultural policy, and climate change are factors cited as contributing to world hunger.[4] Ways to decrease world hunger include decreasing overconsumption, increasing the decline in fertility rates, limiting climate disruption, increasing the efficiency of food production, reducing waste, and changing diets.[8]

## PHYSIOLOGIC NEEDS: CLEAN WATER, SANITATION, AND HOUSING

The provision of safe drinking water is a basic physiologic need and a critical element in preventing disease. More than 780 million people do not have access to safe water and 2.5 billion people lack access to proper toilet facilities. Improved hygiene leads to less disease, increased school attendance, better school performance, and economic growth, particularly in developing countries.[9]

Lack of clean water and poor or nonexistent sanitation predominantly affects children. "More than 800,000 children under age 5 die each year due to diarrhea, more than the number who die due to AIDS, malaria, and measles combined."[10] Diarrhea is the fifth leading cause of death worldwide.[10] Nearly half (47%) of children aged 5 to 9 years in developing countries are infested with soil-transmitted worms.[9] Worm infestations and diarrhea can delay and decrease intellectual development, limit children's growth, and are underlying causes of undernutrition and stunting. "Among all children under age 14, more than 20% of deaths and years lived with illness are attributable to unsafe water, inadequate sanitation or insufficient hygiene."[9]

Clothing and shelter provide essential protection from the elements. Approximately 42.9 million people worldwide are living in substandard temporary housing; millions of others are inadequately housed at their "permanent home site," generally living in substandard temporary housing, often living under a tarp, or in a consumable tent, or even without any roof over their heads. Armed conflicts/wars and disasters may force individuals, many of whom are children, out of their homes. Subsisting under such impoverished and desperate conditions leaves these families and individuals, especially children, extremely vulnerable to poverty, malnutrition, disease, lack of education, violence, exploitation, and abuse.[11]

Lack of an official recording of their birth or birth certificate or birth registration is cited as a rights violation.[12] Without a birth certificate, a child may be denied access to certain services and rights provided to citizens of a country, and this has numerous other consequences. For example, reunification of a child or infant with their family after a disaster or armed conflict/war when there is no formal or legal documentation may create difficult and, perhaps, insurmountable problems. Lack of official documentation of birth may lead to problems with or even denial of legal immigration (see **Box 1**).

## CHILD MALTREATMENT

Child maltreatment, formerly termed child abuse; may take many forms: verbal, physical, or sexual abuse; neglect; or medical child abuse (previous terminology, Munchausen syndrome by proxy, or fabricated or induced illness).[13] Child maltreatment, unfortunately, occurs worldwide.[14,15] Child abuse is not unique to any social, ethnic, religious, political, or economic group; nor to any 1 region or nation.[13]

## PROTECTION FROM VIOLENCE, EXPLOITATION, AND ABUSE

Child protection is the prevention and response to violence, exploitation, and abuse of children in all contexts. Millions of children worldwide experience the worst kinds of rights violations. Millions more are inadequately protected against them. Moreover, these violations are widespread throughout the world, in both underdeveloped and developed countries, and are under-reported and often unrecognized.[16] Examples of the types of violence, exploitation, and abuse that children experience are outlined in **Box 1**.

## VULNERABLE CHILDREN

Certain children are especially vulnerable to violence, abuse, and exploitation.[12,16–20] Children without family support are one group of high-risk children. Displaced and migrant children are at risk. More children are migrating because of family problems, and for social, economic, religious, and political reasons; these may be precipitated by disasters, drought, famine, civil unrest, and armed conflict/war. Children may be exploited and abused if they belong to certain ethnic, religious, political, or social groups, especially minorities (**Box 2**).

Children outside of family care are at high risk for becoming victims of violence, abuse, and exploitations. Children who are outside of family care include children

**Box 2**
**Children particularly vulnerable to violence, exploitation, and abuse**

- Those without family care
- Orphans
- Children living on the streets
- Children in situations of war or armed conflicts
- Children in situations of disasters
- Abandoned children
- Children in institutional care
- Children in detention
- Displaced children
- Migrant children
- Impoverished children or living in slums
- Children with disabilities
- Individuals from ethnic minorities and other marginalized groups
- Gender
- Race
- Age (younger children are at risk for certain types of violence and older children for other types of abuse/exploitation)
- Socioeconomic status

separated or unaccompanied because of disaster or armed conflict/war, children trafficked for forced labor and/or sexual exploitation, child soldiers, children associated with groups or armed forces, children working as live-in domestic servants, abandoned children, children living on the streets, children heading households, children in institutions, and children in detention. A residential facility in which a group of children is cared for by paid personnel is termed residential care, residential institution, or institution.[21]

Children with disabilities are particularly vulnerable to rape, sexual, and physical abuse.[12] Where children live may place them at risk. Living in an area of civil unrest or war, during and after a disaster, in migrant communities, rural areas without adequate law enforcement protection (such as the rural communities where school children were abducted by terrorist groups such as Boko Haram), and in urban slums, especially if an unaccompanied minor, increase the vulnerability of the child to exploitation and abuse.[12,16–20]

## FAMILY SEPARATION

Being lost and alone and separated from family and community is frightening, even more so during a disaster or armed conflict/war. Moreover, such separation from family greatly increases the vulnerability of the child to illness, violence, exploitation, and abuse. More than 1 million children have been orphaned or separated from their families by armed conflict in the last decade. Efforts should be made to identify children separated from their families as soon as possible and to reunite them with their parents, older siblings, or members of their extended families via family tracing and various tracking programs.[21] If reunification is not possible, then alternative arrangements should be made to provide a safe and nurturing environment for the child that does not expose the child to exploitation or abuse.[22]

## CHILD ABANDONMENT

An abandoned child, as defined by the United Nations Children's Fund (UNICEF), is a child who does not live with either their mother or father, who does not know where his or her next meal is coming from, and who does not know where he or she is spending the night.[20] Worldwide, there are 153 million orphans.[23] Greater emotional difficulties and lags in cognitive development have been associated with being an orphan or abandoned.[23] More than 400 million abandoned children live on their own on the streets of cities throughout the world, struggling to survive each day. Every 2 seconds a child becomes an orphan and every 14 seconds a child is orphaned by AIDS.[20] Street children are exposed to all sorts of violence, abuse, and exploitation. In some countries, "Street children are routinely detained illegally, beaten and tortured and sometimes killed by police."[20]

## CHILD LABOR

Although the number of children in child labor declined by about one-third between 2000 and 2012,[24] there are still an estimated 215 million child laborers.[25] Moreover, many of these child laborers, an estimated 115 million, are doing hazardous work.[25] Although the highest number of child laborers are working in Asia and the South Pacific, the highest proportion of children involved in child labor or 1 in 5 children is in sub-Saharan Africa.[24] Most child labor is involved in agriculture; although domestic work, work in factories, mines, and other dangerous occupations are not unusual. Child laborers experience deterioration in their health, a negative impact on their growth and may even have serious limb and/or life-threatening injuries.[24–27] Children are even used as child soldiers.[24–26,28]

Armed conflict/war creates an even greater use of child labor. During the Syrian crisis, children are contributing to the family income in over three-quarters of surveyed households in that country. In Jordan, nearly half of all Syrian refugee children are sole or joint family breadwinners. Children as young as 6 years old are working.[26] The greatest vulnerability for child laborers are those children involved in an armed conflict/war, those who are sexually exploited, and those involved in illegal/illicit activities including child trafficking and organized begging. Children may be forced to plant land mines and other explosives or bombs.[29] Child laborers are generally isolated from contact with their families, often forced to endure a slave-like existence, frequently without adequate food, clothing, or shelter; and are often severely abused.[12,25,26,28,29]

## ARMED CONFLICTS/WARS: CHILD SOLDIERS

Unfortunately, the many armed conflicts/wars around the world create additional avenues for violence toward, and the exploitation and abuse of, children. Around the world, thousands of children; both boys and girls, are recruited or forced to serve as part of a rebel group or government forces during armed conflicts/wars. These children are forced to provide labor, serving as cooks, porters, messengers, spies, or used for sexual purposes, often enduring gang rape, and are even forced to clear or lay landmines and take up arms as child soldiers.[12,26,28,29] Children are not only exposed to the brutalities of war, but may be forced to commit atrocities against their own families, friends, neighbors, and community. Estimates indicate that there may be some 300,000 child (<18 years old) combatants/soldiers with some as young as 7 years old in more than 30 conflicts throughout the world, which is about 10% of the combatants in ongoing conflicts.[28,29]

A study done by the Save the Children organization noted the following: the use of child soldiers in more than 70% of conflict zones studied; 25% of the irregular combatants in Columbia from 1990 to 2000 was a child; girls less than 18 years old participated in armed conflicts in at least 39 countries; and, in Nepal, children aged 13 years or more are recruited as combatants, and children as young as 10 years old are used as porters, spies, informants, and bomb planters by Maoist insurgents.[29]

## MORBIDITY AND MORTALITY FROM ARMED CONFLICTS WORLDWIDE IN RECENT DECADES

Estimates of the morbidity and mortality from armed conflicts/wars since 1990 are as follows: more than 2 million children have died; more than 6 million children have been permanently disabled or seriously injured; and greater than 1 million children have been orphaned or separated from their families. These figures do not include the morbidity and mortality from disasters such as hurricanes, tsunamis, tornadoes, and earthquakes.[29]

## CHILD MARRIAGE/FORCED MARRIAGE

Early marriage is marriage before the age of 18 years.[30,31] Early adolescence, for example, age younger than 15 years, is deemed "too early from any point of view, for transitions such as sexual initiation and marriage."[30] Yet more than 100 million girls will be married as children over the next decade, with 14 million girls are married in early adolescence, that is, less than 15 years of age.[30] The Population Council analysis reported at least 20% of girls in 76 regions or provinces in 22 countries were married before 15 years of age.[30] Child brides as young as 8 years old are not unusual in some regions of the world.[32] In Yemen, for example, more than half (52%) of girls were married before 18 years and 14% before 15 years.[33] Worldwide (excluding China), 34% of girls are married before 18 years and 14% before 15 years.[31,32] In some areas of South Asia and sub-Saharan Africa, up to 50% to 75% of girls, and in South America, Central America, and Eastern Europe 10% to 20% of girls, are married before 18 years of age.[34]

The child bride is usually at a severe disadvantage and experiences significant emotional and sometimes physical trauma. For the girl who is in a child marriage, such an arrangement terminates their childhood and any hope of personal growth and development and a better life.[30,31,35-37] The age difference between child brides and their husbands tends to be large, and their marriages are probably arranged, unwanted, and unexpected. Higher rates of child marriage are associated with higher rates of maternal and infant mortality. Studies indicate that girl child brides have an increased risk of sexually transmitted diseases (STDs) and HIV,[30,31,35,36,38] and intimate partner violence.[30,31,35,36,38] Child marriage increases the risk of mental health disorders.[30,38] Increased rates of suicidal ideation and suicidal attempts have been associated with child marriage.[30]

Child marriage is a sign of the gender inequality that exists and reflects the marginalization of women and the impoverishment of the community.[30,36,37] It is endemic in regions that are remote, rural, underdeveloped, and poor.[30,37] It is usually associated with poor and underdeveloped countries, although a study in the Unites States reported an 8.9% prevalence of child marriage.[38]

Child marriage is not only detrimental to the well-being of the girl child bride but also has a negative impact on the nation: "social and economic development are hindered by child marriage."[36]

The World Health Organization's (WHO's) recent guidelines on preventing early pregnancy includes the prevention of child marriage as 1 of its 6 primary goals.[30] Increased fertility and population growth is associated with child/early marriage because it increases the time girls and women have in childbearing years and decreases the time span between generations.[30,31] The UN Secretary General Ban Ki-moon stated that "the practice of child marriage must be ended everywhere."[32] "Child marriage exposes many more (children) to devastating consequences" than "from poverty, malnutrition, and high rates of illiteracy."[33] Child and/or forced marriage is considered a gender-based health and human rights violation affecting women and girls globally according to UNICEF.[31,34,35]

## FEMALE GENITAL MUTILATION

As defined by the WHO, female genital mutilation pertains to a custom that involves partial or complete removal of external female genitalia or other injury to the female genital organs performed for nonmedical (nontherapeutic) reasons.[39,40] There is no medical benefit from this practice,[41] which has been "euphemistically called female circumcision"[39] or female genital cutting.[42] Moreover, significant immediate and life-long complications can result from this practice including severe pain, significant bleeding or hemorrhage, infections, urination difficulties, difficulties in defecation, increase in viral blood-borne infections, infertility, dysmenorrhea, inability to have sexual intercourse, infertility, sexual dysfunction, childbirth complications, newborn deaths, shock, and death.[42,43]

This procedure is generally carried out by "traditional" nonmedical practitioners. Frequently, no anesthetics are given before, during, or after the procedure and non-sterile nonmedical instruments, such as "a razor blade, a piece of glass, or knife is used to cut the most sensitive part of the body."[41,43] The age of the girls undergoing this procedure ranges from 7 days to puberty or adolescence, contingent on the culture.[41,43] Initially, female genital mutilation was a remote practice, associated only with Africa. Now it is prevalent not only in Africa but also in the Middle East and in Asia, and because of global migration even in Western countries.[40,41] Social and cultural traditions including the perception within the community that men will only marry women who have undergone female genital mutilation are impediments to stopping this practice.[40,41]

The procedure has been described by experts such as Ms Ras-Work, "It is torture. It is inhuman. It is degrading treatment of women. It is against the Convention on the Elimination of All Forms of Discrimination against Woman, the Convention on the Rights of the Child, and so many other conventions... There is no excuse for genital mutilation to live with us."[41]

As with other forms of exploitation and abuse, the actual incidence is unknown because of the hidden nature of the crime. Worldwide, as many as 3 million girls are at high risk of undergoing this brutal procedure, and there are from 100 to 140 million girls and women who are living with the consequences of female genital mutilation.[44] About half a million girls and women who currently reside in Europe, and up to 400,000 girls and women in the United States, have been subjected to this procedure.[41,43]

Although some progress has been made, countries such as Ethiopia have been praised for their efforts that have resulted in a decline in the prevalence of female genital mutilation; and 30 countries (19 African states and 11 European nations) have enacted legislation against the practice of female genital mutilation; there is still a high prevalence in many regions.[41] Of girls and women aged 15 to 49 years, nearly 98% and 91% (prevalence) had been subjected to female genital mutilation in Somalia in 2006 and in Egypt in 2008, respectively.[41]

## CHILD TRAFFICKING

Child trafficking is lucrative, and frequently associated with criminal activity and corruption.[45–47] Thus, child trafficking is generally a hidden crime and because most victims are unable or afraid to come forward, exact numbers are difficult to determine.[47–51] It is estimated that there may be up to 26 million individuals worldwide who are victims of trafficking[52] and 50% of all trafficking victims are children.[47,53]

Child trafficking is increasing exponentially. Worldwide, there are from 5.5 to 13.5 million trafficked children; around 1.2 million children are trafficked on an annual basis. Human trafficking generates some $32 billion in US dollars yearly.[45] On a worldwide basis, human trafficking generates about $10 billion dollars on an annual basis according to UNICEF.[53]

A child may be sold by a family member or acquaintance, or ensnared by false promises of an education, a job or a "better life." Instead, they are trafficked and exploited and held in slavery or bondage with inadequate food, clothing, or shelter; and usually severely abused and cut off from all contact with their families. They may be trafficked for commercial sexual exploitation, child prostitution, used for child labor, whether for domestic servitude, agricultural work, mining, factory work, or even as child soldiers.[53,54]

Child sex trafficking and commercial sexual exploitation are "problems in the United States and throughout the world."[55,56] According to UNICEF, 1 million children enter the sex trade annually. Approximately, 10 million children (90% girls) are working as prostitutes. The conditions in which trafficked children live/survive are deplorable. Without the protection of family or guardians, they are often neglected, malnourished, subjected to violence and sexual abuse, at risk for STDs including HIV, and in constant fear of their traffickers who often control them via threats, violence, rape, and drugs.[45,51–53]

Child trafficking is not unique to the underdeveloped world but also exists in the developed world including the United States.[45,47,51,52,55,56] Children who run away from abusive households may find themselves destitute and on the street and may end up ensnared by a supposedly kind stranger who befriends and entraps them in a brutal cycle of abuse and violence, often exploited for commercial sex including prostitution, pornography, and sex tourism.[55,56] In the United States, every year from 100,000 to 300,000 girls are engaged in sexual trafficking.[45] Human trafficking is the fastest growing and second-largest criminal activity in the world, being second only to drug dealing.[45]

Violence and psychological manipulation are widespread. Victims of child trafficking are subject to a greater risk of physical injury, sexual assault, malnutrition, STDs, infectious diseases, untreated chronic medical conditions, substance abuse, and a host of psychological illnesses ranging from depression, post-traumatic stress disorder to homicide and suicide. Medical providers, law enforcement officers, and other relevant individuals such as social workers, should be aware of these child victims because they may present for medical care and this may be an opportunity to intervene on their behalf. Training is recommended in order to increase identification of these victims and then provide necessary care.[46,47,52,53,56,57]

## STRATEGIES FOR COPING

The importance of early recognition of the psychological stress on the child and referral for psychological "first aid" for children during a disaster is well known. Early intervention and provision of coping mechanisms will aid in the child's recovery. During the disaster itself, allowing children to play and to express themselves during the stressful episode improves the child's ability to fully rebound and to rebound more quickly.[22,58,59]

## SET-UP OF SHELTERS/REFUGEE CAMPS: STRATEGIES TO DETER VIOLENCE

Most survivors of sexual violence in armed conflicts or disasters are children, especially girls. During a disaster or armed conflict/war, preventive measures that may limit the ability of child predators to perpetrate their heinous crime include provision of adequate lighting in shelters or refugee camps, building of toilets inside camps and buildings, having separate toilet facilities for males and females, avoiding separation of children from their families, having mechanisms for early reunification of children with their families, ensuring access to shelters for children, ideally providing separate shelters for families and children away from single adults, especially from child predators, criminals, gangs, and other violent offenders.[18,19,21,29]

## STRATEGIES FOR DEALING WITH CHILD TRAFFICKING

Various steps can be taken to combat child trafficking and help the victims recover and be re-assimilated into society. Medical professionals, child protective services, and law enforcement agencies may have gaps in their knowledge and awareness of child trafficking.[46,49,50,52,57,60] Indeed, "it is likely that the majority of victims are unrecognized."[52] Thus, 1 of the first steps is education and training so that heath care providers, child protective workers, and law enforcement agents are aware of the problem and can recognize and then take action to help the victims.[46,47,50,52,53,60] Dealing with child trafficking could be viewed as a 3-faceted approach (1) establishing a legal framework, (2) assisting the victims and recovery for the victims, and (3) changes in the socioeconomic structure.

Programs for combating sexual trafficking should include adoption of child trafficking legislation (nationally and internationally), enforcement of laws, prosecution of child traffickers, and identification and prosecution of facilitators/exploiters (including corrupt officials). Exploited children should not be criminalized but should be viewed as victims and aided in recovery and re-assimilation into society.[46,49,53,57] Methods for modifying the environment or content in which child trafficking occurs might involve modifying attitudes and prejudices that facilitate abuse, promoting gender equality, altering societal norms so that such practices are condemned, strengthening families and communities, implementing national and international child protection systems, strengthening interdisciplinary communication and collaboration for those treating the victims and those prosecuting the perpetrators, and enhanced economic opportunities within communities.[46,47,61]

## STRATEGIES FOR DEALING WITH PROBLEMS OF VIOLENCE, EXPLOITATION, AND ABUSE

The 3-pronged approach for combating child trafficking could be modified and applied to other problems of violence, exploitation, and abuse that children experience (see **Box 1**; **Box 3**).

| Box 3 |
| :--- |
| **Actions for combating the violence, exploitation, and abuse of children** |

- Advocacy campaigns: increase public awareness
- Increase training for key groups: including law enforcement, teachers, social workers, others
- Prosecute offenders
- Support public policy
- Introduce and adopt legislation and implementation of the laws
- Reintegration of exploited and abused children into communities and society
- Develop programs to change the behaviors of families and communities that create conditions that are conducive to child exploitation and abuse
- Encourage programs that improve the education and health of children and the communities they live in
- Eliminate the poverty, civil unrest that create deplorable conditions in which children can be exploited and abused

## SPECIFIC PROGRAMS FOR MEETING THE PHYSIOLOGIC AND SAFETY NEEDS OF CHILDREN

Specific innovative and cost-effective programs have been shown to positively affect the enormous challenges in providing adequate physiologic and safety needs for all children. Political will and leadership are critical in solving the issues related to the physiologic and safety needs of children. Improvement in the welfare of children can occur through changes in legislation, policies, services, and social norms.[61–65]

Programs, such as "WASH" (for water, sanitation, and hygiene) in schools, have been shown in many countries throughout the world to be an effective and relatively low-cost method for improving sanitation and hygiene.[9]

Projects, such as the "Family Support and Foster Care" project and the "Prevention of Infant Abandonment and De-institutionalisation" project in Eastern Europe have as their goals the prevention of additional residential care and de-institutionalizing children who are already in residential care by dealing with the causes of child abandonment and by providing other options to institutionalized care.[62]

The International Labor Organization and other organizations have been campaigning against the use of child labor, and some progress has been made in that the total number of child laborers has dropped in recent years.[24]

A comprehensive approach to combating human trafficking has been developed. This multifaceted approach involves ensuring child rights via prevention and protection, decreasing demand, strengthening the legal framework via legislation and law enforcement, international instruments/agreements, prosecution of traffickers, destroying the criminal networks that engage in human trafficking, identifying and prosecuting the exploiters and facilitators, improving education/schooling, life skills and economic opportunities, strengthening communities, ensuring safe migration (migrants are often frequent unwitting victims of traffickers), rehabilitating/reintegrating victims, promoting gender equality, implementing national (and international) child protection systems, and improving training for law enforcement and other key personnel.[46]

Recommendations and examples of successful programs for ending violence, exploitation, and abuse against children do exist. Although eliminating the violence, exploitation, and abuse of children is a daunting task, these strategies provide a framework as well as specific methods and programs for addressing the problem.[46,62–65]

## SOME SUCCESS IN DEALING WITH THE GLOBAL PROBLEMS FACING CHILDREN

Since 1990, the mortality rate for children less than 5 years of age has declined by more than one-half, decreasing from 90 per 1000 live births to 43 per 1000 live births. Maternal mortality has decreased by 45%.[65]

In terms of world hunger, there was a 42% decrease in the prevalence of undernourished people between 1990–1992 and 2012–2014, with the greatest success in increasing food security in Latin America and the least progress in sub-Saharan Africa.[4] There are now better sources of drinking water for 2.6 billion people.[65]

## THE RIGHTS OF THE CHILD

The Declaration of the Rights of the Child was adopted in 1959.

The UN Convention on the Rights of the Child is a human rights treaty that enumerates the rights of children: their civil, political, economic, social, health, and cultural rights. A child is defined as any human being under the age of 18 years unless the age of majority is attained earlier under a state's own domestic legislation. Signatories are required to adhere to the Convention as required by international law with compliance monitored by the UN Committee on Rights of the Child. The Convention was adopted by the UN General Assembly and opened for signature on November 20, 1989. After ratification by the required number of countries, it came into existence on September 2, 1990, with 194 countries party to it, all of which were members of the UN except for the United States and Somalia[66] (**Box 4**).

In many countries, common law previously treated children as chattels or possessions and, as such, the ownership of a child could be disputed in court. Therefore, acceptance and implementation of the Convention might necessitate a change in the laws pertaining to child custody and guardianship.

Two additional protocols were adopted by the UN General Assembly on May 25, 2000: "Optional Protocol on the Involvement of Children in Armed Conflict,"

---

**Box 4**
**Tenets in the Convention of the Rights of the Child**

- Every child has basic rights

- These rights include
  - Right to life
  - Right to his/her own identity
  - Right to be raised by his/her parents within a family or cultural grouping
  - Right to have a relationship with both parents even if they are separated
  - Right to express their opinions
  - Right to have their opinions heard and acted on when appropriate
  - Right to be protected from abuse or exploitation
  - Right to have their privacy protected
  - Right not to have their lives subject to excessive interference

- Parents are obligated to exercise their parental responsibilities.

- From the United Nations Convention on the Rights of the Child.

*From* UNICEF. Rights under the Convention on the Rights of the Child. Available at: http://www.unicef.org/crc/index_30177.html.

---

**Box 5**
**Optional protocols adopted by the United Nations general assembly**

*"Optional Protocol on the Involvement of Children in Armed Conflict"*

- Governments should ensure that
  - Children less than 18 years old are not recruited compulsorily into the armed forces
  - Members of their armed forces who are less than 18 years old do not take part in hostilities

*"Optional Protocol on the Sale of Children, Child Prostitution and Child Pornography"*

- Governments should
  - Prohibit the sale of children, child prostitution, and child pornography

*"Optional Protocol to the Convention on the Rights of the Child on a Communications Procedure"*

- Children or their representatives are allowed to file individual complaints for violation of the rights of children

*Adapted from* United Nations Office of the Special Representative of the Secretary-General for Children and Armed Conflict. The optional protocol on the involvement of children in armed conflict. Available at: https://childrenandarmedconflict.un.org/mandate/opac/.

---

and "Optional Protocol on the Sale of Children, Child Prostitution and Child Pornography." One additional protocol, "Optional Protocol to the Convention on the Rights of the Child on a Communications Procedure" was adopted in December 2011[66] (**Box 5**).

## TYPES OF PROTECTION NEEDED BY CHILDREN DURING DISASTERS AND ARMED CONFLICTS/WARS

During disasters and in times of armed conflict/war, the critical types of protection needed by the child identified by the Save the Children organizations are protection from physical harm, protection from exploitation and gender-based violence, protection from psychosocial distress, protection from recruitment into armed groups, protection from family separation, protection from abuses related to forced displacement, and protection from denial of children's access to quality education[29] (**Box 6**).

---

**Box 6**
**Types of protection children need most in disaster areas and during armed conflicts/war zones**

- Protection from physical harm
- Protection form exploitation and gender-based violence
- Protection from psychosocial distress
- Protection from recruitment into armed groups
- Protection from family separation
- Protection from abuses related to forced displacement
- Protection from denial of children's access to quality education

*From* Save the Children. Protecting children in emergencies: escalating threats to children must be addressed policy brief. Available at: www.savethechildren.org/atf/cf/%7B9def2ebe-432c-9bd0-f91d2eba74a%7D/policy_brief_.final.pdf. Accessed July 13, 2015.

## THE FUTURE

Child abuse, more recently termed child maltreatment, has been problematic for centuries, as the writings of Dickens and others have illustrated. The landmark work of C. Henry Kempe on the "Battered-child syndrome" was instrumental in mobilizing forces to mitigate against child maltreatment.[67] We now have laws that make the reporting of child abuse mandatory, and legal and social systems are set up to deal with this issue. Similarly, we can work toward the goal of achieving the "Rights of the Child" for children worldwide. There are multiple steps in this worthwhile objective. First is awareness by the public and recognition of the threats to the safety of children and the problems facing children worldwide. Changes in societal norms, legislative action, legal systems that include the prosecution of those who exploit or abuse children, implementation of policies, and the provision of services to the victimized are all key to achieving success. A concerned public, leadership, and political will are essential to attaining this goal. It is hoped that this article will raise awareness of these issues.

## REFERENCES

1. UN: Global refugee numbers reached alarming levels in 2014, Syria the biggest source. Available at: http://www.usnews.com/news/world/articles/2015/06/18/un-global-refugee-numbers-reach-alarming-levels. Accessed June 15, 2015.
2. UN warns of alarming level in global refugee numbers. Available at: http://www.aljazeera.com/news/2015/06/warns-alarming-level-global-refugee-numbers-150618133734323.html. Accessed June 15, 2015.
3. Global refugee figures highest since WW2, UN says. Available at: http://www.bbc.com/news/world-27921938. Accessed June 15, 2015.
4. 2015 World Hunger and Poverty Facts and Statistics by WHES. Available at: http://worldhunger.org/articles/Learn/world%20hunger%20facts%202002.htm. Accessed July 15, 2015.
5. Maslow AH. A theory of human motivation. Psychol Rev 1943;50(4):370–96.
6. Tang TL, West WB. The importance of human needs during peacetime, retrospective peacetime, and the Persian Gulf War. Int J Stress Manag 1997;4(1):47–62.
7. Singer P, Sukhdev P, Li HL, et al. Quality of life: what does it mean? How should we measure it? World Policy J 2011;28(2):3–6.
8. Ashworth A. Nutrition, food security, and health. In: Kliegman R, Stanton BF, St Geme J, et al, editors. Nelson textbook of pediatrics. Philadelphia: Elsevier; 2016. p. 295–306.e1. chapter 46.
9. Raising even more clean hands: advancing health, learning and equity through WASH in schools. Available at: http://www.unicef.org/wash/schools/files/Raising_Even_More_Clean_Hands_Web_17_October_2012(1).pdf. Accessed July 15, 2015.
10. Sanitation worldwide. Available at: http://www.sanitationworldwide.com. Accessed July 15, 2015.
11. Raise shelter, raise hope. Available at: http://www.worldwideshelters.org. Accessed July 15, 2015.
12. Child protection from violence, exploitation, and abuse. Available at: http://www.unicef.org/protection/57929_57977.html. Accessed July 15, 2015.
13. Mace SE. Behavioral and psychiatric disorders in children and infants. In: Tintinalli JE, Stapczynski JS, Ma OJ, et al, editors. Tintinalli's Emergency Medicine A Comprehensive Study Guide. New York: McGraw-Hill; 2011. p. 967–71.

14. Akmatov MK. Child abuse in 28 developing and transitional countries – results from the Multiple Indicator Cluster surveys. Int J Epidemiol 2011;40:219–27.
15. Barth J, Bermetz L, Helm E, et al. The current prevalence of child sexual abuse worldwide: a systematic review and metanalysis. Int J Public Health 2013;58: 469–83. Child abuse.
16. Children from all walks of life endure violence and millions more are at risk. Global statistics on children's protection from violence, exploitation and abuse. Available at: http://www.data.unicef.org/child-protection/violence. Accessed July 15, 2015.
17. Faul M. (Associated Press) Boko Haram offers to swap kidnapped girls for detainees. Available at: http://abcnews.go.com/International/wireStory/boko-haram-offers-swap-detainees-kidnapped-girls-32299173. Accessed July 15, 2015.
18. Unspeakable crimes against children. Sexual violence in conflict. Available at: www.savethechildren.org/atf/cf/%7B9def2ebe-10ae-432c-abd0-df91d2eba74A%7D/unspeakable_crimes_against_children.pdf. Accessed July 13, 2015.
19. Mello AF, Maciel MR, Fossaluza V, et al. Exposure to maltreatment and urban violence in children working on the streets in Sao Paulo, Brazil: factors associated with street work. Rev Bras Psiquiatr 2014;36:191–8.
20. Statistics on abandoned children. Available at: www.internationalstreetkids.com/statistics.php. Accessed July 13, 2015.
21. Pullum T, Cappa C, Orlando J, et al. Systems and strategies for identifying and enumerating children outside of family care. Child Abuse Negl 2012;36:701–10.
22. Mace SE, Sharieff G, Bern A, et al. Pediatric issues in disaster management, part 2: evacuation centers and family separation/reunification. Am J Disaster Med 2010;5(3):149–61.
23. Escueta M, Whetten K, Ostermann K, et al. Adverse childhood experiences, psychosocial well-being and cognitive development among orphans and abandoned children in five low income countries. BMC Int Health Hum Rights 2014; 14(6):1–13.
24. Child labour drops worldwide: explore the data. Available at: www.theguardian.com/news/datablog/2013/sep/24/child-labour-drops-worldwide-data. Accessed July 15, 2015.
25. Protecting children from exploitation. Available at: www.savethechildren.org/site/c.8rKLIXMGIpIE/b.6192517/k.9ECD/Proteting_Children_from_Exploitation.hmtl. Accessed July 15, 2015.
26. Urgent action needed to tackle child labour caused by Syrian crisis. Available at: http://www.unicef.org/media/media_82462.html.
27. Tiwari RR, Saha A. Morbidity profile of child labor at gem polishing units of Jaipur, India. J Occup Environ Med 2014;5:125–9.
28. Coalition to Stop the Use of Child Soldiers. Guide to the optional protocol on the involvement of children in armed conflict. New York: United Nations Children's Fund (UNICEF); 2003. p. 1–71. Available at: www.unicef.org/publications/index__19025.html. Accessed July 15, 2015.
29. Protecting children in emergencies: escalating threats to children must be addressed. Available at: www.savethechildren.org/atf/cf/%7B9def2ebe-432c-9bd0-df91d2eba74a%7D/policy_brief_.final.pdf. Accessed July 13, 2015.
30. Erulkar A. Adolescence lost: the realities of child marriage. J Adolesc Health 2013;52:513–4.
31. Okonofua F. Prevention of child marriage and teenage pregnancy in Africa: need for more research and innovation. Afr J Reprod Health 2013;17(4):9–10.

32. Machel G, Pires E, Carlsson G. The world we want: an end to child marriage. Lancet 2013;382:1005–6.
33. AlAmodi AA. Child marriage in Yemen. Lancet 2013;382:1979–80.
34. Raj A, Boehmer U. Girl child marriage and its association with national rates of HIV, maternal health, and infant mortality across 97 countries. Violence Against Women 2013;19(4):536–51.
35. Sabbe A, Oulami H, Zekraoui W, et al. Determinants of child and forced marriage in Morocco: stakeholder perspectives on health, policies and human rights. BMC Int Health Hum Rights 2013;13:43–55.
36. Lee-Rife S, Malhotra A, Warner A, et al. What works to prevent child marriage: a review of the evidence. Stud Fam Plann 2012;43(4):287–303.
37. Chatterjee P. India grapples with its child marriage problem. Lancet 2011;378: 1987–8.
38. Le Strat Y, Dubertret C, Le Foll B. Child marriage in the United States and its association with mental health in women. Pediatrics 2011;128:524–30.
39. Rhymer J, O'Flynn N. Female genital mutilation. Br J Gen Pract 2013;63:515–6.
40. Reig Alcaraz MR, Gonzalez JS, Solano Ruiz C. Attitudes toward female genital mutilation: an integrative review. Int Nurs Rev 2013;61:25–34.
41. Cui W. International agencies call for end to female genital mutilation. BMJ 2011; 342:832–4.
42. Perron L, Senikas V, Burnett M, et al. Female genital cutting. J Obstet Gynaecol Can 2013;35(11):1028–45.
43. Hearst AA, Molnar AM. Female genital cutting: an evidenced-based approach to clinical management for the primary care physician. Mayo Clin Proc 2013;88(6): 618–29.
44. Ellsberg M, Arrango DJ, Morton M, et al. Prevention of violence against women and girls: what does the evidence say? Lancet 2015;385(9677):1555–66.
45. O'Connell Davidson J. Telling tales: child migration and child trafficking. Child Abuse Negl 2013;37:1069–79.
46. Rafferty Y. Child trafficking and commercial sexual exploitation: a review of promising prevention policies and programs. Am J Orthopsychiatry 2013;83(4): 559–75.
47. Victory A Sr. Child trafficking. Health Prog 2011;92(3):58–61.
48. Finkel R, Finkel ML. The "dirty downside" of global sporting events: focus on human trafficking for sexual exploitation. Public Health 2015;129:17–22.
49. Swartz MK. Commercial sexual exploitation of minors: overlooked and underreported. J Pediatr Health Care 2014;28:195–6.
50. Beck ME, Lineer MM, Meltzer-Lange M, et al. Medical providers' understanding of sex trafficking and their experience with at-risk patients. Pediatrics 2015; 135(4):e895–902.
51. Testimony of Survivor Leader. Commentary: commercial sexual exploitation – a survivor's perspective: "Can you help me? Do you care?". Curr Probl Pediatr Adolesc Health Care 2014;44:270–1.
52. Greenbaum VJ. Commercial sexual exploitation and sex trafficking of children in the United States. Curr Probl Pediatr Adolesc Health Care 2014;44:245–69.
53. Factsheet: child trafficking. Available at: www.unicef/protecttion/57929_58005. html. Accessed July 15, 2015.
54. McLeigh JD. Protecting children in the context of international migration. Child Abuse Negl 2013;37:1056–68.
55. Smith L, Vardaman S, Snow M. The national report on domestic minor sex trafficking: America's prostituted children. sharedhope International. 2009. Available

at: http://sharedhope.org/wp-content/uploads/2012/09/SHI_National_Report_on_DMST_2009.pdf. Accessed July 15, 2015.

56. Greenbaum J, Crawford-Jakubiak JE. Committee on child abuse and neglect. Child sex trafficking and commercial sexual exploitation: health care needs of victims. Pediatrics 2015;135(3):566–74.
57. Cowell JM. Commercial sexual exploitation and sex trafficking of minors as child abuse. J Sch Nurs 2014;30(2):87. Finding shelter from the shelter – Save the Children.
58. Mace SE, Doyle C, Fuchs S, et al. Pediatric patients in a disaster: part of the all-hazard, comprehensive approach to disaster management. Am J Disaster Med 2012;7(2):111–25.
59. Available at: www.savethechildren.org/site/c.8rKLIXMGIpI4E/b.88437471K.3527/Finding_Shelter_from_Shelter.html. Accessed July 15, 2015.
60. Wise J. Doctors are urged to be alert to signs of child sexual exploitation. BMJ 2014;349:g5934.
61. Malqvist M. Abolishing inequity, a necessity for poverty reduction and the realization of child mortality targets. Arch Dis Child 2015;100(Suppl 1):s5–9.
62. Evaluation Report: 2006 GEO: Evaluation of the Family Support & Foster Care and the Prevention of Infant Abandonment and De-institutionalisation Project. Millions of world's poorest children left behind despite global progress. Available at: http://www.unicef.org/evaldatabase/index_37978.html.    www.unicef.org/media/media_82345.html. Accessed July 15, 2015.
63. Ending violence against children: six strategies for action. UNICEF; 2014.
64. On Universal Children's Day, put violence and abuse in the spotlight. UNICEF. Available at: http://www.unicef.org/media/media_70976.html. Accessed July 15, 2015.
65. Millions of worlds' poorest children left behind despite global progress, new UNICEF report says. Available at: http://www.unicef.org/media/media_82345.html. Accessed July 15, 2015.
66. United Nations Convention on the Rights of the Child. Available at: http://UNcrchttps://treaties.un.org/pages/viewdetails.aspx?src=treaty&mtdsg_no=iv-11&chapter=4&lang=en-title=UNTC-publisher=. Accessed July 15, 2015.
67. Kempe CH, Silverman F, Steele B, et al. The Battered-child Syndrome. JAMA 1962;181:17–24.

# Infectious Diseases of Poverty in Children
## A Tale of Two Worlds

Caitlin Hansen, MD[a], Elijah Paintsil, MD[a,b,c],*

## KEYWORDS

- Infectious diseases • Children • Poverty • HIV/AIDS • Malaria • Tuberculosis
- Neglected tropical diseases

## KEY POINTS

- Poverty is inextricably linked with infectious diseases, including human immunodeficiency virus (HIV) infection, tuberculosis (TB), malaria and neglected tropical diseases (NTDs).
- Advances have been made in HIV treatment; however, access to and management of antiretroviral therapy (ART) in children still lag behind that of adults.
- TB is the leading infectious cause of mortality worldwide; poverty and young age are significant determinants of progression from TB exposure to disease.
- Malaria remains a leading cause of child mortality; access to effective preventive measures and therapy must reach vulnerable populations.
- Clinicians, both in endemic and nonendemic areas, must be familiar with the epidemiology and clinical manifestations of these infections to ensure prompt diagnosis and treatment.

## INTRODUCTION

The phrase "infectious diseases of poverty" (IDoP) is used to describe infectious diseases that are more prevalent among poor and vulnerable populations.[1] IDoP comprises (1) human immunodeficiency virus (HIV) and AIDS, tuberculosis (TB), and malaria—the "big 3" (also referred to as the "Unholy Trinity"); and (2) neglected tropical diseases (NTDs).[2] Poverty has been inextricably linked with infectious diseases since antiquity. Poverty, acting through nongenetic heritable principles, has transformed infectious diseases into "inheritable" conditions. IDoP is seen in pockets of poverty

Disclosures: The authors have nothing to disclose.
[a] Department of Pediatrics, Yale University School of Medicine, 464 Congress Ave, New Haven, CT 06520, USA; [b] Department of Pharmacology, Yale University School of Medicine, 464 Congress Avenue, New Haven, CT 06520, USA; [c] Department of Public Health, Yale University School of Medicine, 464 Congress Avenue, New Haven, CT 06520, USA
* Corresponding author. Departments of Pediatrics, Pharmacology & Public Health, Yale University School of Medicine, 464 Congress Avenue, New Haven, CT 06520.
E-mail address: elijah.paintsil@yale.edu

Pediatr Clin N Am 63 (2016) 37–66
http://dx.doi.org/10.1016/j.pcl.2015.08.002
0031-3955/16/$ – see front matter © 2016 Elsevier Inc. All rights reserved.
pediatric.theclinics.com

in high-income countries as well. IDoP perpetuates poverty by leading to adverse outcomes in pregnancy, child development, and workplace productivity.[3] Gross domestic product, an indicator of the wealth of a country, is the most sensitive surrogate measure of burden of infectious diseases in a country. **Fig. 1** illustrates the positive correlation between poverty and infectious diseases. Substandard housing, lack of access to safe water and sanitation, and inadequate vector control contribute to the efficient transmission of these infections.[4] Other social determinants (eg, gender inequality, unemployment, low educational status, poor nutrition) compound the problem.[5] Strategies to prevent and control infectious diseases require tremendous resources. Therefore, infectious diseases have artificially divided the world into high-income as well as low- and middle-income countries (LMIC), with LMIC bearing the greatest burden of IDoP. However, with globalization and increased interconnectedness of the world, IDoP can transcend this economic divide.

This article provides an overview of IDoP that affect children with a focus on epidemiology, clinical manifestations, diagnosis, management, and prevention. IDoP account for a significant disease burden and high disability-adjusted life-years (**Table 1**).

## HUMAN IMMUNODEFICIENCY VIRUS
### Epidemiology

Thirty-four years into the HIV epidemic, advances in prevention and treatment have been made. However, challenges remain regarding access to and management of antiretroviral therapy (ART), particularly in LMIC. Established modes of HIV transmission are (1) sexual contact, (2) needle injuries, (3) mucous membrane exposure, (4) mother-to-child transmission (MTCT), and (5) transfusion with contaminated blood products. MTCT continues to fuel the pediatric HIV epidemic in LMIC.[6] The use of perinatal antiretroviral drugs to prevent MTCT (PMTCT) of HIV has resulted in a dramatic decrease (to <2%) in the rate of vertical HIV transmission in the United States.[7]

Despite these successes, progress has not been uniform worldwide. At the end of December 2013, only 23% of the 3.2 million children estimated to be living with HIV were receiving ART and in 2013 alone, 240,000 were newly infected and 190,000 (170,000–220,000) died of HIV-related causes.[8] Poverty is related inextricably to the disparity in global coverage of ART, with LMIC reporting low coverage (**Table 2**). Sub-Saharan Africa, with the highest proportion of people living on less than US$2 per day (see **Fig. 1**), is home to 91% of all children living with HIV.[9]

### Clinical Manifestations

The hallmark of HIV infection is progressive depletion of CD4 T cells leading to development of opportunistic infections, AIDS, and death.[7] In acute simian immunodeficiency virus infection, 30% to 60% of all gut-associated CD4 cells become infected, leading to profound depletion within 4 days of infection.[10] Similar CD4 gastroenteropathy occurs with acute HIV infection, albeit at a different pace. During primary infection, HIV infects gut-associated resting and activated memory CD4 cells, leading to breach in the intestinal epithelial barrier with a loss of tight junctions, enterocyte apoptosis, local immune activation, and depletion of CD4 cells.[11] The breach in the mucosal barrier facilitates translocation of pathogenic bacteria and microbial products from the gut lumen to the systemic circulation, leading to chronic immune activation.[12] The time from acute infection to the development of AIDS is defined by a CD4 cell count of less than 200 cells/mm$^3$ or the appearance of AIDS-defining opportunistic infections or cancers (**Box 1**) and ranges from 6 months to 25 years.

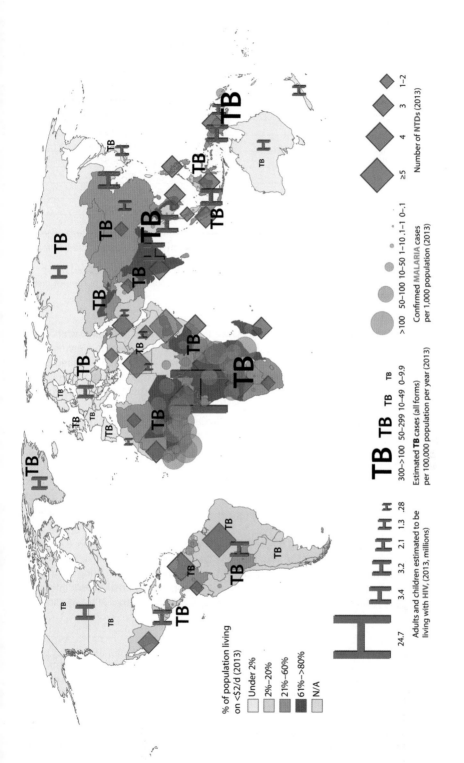

% of population living
on <$2/d (2013)

Under 2%
2%–20%
21%–60%
61%–>80%
N/A

**TB** TB TB TB
300–>100  50–299  10–49  0–9.9

Estimated **TB** cases (all forms)
per 100,000 population per year (2013)

**H** H H H H H
24.7  3.4  3.2  2.1  1.3  .28

Adults and children estimated to be
living with HIV, (2013, millions)

>100  50–100  10–50  1–10  .1–1  0–.1

Confirmed **MALARIA** cases
per 1,000 population (2013)

≥5      4      3      1–2

Number of NTDs (2013)

**Table 1**
**Estimated DALYs of malaria, HIV/AIDS, tuberculosis and NTDs, 2010**

| Disease | DALYs, in Thousands (95% CI) |
| --- | --- |
| HIV/AIDS | 81,547 (75,003–88,367) |
| Tuberculosis | 49,396 (40,065–56,071) |
| Malaria | 82,685 (63,426–109,836) |
| NTDs | |
| Leishmaniasis | 3317 (2180–4890) |
| Schistosomiasis | 3309 (1705–6260) |
| Dengue | 825 (344–1412) |
| Chagas disease | 546 (271–1054) |
| Cysticercosis | 503 (379–663) |
| Other NTDs | 4724 (3525–6351) |

*Abbreviations:* DALY, disability-adjusted life-years (cumulative number of years of life lost from ill health, disability, or premature death); NTD, neglected tropical disease.

*Adapted from* Murray CJ, Vos T, Lozano R, et al. Disability-adjusted life years (DALYs) for 291 diseases and injuries in 21 regions, 1990-2010: a systematic analysis for the global burden of disease study 2010. Lancet 2012;380(9859):2204–05; with permission.

However, in infants, disease progression is rapid; without treatment, 20% and 50% of perinatally infected infants will die by 3 and 24 months of age, respectively.[13]

HIV infection in children results in a wide array of clinical manifestations (see **Box 1**) and has a varied natural history. Early presentations of pediatric HIV infection include unexplained fevers, generalized lymphadenopathy, hepatomegaly, splenomegaly, failure to thrive, oral and diaper candidiasis, recurrent diarrhea, parotitis, hepatitis, central nervous system disease (eg, hyperreflexia, hypertonia, floppiness, developmental delay), recurrent invasive bacterial infections, and other opportunistic infections (see **Box 1**).

### Diagnosis

The HIV nucleic acid test is used for diagnosis of HIV infection. The HIV nucleic acid test includes HIV DNA and RNA polymerase chain reaction (PCR) assays, and related RNA qualitative or quantitative assays.[14,15] HIV culture is not used for routine diagnostic testing.[16] Early HIV testing of all infants born to HIV-infected women is required. Infants born to women with HIV infection will be HIV antibody positive because of transplacental transfer of maternal antibodies. HIV RNA or DNA testing of an HIV-exposed infant should be performed at birth (for infants at high risk of HIV infection), at age 14 to 21 days, at 1 to 2 months, and at age 4 to 6 months. HIV infection can

◄─────────

**Fig. 1.** Global poverty and infectious diseases burden. (*Data from* population living on less than US$2 per day (World Bank: http://data.worldbank.org/indicator/SI.POV.2DAY/ countries); adults and children estimated to be living with human immunodeficiency virus (HIV; available from the World Health Organization [WHO]: http://www.who.int/hiv/data/ en/); estimated tuberculosis (TB) cases per year (available from the WHO: http://www.who.int/tdr/publications/global_report/en/); confirmed malaria cases in 2013 (available from the WHO: http://www.who.int/malaria/publications/world_malaria_report_2013/en/); number of neglected tropical diseases (NTDs; available from the US Centers for Disease Control and Prevention: http://www.cdc.gov/globalhealth/ntd/diseases/ntd-worldmap-table.html).)

**Table 2**
**ART coverage among human immunodeficiency virus–infected children in low- and middle-income countries and by WHO region, December 2013**

| WHO Region | Number on ART | Percent Coverage (Range) |
|---|---|---|
| Africa region | 630,300 | 22 (20–24) |
| The Americas | 26,400 | 51 (38–62) |
| South-East Asia region | 13,900 | >95 (94–>95) |
| Eastern Mediterranean region | 1100 | 7 (5–9) |
| Western Pacific region | 13,200 | 61 (56–67) |
| Total | 684,900 | 47.2 (7–>95%) |

*Abbreviations:* ART, Antiretroviral therapy; WHO, World Health Organization.
*Adapted from* Global AIDS Response Progress Reporting (WHO/UNICEF/UNAIDS). 2014. Available at: http://www.who.int/hiv/data/pedartmap2014.png?ua51.

**Box 1**
**Common HIV-related manifestation in HIV-infected children**

*Mild HIV-related symptoms*

Children with 2 or more of the conditions listed but none of the conditions listed in Moderate Symptoms category
- Lymphadenopathy ($\geq$0.5 cm at >2 sites; bilateral at 1 site)
- Hepatomegaly
- Splenomegaly
- Dermatitis
- Parotitis
- Recurrent or persistent upper respiratory tract infection, sinusitis, or otitis media

*Moderate HIV-related symptoms*

- Anemia (hemoglobin <8 g/dL [normal, <80 g/L]), neutropenia (white blood cell count <1000/$\mu$L [normal, <1.0 $\times$ 109/L]), and/or thrombocytopenia (platelet count <100 $\times$ 103/$\mu$L [normal, <100 $\times$ 109/L]) persisting for $\geq$30 days

- Bacterial meningitis, pneumonia, or sepsis (single episode)

- Candidiasis, oropharyngeal (thrush), persisting (>2 months) in children older than age 6 months

- Cardiomyopathy

- Cytomegalovirus infection, with onset before 1 month

- Diarrhea, recurrent or chronic

- Hepatitis

- Herpes simplex virus stomatitis, recurrent (>2 episodes within 1 year)

- Herpes simplex virus bronchitis, pneumonitis, or esophagitis with onset before 1 month

- Herpes zoster (shingles) involving at least 2 distinct episodes or more than 1 dermatome

- Leiomyosarcoma

- Lymphoid interstitial pneumonia or pulmonary lymphoid hyperplasia complex

- Nephropathy

- Nocardiosis

- Persistent fever (lasting >1 month)

- Toxoplasmosis, onset before 1 month
- Varicella, disseminated (complicated chickenpox)

*Stage 3–defining opportunistic illnesses in HIV infection*

- Bacterial infections, multiple or recurrent
- Candidiasis of bronchi, trachea, or lungs
- Candidiasis of esophagus
- Cervical cancer, invasive
- Coccidioidomycosis, disseminated or extrapulmonary
- Cryptococcosis, extrapulmonary
- Cryptosporidiosis, chronic intestinal (>1 month duration)
- Cytomegalovirus disease (other than liver, spleen, or nodes), onset at age greater than 1 month
- Cytomegalovirus retinitis (with loss of vision)
- Encephalopathy attributed to HIV
- HSV: chronic ulcers (>1 month duration) or bronchitis, pneumonitis, or esophagitis (onset at age >1 month)
- Histoplasmosis, disseminated or extrapulmonary
- Isosporiasis, chronic intestinal (>1 month duration)
- Kaposi sarcoma
- Lymphoma, Burkitt (or equivalent term)
- Lymphoma, immunoblastic (or equivalent term)
- Lymphoma, primary, of the brain
- Mycobacterium avium complex or *Mycobacterium kansasii*, disseminated or extrapulmonary
- *Mycobacterium tuberculosis* of any site, pulmonary, disseminated, or extrapulmonary
- Mycobacterium, other species or unidentified species, disseminated or extrapulmonary
- Pneumocystis jirovecii (previously known as Pneumocystis carinii) pneumonia
- Pneumonia, recurrent
- Progressive multifocal leukoencephalopathy
- Salmonella septicemia, recurrent
- Toxoplasmosis of brain, onset at age greater than 1 month
- Wasting syndrome attributed to HIV

*Abbreviations:* HIV, human immunodeficiency virus; HSV, herpes simplex virus.
*Adapted from* Centers for Disease Control and Prevention. Revised surveillance case definition for HIV infection—United States, 2014. MMWR Recomm Rep 2014;63(No. RR-3):10.

be excluded in a non-breastfed infant with 2 or more negative virologic tests (ie, negative RNA or DNA), one at age 1 month or older and one at age 4 months or older, or 2 negative antibody tests from separate specimens obtained at age 6 months or older. The World Health Organization (WHO) recommends that all HIV-exposed infants have HIV virologic testing at 4 to 6 weeks of age and HIV serologic testing at 9 months to identify infants with persisting HIV antibody or who have seroreverted.[17] Furthermore, serologic testing followed by virologic testing (if seroreverted) is recommended at least 6 weeks after breastfeeding cessation in children less than 18 months of age. For infants and children greater than 18 to 24 months of age who present with symptoms consistent with HIV infection (see **Box 1**) and unknown maternal HIV status, HIV diagnosis relies on antibody tests and a confirmatory PCR test.

### Management

The goal of combination ART (cART) is to suppress HIV viral replication and restore immune function. Current treatment strategies focus on timely initiation of cART regimens capable of maximally suppressing viral replication to prevent disease progression. There are emerging reports that very early cART is associated with very small proviral reservoirs and restricted HIV-specific immune responses in perinatal infection.[18–20] However, when to start (**Box 2**) and what ART regimen to start a patient on (**Table 3**) vary from country to country. The management of patients failing first-line regimens and treatment options for multiple drug resistant HIV is complicated and should involve an expert in HIV medicine.

The standard of care for monitoring treatment in HIV-infected children is routine laboratory monitoring of CD4 absolute count or percentage and HIV viral load.[21] The WHO recommends viral load surveillance as the preferred monitoring of HIV treatment; if not routinely available, CD4 count and clinical monitoring are used.[17]

### Prevention

HIV prevention in children can be categorized into (1) primary prevention, mainly by PMTCT, and (2) secondary prevention of morbidity and mortality of HIV. PMTCT rates as low as 1% have been achieved as a result of the use of the PACTG 076 regimen,[22] cART, and appropriate management of labor and delivery. The birth of an infected child in a high-income countries is now rare and represents systems failure and missed opportunities during pregnancy, labor, and delivery.[23] The WHO recommends Option B+ as the main strategy to eliminate MTCT: Option B+ proposes that all HIV-infected women receive lifelong ART beginning at their first pregnancy, regardless of CD4 count.[2] This strategy may improve maternal health through reduced morbidity and mortality, and reduce overall MTCT, especially in settings with high fertility rates.[2] The cost effectiveness of Option B+ has been reported by several studies.[24–26]

In the era of expanded access to ART, millions of children with perinatally acquired HIV infection are now living longer. However, pediatric HIV faces new challenges related to adherence, drug resistance, reproductive health planning, transition to adult medical care, and the potential for long-term complications from HIV and the treatment thereof.[21,27]

## TUBERCULOSIS
### Epidemiology

TB is caused by the bacillus *Mycobacterium tuberculosis* and is the leading infectious cause of death worldwide. Childhood TB accounts for approximately 10% to 20% of the global burden of TB disease. In 2013, there were an estimated 9.0 million incident cases and 1.5 million deaths,[28] including 550,000 cases and 80,000 deaths among children. In the same year, TB case rates in the United States continued to decline in all age groups except among children aged 14 years or younger (0.8 cases per 100,000).[29] Moreover, poor case ascertainment, absence of active case finding, and limited surveillance data in TB-endemic areas contribute to underestimation of global burden of pediatric TB disease.[30] Incidence of pediatric TB is an accurate measure of ongoing transmission of TB within a community.

**Box 2**
**When to start ART in children**

*WHO Guidelines on when to start ART in children*

ART should be initiated among *all children younger than 10 years of age* living with HIV, regardless of WHO clinical stage or at any CD4 cell count
- As a priority, ART should be initiated among all children <2 years old or with WHO stage 3 or 4 or CD4 count $\leq$750 cells/mm$^3$ or CD percentage <25% among children younger than 5 years and CD4 count $\leq$350 cells/mm$^3$ among children 5 years and older

ART should be initiated among *all adolescents (i.e., 10 to 19 years)* living with HIV regardless of WHO clinical stage and at any CD4 cell count
- As a priority, ART should be initiated among all adolescents with severe or advanced HIV clinical disease (WHO clinical stage 3 or 4) and adolescents with CD4 count $\leq$350 cells/mm$^3$

*US Department of Health and Human Services Guidelines on when to start ART in children*

cART should be initiated urgently in all HIV-infected children with any of the following:
- Age younger than 12 months
- Age 1 year or older (with CDC stage 3-defining opportunistic illnesses or CDC stage 3 immunodeficiency)
- Aged 1 to younger than 6 years, CD4 less than 500 cells/mm$^3$
- Aged 6 years or older, CD4 less than 200 cells/mm$^3$

cART should be initiated in HIV-infected children aged 1 year or older with any of the following:
- Moderate HIV-related symptoms (see **Box 1**)
- Plasma HIV RNA greater than 100,000 copies/mL
- CDC stage 2

  Age 1 to younger than 6 years, CD4 count 500 to 999 cells/mm$^3$.

  Age 6 years or older, CD4 count 200 to 499 cells/mm$^3$.

  If CD4 count is less than 350 cells/mm$^3$.

  If CD4 count is 350 to 499 cells/mm$^3$.

cART should be considered for HIV-infected children aged 1 year or older with:
- Mild HIV-related symptoms (see **Box 1**) or asymptomatic and CDC stage 1

  Ages 1 to younger than 6 years, CD4 count 1000 cells/mm$^3$ or greater.

  Age 6 years or older, CD4 count of 500 cells/mm$^3$ or greater.

*Pediatric European Network for Treatment of AIDS guidelines for ART initiation*

ART is recommended
- In all children under 1 year of age;
- In all children with significant disease [WHO stage 3 or 4 or CDC stage B or C];
- In asymptomatic children over 1 year of age based on age-specific CD4 count; and
- In those with hepatitis C virus or active tuberculosis coinfection.

ART should be considered:
- In asymptomatic children over 5 years of age at CD4 counts of 350 to 500 cells/mm$^3$;
- In children with high VL (>100,000 copies/mL);
- In asymptomatic children aged 1 to 3 years irrespective of immune status and VL;
- In sexually active adolescents, to minimize the risk of onward transmission;
- In the presence of any significant HIV-related clinical symptoms; and
- In hepatitis B virus coinfection irrespective of immune status.

*Abbreviations:* ART, antiretroviral therapy; cART, combination antiretroviral therapy; CDC, US Centers for Disease Control and Prevention; HIV, human immunodeficiency virus: VL, viral load; WHO, World Health Organization.

*Adapted from* WHO Early Release Guidelines on when to start antiretroviral therapy and on pre-exposure prophylaxis for HIV. September 2015. Available at: www.who.int. Accessed October 3, 2015. US Department of Health and Human Services (HHS) Guidelines on Antiretroviral Agents in Pediatric HIV Infection (2013, revised in 2015); Available at https://aidsinfo.nih.gov/guidelines. Accessed June 2, 2015. Paediatric European Network for Treatment of AIDS (PENTA) guidelines for ART initiation (2015). Available at http://penta-id.org/hiv/penta-trials-treatment-guidelines.html. Accessed June 2, 2015.

**Table 3**
**Overview of current pediatric first-line HIV treatment regimens**

| Organization (Source) | Age (y) | Preferred Regimen | Alternate Regimen |
|---|---|---|---|
| WHO (2013) | Children <3 y | LPV/r + ABC + 3 TC or<br>LPV/r + AZT + 3 TC | NVP[a] + ABC + 3 TC<br>or<br>NVP[a] + AZT + 3 TC (ABC + 3 TC + AZT)[b] |
| | 3–10 y (<35 kg) | EFV + ABC + 3 TC<br>or<br>EFV + AZT (or TDF) + 3 TC (or FTC) | NVP + ABC + 3 TC<br>or<br>NVP + AZT (or TDF) + 3 TC (or FTC) |
| | 10–19 y (≥35 kg) | EFV + TDF + 3 TC (or FTC)<br>or<br>EFV + AZT + 3 TC<br>EFV + ABC + 3 TC | NVP + TDF + 3 TC (or FTC)<br>or<br>NVP + AZT + 3 TC<br>NVP + ABC + 3 TC |
| US HHS (2015) | Children aged ≥14 d to <3 y | 2 NRTIs + LPV/r | 2 NRTIs + NVP |
| | Children aged ≥3–6 y | 2 NRTIs + EFV (or LPV/r) | 2 NRTIs + ATV/r (≥3 mo to <6 y)<br>2NRTIs + RAL (≥2 y) |
| | Children aged ≥6 y | 2 NRTIs + ATV/r or EFV or LPV/r | 2NRTIs + DRV/r (≥3 to <12 y)<br>2 NRTIs + DRV/r (≥12 y)<br>2 NRTIs + DTG (≥12 y and weighing ≥40 kg) |

*(continued on next page)*

**Table 3**
*(continued)*

| Organization (Source) | Age (y) | Preferred Regimen | Alternate Regimen |
|---|---|---|---|
| PENTA (2015) | Children <1 y | ABC[c] + 3 TC + LPV/r<br>Or<br>(ABC + 3 TC + AZT + NVP)[d] | NNRTI backbone: AZT + 3 TC |
| | Children 1–3 y | ABC + 3 TC + LPV/r<br>Or<br>(ABC + 3 TC + AZT + NVP)[e] | NRTI backbone: AZT + 3 TC |
| | Children 3–6 y | ABC + 3 TC + LPV/r or EFV | AZT + 3 TC + NVP or DRV/r<br>or<br>TDF + 3 TC (FTC) + NVP or DRV/r |
| | Children 6–12 y | ABC + 3 TC + ATV/r<br>or<br>ABC + 3 TC + EFV<br>or<br>TDF + FTC + ATV/r or DRV/r or EFV | AZT + 3 TC + NVP (or LPV/r or DRV/r)<br>or<br>TDF + 3 TC (FTC) + NVP or LPV/r or DRV/r |
| | Children >12 y | ABC + 3 TC + ATV/r or DRV/r or EFV | ABC + 3 TC + NVP or LPV/r or RAL[f] or DTG |

*Abbreviations:* 3TC, lamivudine; ABC, abacavir; ARV, antiretroviral; ATV, atazanavir; ATV/r, atazanavir plus ritonavir; AZT, zidovudine; d4T, stavudine; DRV, darunavir; DRV/r, darunavir plus ritonavir; DTG, dolutegravir; EFV, efavirenz; FTC, emtricitabine; HHS, US Department of Health and Human Services; LPV/r, fixed dose formulation lopinavir/ritonavir; NNRTI, nonnucleoside reverse transcriptase inhibitor; NRTI, nucleoside reverse transcriptase inhibitor; NVP, nevirapine; PENTA, Pediatric European Network for Treatment of AIDS; PI, protease inhibitor; RAL, raltegravir; RTV, ritonavir; TDF, tenofovir; WHO, World Health Organization.

[a] NVP-based regimen if LPV/r is not feasible.

[b] As an option for children who develop tuberculosis while on ART regimen containing NVP or LPV/r. Once tuberculosis therapy is completed, a switch to initial regimen is recommended.

[c] Before starting abacavir (ABC), test for HLA B*5701. If positive, then ABC should not be prescribed.

[d] In children less than 3 years, consider adding AZT to NVP-based regimens if there is a very high viral load or central nervous system involvement until viral load has been suppressed for at least 3 months.

[e] Four-drug induction for infants on NVP-based therapy may be considered until viral load has been suppressed for at least 3 months, followed by 3-drug maintenance therapy.

[f] In rare instances (eg, transmitted resistance or toxicity), raltegravir may be used as first-line therapy in children <12 years of age.

*Data from* the WHO consolidated guidelines on the use of antiretroviral drugs for treating and preventing HIV infection: recommendations for a public health approach (2013). Available at: http://www.who.int/hiv/pub/guidelines/arv2013/download/en/. Accessed June 2, 2015; US Department of Health and Human Services (HHS) Guidelines on Antiretroviral Agents in Pediatric HIV Infection (2013, revised in 2015). Available at: https://aidsinfo.nih.gov/guidelines. Accessed June 2, 2015; and Paediatric European Network for Treatment of AIDS (PENTA) guidelines for ART initiation (2015). Available at: http://penta-id.org/hiv/penta-trials-treatment-guidelines.html. Accessed June 2, 2015.

The natural history of TB in children can be quite different from that of adults. Duration from TB exposure to infection to disease is much shorter owing to several factors, by far the most important of which is poverty. Poverty increases a child's risk of TB exposure through cultural practices around child care,[31] overcrowding in school and at home,[32–36] poor housing with inadequate ventilation,[37,38] adults in household with comorbidities such as HIV,[39] seasonal and environment-related exposure,[40–42] and lack of public health infrastructure.[43] After TB exposure, risk of a child developing infection is influenced by the acid fast bacilli sputum positivity of the source case,[33] duration and intensity of exposure,[35,44] infectiousness of the TB strain,[45,46] coinfections,[47,48] and the child's immune and genetic makeup.[49,50]

## Clinical Manifestations

TB infection could be asymptomatic in children for several years. When disease occurs, signs and symptoms may be nonspecific, leading to diagnostic delay.[51] TB disease could manifest as pulmonary or extrapulmonary. Clinical manifestations of pulmonary TB in children include fever, weight loss, cough, and night sweats. Pulmonary TB is the most common manifestation of TB in children, accounting for 60% to 80% of all cases.[52] Manifestations of extrapulmonary TB include lymphadenopathy (67%), central nervous system involvement (13%), miliary and/or disseminated disease (5%), and musculoskeletal (4%).[53] TB can affect any organ and presentation may be nonspecific or unusual; therefore, in TB-endemic areas physicians should have a high index of suspicion for TB.[51] In a TB-endemic area, the use of a symptom-based diagnostic approach provided a fairly accurate diagnosis of pulmonary TB in HIV-uninfected children 3 years and older (sensitivity, 68.3%; specificity, 80.1%; positive predictive value, 82.1%).[54] The symptom-based diagnostic approach comprised 3 well-defined symptoms at presentation: (1) persistent, nonremitting cough of greater than 2 weeks' duration, (2) weight loss during the preceding 3 months, and (3) fatigue.[54]

## Diagnosis

Positive culture of *M tuberculosis* complex from gastric aspirates, sputum, bronchial lavage, pleural fluid, cerebrospinal fluid, urine, or other body fluid or tissue biopsy specimen establishes the diagnosis of TB. TB in children is usually paucibacillary; therefore, often acid fast bacilli negative on microscopy (sputum smears are positive in <10%–15% of children diagnosed with TB)[55,56] and culture negative (confirmation by culture in only 30%–40% of cases).[57,58] In nonendemic areas, in the absence of bacteriologic confirmation, diagnosis of TB in children is based on a triad of (1) close contact with an infectious index patient, (2) positive tuberculin skin test (TST) result, and (3) abnormal chest x-ray findings.[59] The best specimen for diagnosis of pulmonary TB in a child with nonproductive cough is an early morning gastric aspirate obtained before ambulation or feeding; 3 gastric aspirates on 3 consecutive mornings are required. There are innovative ways of obtaining swallowed respiratory samples for TB diagnosis in children who cannot produce sputum, such as induction of sputum with aerosolized hypertonic saline[58] and the string test.[60,61] Nucleic acid amplification tests for the detection of mycobacterial DNA or RNA are in clinical use. Their sensitivities are low in paucibacillary TB, which includes most cases of childhood TB and extrapulmonary TB.[62]

The TST is the most common method for diagnosing latent TB infection in asymptomatic patients. TST is an immune-based test driven by interferon-gamma production by T lymphocytes. Of immunocompetent children with culture-proven TB, 10% to 15% may have a negative TST initially.[63] Moreover, previous Bacille Calmette-Guérin (BCG) vaccination or infection with nontuberculous mycobacteria may give a false-positive TST.[64] In most high-income countries with low TB incidence such as the United Kingdom, a TST is regarded as positive with induration of greater than 5 mm in those without prior BCG vaccination and greater than 15 mm for those with prior BCG vaccination.[62] In the United States, TST results are interpreted based on an individual's risk of contracting TB and clinical factors: 5 mm or greater (close contacts, TB disease, immunosuppression), 10 mm or greater (increased risk of disseminated disease or increased exposure to TB disease), and 15 mm or greater (children >4 years of age with no risk factors).[65] The WHO guidelines differ slightly, with a positive TST being greater than 5 mm for those with risk factors (eg, HIV infection, malnutrition) and greater than 10 mm for all others.[66]

Alternate tests to TST are the in vitro T-cell–based interferon-gamma release assays (IGRA). In these assays (eg, QuantiFERON-TB Gold, T-SPOT.TB, and Gold In-Tube), interferon-gamma is produced in response to stimulation of mononuclear cells or whole blood by specific *M tuberculosis* antigens.[62] These antigens are present only in *M tuberculosis* complex and absent from all strains of *Mycobacterium bovis* BCG and almost all environmental mycobacteria. They do not have significant advantages over the TST for the diagnosis of active TB disease but may be useful in excluding false-positive TST. In 2011, the WHO's Stop TB Department published new recommendations on the use of IGRAs and TST to detect latent TB in LMIC: (1) IGRAs and TST cannot accurately predict the risk of infected individuals developing active TB disease; (2) neither IGRAs nor TST should be used for the diagnosis of active TB disease; (3) IGRAs are more costly and technically complex than TST; and (4) given comparable performance but increased cost, replacing the TST by IGRAs in resource-constrained settings is not recommended.[67]

## Management

Latent TB infection can be treated effectively to prevent progression to active TB. The following regimens are recommended by WHO: 6 or 9 months of isoniazid daily; 3 months of rifapentine plus isoniazid weekly; 3 or 4 months of isoniazid plus rifampicin daily; and 3 or 4 months of rifampicin daily. Treatment of most forms of childhood TB disease (eg, pulmonary and extrapulmonary) consists of a 6-month chemotherapy regimen with 4 drugs (isoniazid, rifampin, ethambutol, and pyrazinamide) in the initial intensive phase, followed by 2 drugs in the continuation phase (**Fig. 2**). For miliary, meningeal, bone/joint, or disseminated TB, treatment is extended to 9 to 12 months. Directly observed therapy is highly recommended.

Limited data exist on the prevalence and management of drug-resistant TB in children. Studies from South Africa report an increasing proportion of drug resistant TB isolates in children (7%–15%).[68,69] Drug-resistant TB is categorized into 2 categories: (1) multidrug resistant TB, defined as resistance to isoniazid and rifampin, the 2 most important first-line anti-TB drugs; and (2) extensively drug-resistant TB, defined as multidrug resistant TB with additional resistance to a fluoroquinolone and one of either amikacin, capreomycin, or kanamycin.[70] The management of drug-resistant TB is complicated and should involve an expert with experience in treating drug-resistant TB. Four or 5 anti-TB drugs that the child's resistant isolate or that of an adult contact's resistant isolate is susceptible to are used.[71] These may include second-line anti-TB drugs that are usually expensive and cause more side effects that can affect compliance to treatment (**Table 4**).

## Prevention

Prevention strategies of childhood TB include (1) immunization in high burden countries and improvement of housing and sanitation, (2) chemoprophylaxis of latent TB

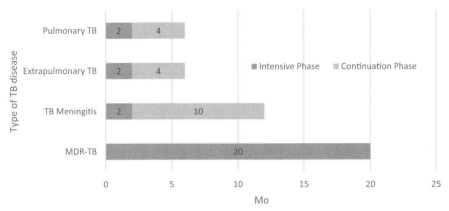

**Fig. 2.** Treatment of tuberculosis (TB) in children. Treatment duration composed of intensive and continuation phases. For most forms of pulmonary TB and extrapulmonary TB, a 6-month course of chemotherapy regimen with 4 drugs (isoniazid [INH], rifampin [RMP], ethambutol [EMB], and pyrazinamide [PZA]) in the 2-month intensive phase, followed by 2 drugs (INH and RMP) in the 4-month continuation phase. For TB meningitis, the continuation phase is extend to a least 10 months using the same drugs. Recommended treatment duration of multidrug resistant (MDR)-TB is at least 20 months with 4 second-line drugs likely to be effective plus PZA.

infection and efficient surveillance programs, and (3) discovery of more efficacious and tolerable anti-TB drugs to shorten treatment duration, improve compliance, and decrease community TB bacilli burden.

## MALARIA
### *Epidemiology*

Malaria, a mosquito-borne parasitic disease, is a leading cause of child mortality. Worldwide, an estimated 3.2 billion people are at risk for malaria; as an IDoP, the geographic distribution of endemic malaria closely mirrors that of the world's population residing in extreme poverty (see **Fig. 1**).[72,73] Progress has been made in malaria control and elimination. From 2000 to 2013, a 46% relative decrease in malaria infection prevalence occurred among children aged 2 to 10 years, and an estimated 4.3 million deaths were averted worldwide.[72] Despite these gains, annually there are 200 million cases of malaria and more than 500,000 deaths, the majority of which occur in sub-Saharan Africa and in young children.[74] Mortality owing to malaria disproportionately affects children aged less than 5 years, who comprise 78% of deaths.[72]

Malaria is caused by the *Plasmodium* parasite transmitted by the bite of an infected female Anopheles mosquito. Five species of *Plasmodium* typically cause disease in humans: *P falciparum, P vivax, P ovale, P malariae*, and *P knowlesi*. The *Plasmodium* life cycle includes stages in both mosquitoes and humans. When an infected mosquito bites a human, *Plasmodium* sporozoites are passed into the bloodstream and travel to the liver. There, sporozoites enter hepatocytes, where they replicate asexually and develop into schizonts. This stage, known as hepatic schizogeny, takes approximately 7 to 10 days for *P falciparum* and *P vivax* and approximately 2 weeks for *P malariae*. Then infected hepatocytes rupture, releasing merozoites into the bloodstream to infect red blood cells. In the erythrocyte, merozoites either undergo a cycle of asexual reproduction and lysis, subsequently infecting other erythrocytes, or they differentiate

**Table 4**
**Dosages and side effects of antituberculous drugs**

| Drug | Total Dose (mg/kg/d) | Routes of Administration | Side Effects |
|---|---|---|---|
| Isoniazid | 10–15 | PO/IV/IM | Hepatotoxicity, peripheral neuropathy, myelosuppression |
| Rifampin | 10–20 | PO/IV | Hepatotoxicity, myelosuppression, rash |
| Pyrazinamide | 30–40 | PO | Hepatotoxicity, arthralgia, rash |
| Ethambutol | 15–25 | PO | Optic neuritis |
| Amikacin | 12–30 | IV/IM | Nephrotoxicity, ototoxicity, hypokalemia |
| Kanamycin | 15–20 | IV/IM | Nephrotoxicity, ototoxicity, rash |
| Capreomycin | 15–30 | IV/IM | Nephrotoxicity, ototoxicity |
| Ofloxacin | 15–20 | PO/IV | Gastrointestinal disturbance, arthralgia, insomnia |
| Levofloxacin | 7.5–10 | PO/IV | Gastrointestinal disturbance, arthralgia, insomnia |
| Moxifloxacin | 7.5–10 | PO/IV | Gastrointestinal disturbance, arthralgia, insomnia |
| Ethionamide | 15–20 | PO | Gastrointestinal disturbance, hepatotoxicity, hypothyroidism |
| Protionamide | 15–20 | PO | Gastrointestinal disturbance, hepatotoxicity, hypothyroidism |
| Cycloserine | 15–20 | PO | Psychosis, convulsions |
| Terizidone | 15–20 | PO | Psychosis, convulsions |
| Para-aminosalicylic acid | 150–200 | PO | Anorexia, diarrhea, hypothyroidism |
| Thioacetazone | 150 | PO | Severe skin rash, myelosuppression |
| Clofazimine | 300 | PO | Reversible discoloration of skin, hair, etc. |
| Linezolid | 15–20 | PO/IV | Myelosuppression, lactic acidosis, peripheral neuropathy, pancreatitis |
| Imipenem + cilastatin | 40–80 | IV/IM | Gastrointestinal disturbance, phlebitis, convulsion, encephalopathy |

*Abbreviations:* IM, intramuscularly; IV, intravenously; PO, by mouth.

into male and female gametocytes, which are ingested by biting mosquitoes to undergo a sexual reproductive cycle in the mosquito's gut. In *P vivax* and *P ovale* malaria, a subset of infected hepatocytes develop into hypnozoites, which can remain dormant for weeks to years, causing relapse of disease upon reactivation.

### Clinical Manifestations

Clinical presentation of malaria depends on the infecting species, parasite burden, and immune status of the patient. Acute malaria commonly presents with nonspecific symptoms of fever, chills, headache, and myalgias. Gastrointestinal symptoms such as nausea, vomiting, and diarrhea can also occur.

Severe malaria is generally owing to infection with *P falciparum* and is characterized by 1 or more of the following: impaired consciousness, severe anemia, renal impairment, pulmonary edema, spontaneous bleeding, acidosis, hypoglycemia, jaundice, shock, or hyperparasitemia. Additional clinical and laboratory features of severe malaria can be found in **Box 3**. Manifestations of severe malaria vary by age, with severe

---

**Box 3**
**Features of severe malaria**

Clinical
    Impaired consciousness (including coma)
    Prostration (inability to sit, stand, or walk without assistance)
    Multiple convulsions (>2 episodes in 24 hours)
    Deep breathing and respiratory distress (acidotic breathing)
    Acute pulmonary edema and acute respiratory distress syndrome
    Circulatory collapse or shock (systolic blood pressure <50 mm Hg in children)
    Acute kidney injury
    Jaundice
    Abnormal bleeding

Laboratory
    Hypoglycemia (<40 mg/dL)
    Metabolic acidosis (plasma bicarbonate <15 mmol/L)
    Severe normocytic anemia (<5 mg/dL in children)
    Hemoglobinuria
    Hyperlactatemia (lactate >5 mmol/L)
    Renal impairment (serum creatinine >265 μmol/L)
    Pulmonary edema (radiographic)

*From* WHO. Management of severe malaria. 2012. Available at: http://apps.who.int/iris/bitstream/10665/79317/1/9789241548526_eng.pdf. Accessed June 2, 2015; with permission.

---

anemia and hypoglycemia seen more commonly in children.[74] In endemic regions, recurrent infections in young children can lead to chronic anemia and splenomegaly.[74]

## Diagnosis

Diagnosis of malaria can be made by examination of Giemsa-stained thick and thin blood smears and rapid diagnostic tests. Microscopic examination remains the gold standard of diagnosis. Examination of a thick smear allows for detection of parasites present in small numbers, and thin smears aid in species identification. Classic features of *P falciparum* on microscopy include ring forms in normal-sized erythrocytes (commonly multiply infected) and extracellular crescent- or banana-shaped gametocytes. In *P vivax* and *P ovale* infections, erythrocytes are commonly enlarged with Schuffner's dots, or eosinophilic stippling, seen on the infected erythrocyte. Rapid diagnostic tests detect various antigens or enzymatic activities from malaria parasites and provide results in minutes. However, they may be less sensitive in nonfalciparum malaria (depending on the type of test used) or low levels of parasitemia.[75]

## Management

Treatment depends on the *Plasmodium* species causing infection, as well as the geographic location where infection was acquired, owing to varying antimalarial resistance. For uncomplicated malaria, the WHO guidelines recommend artemisinin-based combination therapy (ACT) as the treatment of choice for *falciparum* malaria; ACT is effective in the treatment of all other human malarias as well.[74,76] ACT consists of a rapidly acting artemisinin component (artesunate, artemether, or dihydroartemisinin) with a longer acting antimalarial for 3 days; fixed-dose combination formulations are available.[74] For patients diagnosed within the United States, the Centers for Disease Control and Prevention provide clinicians with guidance in selection of appropriate antimalarial therapy.[77]

Individuals with *P vivax* or *P ovale* infections can be treated with ACT or chloroquine (if susceptible). Patients should also receive a 14-day course of primaquine to prevent relapse from the liver stage. Primaquine causes hemolysis in patients with G6PD deficiency; therefore, testing for G6PD deficiency is necessary before starting therapy.

Severe malaria is a medical emergency and patients with manifestations of severe disease (see **Box 3**) require aggressive treatment with parenteral antimalarials and careful supportive care. Intravenous artesunate is the treatment of choice in severe disease because it decreases mortality in children hospitalized with severe falciparum malaria as compared with intravenous quinine.[74] After intravenous therapy, a course of ACT can be administered once oral tablets can be given. Supportive care for severe malaria may include infusion of dextrose to maintain euglycemia, blood transfusions for bleeding and severe anemia, hemodialysis in cases of acute renal failure, and treatment of seizures with benzodiazepines.[74] Unfortunately, the linkage between poverty and malaria extends to treatment access, with poorer groups more likely to self-treat than access trained health care providers.[78]

### Prevention

Vector control is of the utmost importance in the prevention of malaria. Strategies include use of insecticide-treated bed nets to prevent mosquito bites while sleeping, indoor residual spraying of long-lasting insecticide to kill mosquitoes, and treatment of water sources to kill mosquito larvae.[73] Although these interventions are effective in interrupting the transmission of malaria, socioeconomic disparities exist in access to preventive measures.[78]

Travelers to malaria endemic areas are at risk of infection, and chemoprophylaxis is recommended for travelers to these regions. Selection of appropriate prophylaxis depends on local antimalarial susceptibility patterns (eg, prevalence of chloroquine resistance), and prevalent malarial species (to determine the need for liver stage prophylaxis in areas where P vivax and P ovale are the predominant malarial species). In addition, clinicians should consider malaria in the differential diagnosis of any febrile illness in a traveler who has recently returned from an endemic region, even if chemoprophylaxis was given.

Insecticide and drug resistance remain major concerns to malaria control. A vaccine against malaria is not yet available. The most advanced vaccine candidate to date targets the pre-erythrocytic stage of P falciparum; data from ongoing phase III trials demonstrated 30% to 50% efficacy of the vaccine against clinical malaria in children, although efficacy waned over time.[79–81]

### NEGLECTED TROPICAL DISEASES

The WHO defines NTDs as medically diverse infections that form a group because of their association with poverty.[82] NTDs comprise 17 parasitic, viral, and bacterial infections (**Box 4**) that affect 1 billion people worldwide.[1] In recognition of the association between neglected parasitic infections and child poverty in the United States,[83] the Centers for Disease Control and Prevention have targeted 5 parasitic diseases, namely, Chagas disease, cysticercosis, toxocariasis, toxoplasmosis, and trichomoniasis, for public health action.[84] A description of selected NTDs that may be encountered by pediatricians, even in high-income countries, is presented herein; a summary of these selected NTDs is presented in **Table 5**.

### Chagas Disease

#### Epidemiology

Chagas disease, caused by the parasite Trypanosoma cruzi, is found only in the Americas and often in rural areas of widespread poverty. Most infections are vector borne

---

**Box 4**
**Neglected tropical diseases prioritized by the World Health Organization, by causative pathogen**

Protozoa
  Chagas disease
  Human African trypanosomiasis (sleeping sickness)
  Leishmaniasis

Bacteria
  Buruli ulcer
  Leprosy (Hansen disease)
  Trachoma
  Yaws

Helminth
  Cysticercosis/taeniasis
  Dracunculiasis (guinea worm disease)
  Echinococcosis
  Foodborne trematodiases
  Lymphatic filariasis
  Onchocerciasis (river blindness)
  Schistosomiasis
  Soil-transmitted helminths (Ascaris, hookworm, whipworm)

Virus
  Dengue
  Rabies

*From* WHO. Neglected tropical diseases. Available at: http://www.who.int/neglected_diseases/ diseases/en/. Accessed June 6, 2015; with permission.

---

and result from contact with an infected triatomine bug; however, transmission can occur from mother to child,[90] blood transfusion, and organ transplantation.[91] Worldwide, an estimated 8 million people are infected with Chagas disease, including about 300,000 in the United States.[91,92] Congenital Chagas disease occurs in approximately 1% to 10% of children born to infected mothers, with an estimated 63 to 315 infants congenitally infected in the United States each year.[92]

*Clinical manifestations*
Acute Chagas disease occurs immediately after infection, concurrent with parasitemia, lasting about 4 to 8 weeks. Often asymptomatic, mild nonspecific symptoms such as fever or, rarely, acute myocarditis or meningoencephalitis may occur.[91,93] In the absence of treatment, parasitemia declines after 8 to 12 weeks and lifelong chronic infection ensues. Although most chronically infected individuals remain asymptomatic, 20% to 30% develop chronic Chagas disease[93] characterized by cardiac and gastrointestinal manifestations (see **Table 5**).

Congenital Chagas disease often has no overt clinical manifestations; symptomatic newborns may present with low birth weight, low Apgar scores, organomegaly, anasarca, respiratory distress, hematologic abnormalities, or meningoencephalitis.[74,91] Although congenital Chagas disease can be potentially life threatening, affected infants may go unrecognized owing to nonspecific symptoms or because the diagnosis was not considered.

*Diagnosis*
In acute or congenital Chagas disease, parasites may be visualized on blood smear; PCR tests are also available. In chronic disease, serology is the mainstay of

**Table 5**
Key points on selected neglected tropical diseases affecting children

| Disease | Transmission | Diagnosis | Clinical Manifestations | Interventions | Key WHO 2020 Targets |
|---|---|---|---|---|---|
| Chagas disease | Vector-borne (triatomine bug), congenital, via blood transfusion or organ transplantation | Acute/congenital infection: blood smear examination for parasites, PCR. Chronic infection: serology (≥2 positive tests required for diagnosis) | Cardiomyopathy, megacolon, megaesophagus | Case detection and management, nifurtimox, benznidazole, vector control, screening of blood donors | Elimination of peridomiciliary infestation in Latin America by 2020 |
| Toxocariasis | Ingestion of *Toxocara* eggs in contaminated soil | Serologic testing; stool examination not useful (eggs are not excreted by humans) | Visceral infection: Abdominal pain, fever, hepatomegaly, cough, wheezing, meningoencephalitis. Ocular infection: strabismus, unilateral vision loss | Albendazole, mebendazole, ophthalmology referral ± steroids for ocular disease | Reach 75% of all school-age children for deworming by 2020 |
| Cysticercosis | Ingestion of eggs excreted in the feces of tapeworm carrier | Neurocysticercosis: serologic testing, neuroimaging | Neurocysticercosis: seizures, headaches, increased intracranial pressure | Hand hygiene, symptom control, consider antihelminths/steroids. Screening of close contacts for tapeworm infection | Validated strategy for control and elimination of *Taenia solium* taeniasis/cysticercosis available by 2015. Interventions for control and elimination scaled up in selected countries in Asia, Africa, and Latin America by 2020 |

| | Transmission | Diagnosis | Clinical manifestations | Treatment/Prevention | WHO goals |
|---|---|---|---|---|---|
| Dengue | Vector-borne (*Aedes* mosquito) | Serologic testing; RT-PCR | Fever, headache, arthralgia, myalgia, retroorbital pain, hemorrhagic manifestations, vascular permeability, shock | Supportive care, fluid repletion, vector control | Reduction of rates of morbidity by at least 25% and of mortality by 50% by 2020 by using an integrated vector management approach |
| Leishmaniasis | Vector-borne (sandfly) | Biopsy (visualization of parasites in tissue or aspirate material gold standard); culture, PCR | Cutaneous: skin papules → nodules → large, painless ulcers Mucosal: nasal stuffiness or bleeding, ulcerative destruction of nasooropharyngeal mucosa Visceral: Fever, weight loss, hepatosplenomegaly | Case detection and management, antimonials, amphotericin B, miltefosine, azoles, vector control | Detection of at least 70% of all cases of cutaneous leishmaniasis and treatment of at least 90% of all detected cases in the Eastern Mediterranean Region by 2015 100% case detection and treatment of visceral leishmaniasis on the Indian subcontinent by 2020 |
| Schistosomiasis | *Schistosoma* worms spread by infected snails in contaminated fresh water, | Detection of *Schistosoma* eggs in urine or feces, serologic testing | Hematuria, genitourinary tract disease, intestinal and liver fibrosis, growth and cognitive delays | Praziquantel, clean water and sanitation | Elimination as a public health problem in multiple countries in Africa by 2020, and globally by 2025 |

*Abbreviations:* PCR, polymerase chain reaction; RT-PCR, reverse transcription polymerase chain reaction; WHO, World Health Organization.
*Adapted from Refs.*[85–89]

diagnosis.[91] Owing to limitations of serologic testing, at least 2 different tests based on different antigens or formats are required for accurate diagnosis.[91]

### Management/prevention

Benznidazole and nifurtomox are available for the treatment of Chagas disease. Both are effective in acute disease, but less effective in chronic disease; benznidazole tends to be better tolerated.[94] Treatment is recommended in all cases of acute infection, congenitally infected infants, and chronic disease in children 18 years of age or younger.[94]

In endemic areas, prevention has focused on reducing disease transmission from the triatomine vector by insecticide spraying and improved housing. Control efforts in the United States center on preventing transmission through blood products (via donor screening since 2007), organ transplantation, and congenital infection.[95,96]

## Neurocysticercosis

### Epidemiology

Neurocysticercosis is a central nervous system infection with the larval form of the pork tapeworm, *Taenia solium*. Humans can become *T solium* carriers by consuming undercooked pork. The adult *T solium* worm produces infective eggs in the host intestine, which spread in the environment to humans via food contaminated with feces or by autoinoculation. Ingested eggs invade the intestine and migrate to distant tissues, where they develop into cystcerci. In endemic regions of Central and South America, prevalence estimates of neurocysticercosis range from 15% to 38%.[97] In the United States, population-level estimates of neurocysticercosis are incomplete, but regional data put the prevalence at 0.2 to 5.5 per 100,000 population.[98]

### Clinical manifestations

Although many individuals infected with *T solium* are asymptomatic, serious sequelae result when cysts localize to the brain, resulting in neurocysticercosis. Symptoms include seizures, headaches, hydrocephalus, or focal neurologic signs.[98]

### Diagnosis

Diagnosis is made with neuroimaging and serologic testing. The hallmark of neurocysticercosis on neuroimaging is cerebral calcifications; if the tapeworm scolex is visualized, this is diagnostic.[98] Enzyme-linked immunoelectrotransfer blot is the preferred serologic test for diagnosis of cysticercosis, although sensitivity is reduced in the presence of a single cyst or calcified cysts.[98]

### Treatment/prevention

Treatment of neurocysticercosis is multifactorial, and because neurocysticercosis represents a spectrum of disease, treatment must often be individualized.[99] The initial goal of therapy is to control symptoms. Antiparasitic therapy can be considered after symptom control; however, it may exacerbate symptoms owing to the inflammatory response provoked by killing the cysts. Therefore, steroids are often coadministered. Albendazole is the drug of choice, with praziquantel used as second-line therapy.[99]

Hand hygiene is important in preventing cysticercosis. In addition, infected individuals and their close contacts should be screened for *T solium* carriage, owing to asymptomatic household tapeworm carriers being a common source of infective eggs.[100] Elimination of cysticercosis requires improvement in sanitary conditions worldwide.[101]

## Toxocariasis

### Epidemiology
Toxocariasis is caused by the roundworms *Toxocara canis* or *Toxocara cati* that are associated with dogs and cats, respectively. In the United States, *Toxocara* seroprevalence is 13.9% among individuals aged 6 years and older.[102] *Toxocara* eggs are shed in the feces of the host dog or cat. Human infection occurs upon ingestion of infective eggs in contaminated soil. Infections typically occur in young children who may play in contaminated sandboxes or playgrounds. After ingestion, *Toxocara* larvae hatch from eggs in the gastrointestinal tract, penetrate the intestinal wall, and hematogenously disseminate to distal organs.

### Clinical manifestations
Three major clinical syndromes of toxocariasis have been described: visceral, ocular, and covert toxocariasis. Most patients with *Toxocara* infection, however, are asymptomatic. Visceral toxocariasis typically affects young children and occurs when larvae migrate to organs and tissues, most commonly the liver or lung, with resulting inflammatory response leading to location-specific symptoms (see **Table 5**).[102]

Ocular toxocariasis results from larval migration to the eye. Inflammation and scarring can be severe and lead to blindness. A national survey of ophthalmologists, reported 68 cases of ocular toxocariasis, of whom 68% were reported to have experienced visual loss.[102] Each year, at least 70 people (mostly children) are blinded from *Toxocara* infection.[84]

In covert toxocariasis, symptoms are typically mild and nonspecific, and can include wheezing and eosinophilia, but not all signs and symptoms of visceral disease.

### Diagnosis
*Toxocara* diagnosis is made by serology, the utility of which is limited because titers can remain elevated for years. Serology can be unreliable in cases of ocular toxocariasis. Other laboratory findings in acute infection may include eosinophilia, anemia, and hypergammaglobulinemia.

### Management/prevention
Albendazole or mebendazole is recommended for treatment of visceral and ocular toxocariasis. In ocular disease, steroids are beneficial in reducing inflammation to prevent scarring and vision loss. Prevention measures include regular deworming of dogs and cats, proper disposal of pet feces, and hand hygiene.

## Schistosomiasis

### Epidemiology
Schistosomiasis is a common parasitic disease caused by *Schistosoma* worms spread by contact with infected freshwater snails. Five species infect humans; the 3 most common are *S haematobium, S mansoni,* and *S japonicum.* More than 200 million people worldwide are affected; most infections occur in sub-Saharan Africa, with children carrying a substantial burden.

### Clinical manifestations
*Schistosoma* infection results from contact with cercariae, the free-swimming larval form of the worm, in contaminated fresh water. Cercariae penetrate skin; a maculopapular rash may occur after exposure. Over several weeks, parasites migrate through host tissues and develop into adult worms. Symptoms result from host response to egg deposition into tissues and may include fever, headache, myalgias, right upper quadrant abdominal pain, and diarrhea.[103] Tender hepatomegaly and splenomegaly

may also be present. Chronic schistosomiasis results from granuloma formation at sites of maximal egg accumulation and leads to site-specific symptoms (see **Table 5**): for *S mansoni* and *S japonicum* the intestine and liver are affected, whereas for *S haematobium* genitourinary tract involvement is seen.[103] Chronic infections can result in impaired growth and development, chronic inflammation, anemia, and nutritional deficiencies.[104] Furthermore, infections acquired in childhood can progress to long-term consequences, including bladder cancer, liver damage, reproductive issues, and heightened susceptibility to HIV, if treatment is delayed or not given.[105]

### Diagnosis

Detection of *Schistosoma* eggs in urine or feces is diagnostic. Location of the spine— terminal (*S haematobium*) or lateral (*S mansoni*) —can aid in species identification. Serologic testing aids in diagnosing patients who are infected but not yet shedding eggs. Other supportive laboratory findings include eosinophilia, anemia, hypoalbuminemia, and increased urea and creatinine.[106]

### Treatment/prevention

Praziquantel is effective in achieving egg reduction rates and cures in 60% to 90% of patients.[103,105] In endemic areas, regular school-based deworming is a common control measure; however, preschool-age children, who may have prevalence of disease similar to older children and adults, are often excluded from these programs.[105] Access to clean water and adequate sanitation are essential to prevention of schistosomiasis; travelers to endemic areas should be advised to avoid swimming or bathing in fresh water and to drink water from a safe source. A vaccine against *Schistosoma* is not yet available.

## Dengue

### Epidemiology

Dengue is caused by a flavivirus transmitted by *Aedes* mosquitoes. Four serotypes (DENV 1–4) exist. Dengue is endemic in more than 100 countries in Africa, the Americas, the Mediterranean, and Asia, with an estimated 390 million dengue infections annually, 96 million of which are clinically apparent.[85,107,108] The incidence of dengue is increasing, likely owing to increased urbanization and ineffective vector control; dengue infection is closely associated with poor populations and urban crowding.[107] The majority of dengue infections occur in children aged less than 15 years, who tend to suffer from greatest morbidity and mortality.[83,109]

### Clinical manifestations

Dengue may present with a wide range of symptoms from inapparent asymptomatic infection, to mild febrile illness, to life-threatening shock. Symptomatic illness begins with abrupt onset of fever accompanied by headache, arthralgia, myalgia, retroorbital pain, and hemorrhagic manifestations.[107] Severe dengue, also known as dengue shock syndrome, is associated with rapid increase in (and reversal of) vascular permeability occurring toward the end of the febrile phase of illness that can lead to shock, severe bleeding, and organ failure.[107,109]

### Diagnosis

Acute and convalescent serology is the mainstay of diagnosis. In primary infection, immunoglobulin (Ig)M antibody appears by day 3 to 5 of illness and IgG antibody is detectable by day 5.[109] Infection is confirmed with seroconversion of IgM antibody or a 4-fold increase in IgG titers. RT-PCR of blood or tissue can also be used; viremia typically correlates with fever, and lasts approximately 4 to 5 days after fever onset.[85]

*Management/prevention*
No specific antiviral therapy for dengue is available; treatment is supportive and consists of volume repletion, monitoring of hematologic parameters, and close observation for signs of severe disease.[109] Presently, the most effective method for prevention of dengue infection is vector control. Travelers to endemic areas should be counseled to avoid mosquito bites through the use of DEET-containing insect repellent, protective clothing, and bed nets. Although no licensed vaccine is available, an investigational tetravalent vaccine demonstrated 61% efficacy against virologically confirmed dengue infection in Latin American children in a phase III trial.[110]

### Cutaneous Leishmaniasis

*Epidemiology*
Cutaneous leishmaniasis (CL) is the most common presentation of disease caused by infection with several species of *Leishmania*, a vector-borne parasite spread by the bite of the sandfly. CL is endemic in more than 70 countries, with the majority of cases occurring in the Eastern Mediterranean region, Americas, and East Asia; globally, children have the greatest burden of disease.[111-113] Infections, including those related to travel, are increasing.[112,114]

*Clinical manifestations*
CL is characterized by the development of skin lesions on exposed areas that develop weeks to months after a bite by an infected sandfly. Skin lesions typically evolve from firm papules to nodular lesions to large, nonpainful ulcers over the course of 2 weeks to 6 months.[111]

*Diagnosis*
Parasitologic diagnosis, by visualization of *Leishmania* parasites in tissue biopsy or aspirate, is the gold standard. Culture of biopsy material can aid in species identification, but is time consuming and may be of low yield. PCR is available to make species-level diagnosis, which helps to guide therapy. The Centers for Disease Control and Prevention provide diagnostic testing and a guide to assist clinicians with specimen collection.[115]

*Treatment/prevention*
There is debate over the need for treatment of CL, which usually resolves spontaneously over several months. However, owing to potential scarring, and to speed recovery, therapy is often given. Indications for treatment include (1) infection acquired in South or Central America (where *L braziliensis* predominates, which can progress to potentially disfiguring mucosal disease), (2) lesion on the face, hands, or feet, or over the joints, (3) lesions present for longer than 6 months, (4) multiple (>2–5) or large (>4–5 cm) lesions, (5) evidence of local dissemination, or (6) an immunocompromised host.[111]

Several treatment options for CL exist (see **Table 5**); the causative *Leishmania* species and strain, which depends on geography, likely affects drug efficacy. With any treatment, response can be slow, but a reduction in lesion size and inflammation is generally seen after 4 to 6 weeks.[111] Prevention of CL focuses on avoiding sandfly bites in endemic areas and vector control through the use of insecticides and bed nets. As a disease of poverty, there has been limited investment in a vaccine against *Leishmania*.[113]

### PREVENTION AND CONTROL OF INFECTIOUS DISEASES OF POVERTY IN LOW- AND MIDDLE-INCOME COUNTRIES: IMPLEMENTATION CHALLENGES AND FUTURE RESEARCH PRIORITIES

Although progress has been made in tackling major IDoP worldwide, significant challenges remain to reach the WHO control and elimination targets set for 2020 (see

**Table 6**
Implementation challenges and future research needs for prevention and control of infectious diseases of poverty in low- and middle-income countries

| Disease | Examples of Current Interventions | Implementation Challenges/ Future Research Needs |
|---|---|---|
| Helminthic NTDs | School-based platforms | Evaluation of large-scale integrated programs in resource-limited settings |
| Nonhelminthic NTDs | Insecticide-treated bed nets, community education and cleanliness campaigns, mass drug administration, treatment | Evaluation of effectiveness of various community delivery models Simultaneous improvements in water and sanitation are needed |
| Malaria | Insecticide-treated bed nets, indoor residual spraying | Integration of interventions with existing antenatal care and immunization campaigns to lower cost Prevention of drug resistance |
| HIV/AIDS | Community-based awareness and risk reduction interventions | Evaluation of effectiveness of community delivery platforms for PMTCT and models of care for improving morbidity and mortality |
| Tuberculosis | Treatment delivery through community health workers (coupled with DOT) | Comparative evaluation of various community-based delivery models for relative effectiveness |

*Abbreviations:* DOT, directly observed therapy; HIV, human immunodeficiency virus; NTD, neglected tropical disease; PMTCT, prevention of mother to child transmission; TB, tuberculosis.
*Data from* Bhutta ZA, Salam RA, Das JK, et al. Tackling the existing burden of infectious diseases in the developing world: existing gaps and the way forward. Infect Dis Poverty 2014;3:28.

**Table 5**).[116] Effective preventative or treatment interventions exist for a majority of IDoP in LMIC.[2] Many neglected parasitic infections can be treated with a US$0.50 treatment package.[117] Although evidence-based interventions exist to tackle various IDoP, coverage remains poor in many LMIC warranting development of innovative strategies (**Table 6**). Integrated, community-based interventions for prevention and control of IDoP are an area of active research.[118] Because transmission of IDoP is closely linked to social and economic inequalities, social science research may contribute to our understanding of implementation gaps and improve outcomes.[119]

## SUMMARY

IDoP, including HIV/AIDS, TB, malaria, and NTDs, impact children worldwide. Clinicians must be familiar with the epidemiology and clinical manifestations of these infections to ensure prompt diagnosis and treatment.

## REFERENCES

1. Global report for research on infectious diseases of poverty. Available at: http://whqlibdoc.who.int/publications/2012/9789241564489_eng.pdf. Accessed June 2, 2015.
2. Bhutta ZA, Sommerfeld J, Lassi ZS, et al. Global burden, distribution, and interventions for infectious diseases of poverty. Infect Dis Poverty 2014;3:21.

3. Barry MA, Bezek S, Serpa JA, et al. Neglected infections of poverty in Texas and the rest of the united states: management and treatment options. Clin Pharmacol Ther 2012;92(2):170–81.
4. Alsan MM, Westerhaus M, Herce M, et al. Poverty, global health, and infectious disease: lessons from Haiti and Rwanda. Infect Dis Clin North Am 2011;25(3): 611–22.
5. Manderson L, Aagaard-Hansen J, Allotey P, et al. Social research on neglected diseases of poverty: continuing and emerging themes. PLoS Negl Trop Dis 2009;3(2):e332.
6. Paintsil E, Andiman WA. Update on successes and challenges regarding mother-to-child transmission of HIV. Curr Opin Pediatr 2009;21(1):94–101.
7. Brady MT, Oleske JM, Williams PL, et al. Declines in mortality rates and changes in causes of death in HIV-1-infected children during the HAART era. J Acquir Immune Defic Syndr 2010;53(1):86–94.
8. Optimizing treatment options and improving access to priority products for children living with HIV brief. World Health Organization. Available at: http://www.who.int/hiv/pub/toolkits/paediatric_art_optimisation-brief/en/. Accessed May 20, 2015.
9. UNAIDS. Global report. UNAIDS report on the global AIDS epidemic 2013. Available at: http://www.unaids.org/sites/default/files/en/media/unaids/contentassets/documents/epidemiology/2013/gr2013/UNAIDS_Global_Report_2013_en.pdf. Accessed April 30, 2015.
10. Veazey RS, DeMaria M, Chalifoux LV, et al. Gastrointestinal tract as a major site of CD4+ T cell depletion and viral replication in SIV infection. Science 1998; 280(5362):427–31.
11. Brenchley JM, Schacker TW, Ruff LE, et al. CD4+ T cell depletion during all stages of HIV disease occurs predominantly in the gastrointestinal tract. J Exp Med 2004;200(6):749–59.
12. Marchetti G, Tincati C, Silvestri G. Microbial translocation in the pathogenesis of HIV infection and aids. Clin Microbiol Rev 2013;26(1):2–18.
13. Newell ML, Coovadia H, Cortina-Borja M, et al. Mortality of infected and uninfected infants born to HIV-infected mothers in Africa: a pooled analysis. Lancet 2004;364(9441):1236–43.
14. Burgard M, Blanche S, Jasseron C, et al. Performance of HIV-1 DNA or HIV-1 RNA tests for early diagnosis of perinatal HIV-1 infection during anti-retroviral prophylaxis. J Pediatr 2012;160(1):60–6.e1.
15. Stevens WS, Noble L, Berrie L, et al. Ultra-high-throughput, automated nucleic acid detection of human immunodeficiency virus (HIV) for infant infection diagnosis using the gen-probe aptima HIV-1 screening assay. J Clin Microbiol 2009; 47(8):2465–9.
16. McIntosh K, Pitt J, Brambilla D, et al. Blood culture in the first 6 months of life for the diagnosis of vertically transmitted human immunodeficiency virus infection. The women and infants transmission study group. J Infect Dis 1994;170(4):996–1000.
17. Consolidated guidelines on the use of antiretroviral drugs for treating and preventing HIV infection World Health Organization. Available at: http://www.who.int/hiv/pub/guidelines/arv2013/en/. Accessed April 30, 2015.
18. Rainwater-Lovett K, Luzuriaga K, Persaud D. Very early combination antiretroviral therapy in infants: prospects for cure. Curr Opin HIV AIDS 2015;10(1):4–11.
19. Luzuriaga K, Tabak B, Garber M, et al. HIV type 1 (HIV-1) proviral reservoirs decay continuously under sustained virologic control in HIV-1-infected children who received early treatment. J Infect Dis 2014;210(10):1529–38.

20. Persaud D, Patel K, Karalius B, et al. Influence of age at virologic control on peripheral blood human immunodeficiency virus reservoir size and serostatus in perinatally infected adolescents. JAMA Pediatr 2014;168(12): 1138–46.

21. Hazra R, Siberry GK, Mofenson LM. Growing up with HIV: children, adolescents, and young adults with perinatally acquired HIV infection. Annu Rev Med 2010; 61:169–85.

22. Mofenson LM. Can perinatal HIV infection be eliminated in the united states? JAMA 1999;282(6):577–9.

23. Paintsil E, Andiman WA. Care and management of the infant of the HIV-1-infected mother. Semin Perinatol 2007;31(2):112–23.

24. Gopalappa C, Stover J, Shaffer N, et al. The costs and benefits of option B+ for the prevention of mother-to-child transmission of HIV. AIDS 2014;28(Suppl 1): S5–14.

25. VanDeusen A, Paintsil E, Agyarko-Poku T, et al. Cost effectiveness of option B plus for prevention of mother-to-child transmission of HIV in resource-limited countries: Evidence from Kumasi, Ghana. BMC Infect Dis 2015;15:130.

26. Shah M, Johns B, Abimiku A, et al. Cost-effectiveness of new who recommendations for prevention of mother-to-child transmission of HIV in a resource-limited setting. AIDS 2011;25(8):1093–102.

27. Committee On Pediatric Adolescence. Transitioning HIV-infected youth into adult health care. Pediatrics 2013;132(1):192–7.

28. Global tuberculosis report. World Health Organization. Available at: http://www.who.int/tb/publications/global_report/en/. Accessed April 20, 2015.

29. Reported tuberculosis in the United States 2013. Centers for Disease Control and Prevention. Available at: http://www.cdc.gov/tb/statistics/reports/2013/pdf/report2013.pdf. Accessed April 20, 2015.

30. Newton SM, Brent AJ, Anderson S, et al. Paediatric tuberculosis. Lancet Infect Dis 2008;8(8):498–510.

31. Teo SS, Riordan A, Alfaham M, et al. Tuberculosis in the United Kingdom and Republic of Ireland. Arch Dis Child 2009;94(4):263–7.

32. Wood R, Racow K, Bekker LG, et al. Indoor social networks in a South African township: Potential contribution of location to tuberculosis transmission. PLoS One 2012;7(6):e39246.

33. Singh M, Mynak ML, Kumar L, et al. Prevalence and risk factors for transmission of infection among children in household contact with adults having pulmonary tuberculosis. Arch Dis Child 2005;90(6):624–8.

34. Lienhardt C, Fielding K, Sillah JS, et al. Investigation of the risk factors for tuberculosis: a case-control study in three countries in West Africa. Int J Epidemiol 2005;34(4):914–23.

35. Lienhardt C, Sillah J, Fielding K, et al. Risk factors for tuberculosis infection in children in contact with infectious tuberculosis cases in The Gambia, West Africa. Pediatrics 2003;111(5 Pt 1):e608–14.

36. Rutherford ME, Hill PC, Maharani W, et al. Risk factors for mycobacterium tuberculosis infection in Indonesian children living with a sputum smear-positive case. Int J Tuberc Lung Dis 2012;16(12):1594–9.

37. Lygizos M, Shenoi SV, Brooks RP, et al. Natural ventilation reduces high TB transmission risk in traditional homes in rural Kwazulu-Natal, South Africa. BMC Infect Dis 2013;13:300.

38. Escombe AR, Oeser CC, Gilman RH, et al. Natural ventilation for the prevention of airborne contagion. PLoS Med 2007;4(2):e68.

39. Cruciani M, Malena M, Bosco O, et al. The impact of human immunodeficiency virus type 1 on infectiousness of tuberculosis: a meta-analysis. Clin Infect Dis 2001;33(11):1922–30.
40. Koh GC, Hawthorne G, Turner AM, et al. Tuberculosis incidence correlates with sunshine: an ecological 28-year time series study. PLoS One 2013;8(3):e57752.
41. Lienhardt C. From exposure to disease: the role of environmental factors in susceptibility to and development of tuberculosis. Epidemiol Rev 2001;23(2):288–301.
42. Gao L, Tao Y, Zhang L, et al. Vitamin D receptor genetic polymorphisms and tuberculosis: updated systematic review and meta-analysis. Int J Tuberc Lung Dis 2010;14(1):15–23.
43. Seddon JA, Shingadia D. Epidemiology and disease burden of tuberculosis in children: a global perspective. Infect Drug Resist 2014;7:153–65.
44. Gillman A, Berggren I, Bergstrom SE, et al. Primary tuberculosis infection in 35 children at a Swedish day care center. Pediatr Infect Dis J 2008;27(12):1078–82.
45. Gessner BD, Weiss NS, Nolan CM. Risk factors for pediatric tuberculosis infection and disease after household exposure to adult index cases in Alaska. J Pediatr 1998;132(3 Pt 1):509–13.
46. Hanekom M, van der Spuy GD, Streicher E, et al. A recently evolved sublineage of the Mycobacterium tuberculosis Beijing strain family is associated with an increased ability to spread and cause disease. J Clin Microbiol 2007;45(5):1483–90.
47. Verhagen LM, Hermans PW, Warris A, et al. Helminths and skewed cytokine profiles increase tuberculin skin test positivity in Warao Amerindians. Tuberculosis 2012;92(6):505–12.
48. van Soelen N, Mandalakas AM, Kirchner HL, et al. Effect of Ascaris lumbricoides specific IgE on tuberculin skin test responses in children in a high-burden setting: a cross-sectional community-based study. BMC Infect Dis 2012;12:211.
49. Qu HQ, Fisher-Hoch SP, McCormick JB. Knowledge gaining by human genetic studies on tuberculosis susceptibility. J Hum Genet 2011;56(3):177–82.
50. Moller M, de Wit E, Hoal EG. Past, present and future directions in human genetic susceptibility to tuberculosis. FEMS Immunol Med Microbiol 2010;58(1):3–26.
51. Hertting O, Shingadia D. Childhood TB: when to think of it and what to do when you do. J Infect 2014;68(Suppl 1):S151–4.
52. Marais BJ, Gie RP, Schaaf HS, et al. The clinical epidemiology of childhood pulmonary tuberculosis: a critical review of literature from the pre-chemotherapy era. Int J Tuberc Lung Dis 2004;8(3):278–85.
53. Marais BJ, Gie RP, Schaaf HS, et al. The spectrum of disease in children treated for tuberculosis in a highly endemic area. Int J Tuberc Lung Dis 2006;10(7):732–8.
54. Marais BJ, Gie RP, Hesseling AC, et al. A refined symptom-based approach to diagnose pulmonary tuberculosis in children. Pediatrics 2006;118(5):e1350–9.
55. Osborne CM. The challenge of diagnosing childhood tuberculosis in a developing country. Arch Dis Child 1995;72(4):369–74.
56. Eamranond P, Jaramillo E. Tuberculosis in children: reassessing the need for improved diagnosis in global control strategies. Int J Tuberc Lung Dis 2001;5(7):594–603.
57. Starke JR. Pediatric tuberculosis: time for a new approach. Tuberculosis 2003;83(1–3):208–12.

58. Zar HJ, Hanslo D, Apolles P, et al. Induced sputum versus gastric lavage for microbiological confirmation of pulmonary tuberculosis in infants and young children: a prospective study. Lancet 2005;365(9454):130–4.

59. Swaminathan S, Rekha B. Pediatric tuberculosis: global overview and challenges. Clin Infect Dis 2010;50(Suppl 3):S184–94.

60. Vargas D, Garcia L, Gilman RH, et al. Diagnosis of sputum-scarce HIV-associated pulmonary tuberculosis in Lima, Peru. Lancet 2005;365(9454):150–2.

61. Chow F, Espiritu N, Gilman RH, et al. La cuerda dulce–a tolerability and acceptability study of a novel approach to specimen collection for diagnosis of paediatric pulmonary tuberculosis. BMC Infect Dis 2006;6:67.

62. Shingadia D. The diagnosis of tuberculosis. Pediatr Infect Dis J 2012;31(3):302–5.

63. Starke JR, Taylor-Watts KT. Tuberculosis in the pediatric population of Houston, Texas. Pediatrics 1989;84(1):28–35.

64. Larsson LO, Bentzon MW, Lind A, et al. Sensitivity to sensitins and tuberculin in Swedish children. Part 5: a study of school children in an inland rural area. Int J Tuberc Lung Dis 1993;74(6):371–6.

65. American Academy of Pediatrics. Tuberculosis. In: Pl K, editor. Red book: 2012 report of the committee on infectious diseases. 27th edition. Elk Grove Village (IL): American Academy of Pediatrics 2012. p. 737–60.

66. Guidance for national tuberculosis programmes on the management of tuberculosis in children. 2nd edition. Available at: http://apps.who.int/medicinedocs/documents/s21535en/s21535en.pdf. Accessed May 20, 2015.

67. New who recommendations on use of commercial TB interferon-gamma release assays (IGRAS) in low- and middle-income countries. World Health Organization. Available at: http://www.who.int/tb/features_archive/igra_policy24oct/en/. Accessed May 20, 2015.

68. Schaaf HS, Marais BJ, Hesseling AC, et al. Surveillance of antituberculosis drug resistance among children from the Western Cape Province of South Africa–an upward trend. Am J Public Health 2009;99(8):1486–90.

69. Fairlie L, Beylis NC, Reubenson G, et al. High prevalence of childhood multidrug resistant tuberculosis in Johannesburg, South Africa: a cross sectional study. BMC Infect Dis 2011;11:28.

70. Multidrug and extensively drug-resistant TB (M/XDR-TB); 2010 global report on surveillance and response. Who/htm/tb/2010.3. World Health Organization. Available at: http://www.who.int/tb/features_archive/m_xdrtb_facts/en/. Accessed April 30, 2015.

71. Al-Dabbagh M, Lapphra K, McGloin R, et al. Drug-resistant tuberculosis: pediatric guidelines. Pediatr Infect Dis J 2011;30(6):501–5.

72. WHO world malaria report 2014. Available at: http://www.who.int/malaria/publications/world_malaria_report_2014/report/en/. Accessed June 2, 2015.

73. Owens S. Malaria and the millennium development goals. Arch Dis Child 2015;100(Suppl 1):S53–6.

74. White NJ, Pukrittayakamee S, Hien TT, et al. Malaria. Lancet 2014;383(9918):723–35.

75. Nadjm B, Behrens RH. Malaria: an update for physicians. Infect Dis Clin North Am 2012;26(2):243–59.

76. WHO guidelines for the treatment of malaria, 2nd edition. Available at: http://whqlibdoc.who.int/publications/2010/9789241547925_eng.pdf. Accessed June 2, 2015.

77. Treatment of malaria (guidelines for clinicians). Available at: http://www.cdc.gov/malaria/resources/pdf/clinicalguidance.pdf. Accessed May 28, 2015.

78. Worrall E, Basu S, Hanson K. Is malaria a disease of poverty? A review of the literature. Trop Med Int Health 2005;10(10):1047–59.
79. Ouattara A, Laurens MB. Vaccines against malaria. Clin Infect Dis 2015;60(6): 930–6.
80. Agnandji ST, Lell B, Fernandes JF, et al. A phase 3 trial of RTS,S/AS01 malaria vaccine in African infants. N Engl J Med 2012;367(24):2284–95.
81. Olotu A, Fegan G, Wambua J, et al. Four-year efficacy of RTS,S/AS01e and its interaction with malaria exposure. N Engl J Med 2013;368(12): 1111–20.
82. Accelerating work to overcome the global impact of neglected tropical diseases roadmap for implementation. Available at: http://www.who.int/neglected_diseases/NTD_RoadMap_2012_Fullversion.pdf. Accessed April 20, 2015.
83. Hotez P. Pediatric tropical diseases and the world's children living in extreme poverty. Available at: http://digitalcommons.library.tmc.edu/childrenatrisk/vol4/iss2/10. Accessed January 14, 2015.
84. Neglected parasitic infections (NPIS) in the United States. Available at: http://www.cdc.gov/parasites/npi/. Accessed June 2, 2015.
85. Guzman MG, Harris E. Dengue. Lancet 2015;385(9966):453–65.
86. Murray CJ, Vos T, Lozano R, et al. Disability-adjusted life years (DALYs) for 291 diseases and injuries in 21regions, 1990-2010: a systematic analysis for the global burden of disease study 2010. Lancet 2012;380(9859):2197–223.
87. Hotez PJ, Molyneux DH, Fenwick A, et al. Control of neglected tropical diseases. N Engl J Med 2007;357(10):1018–27.
88. Woodhall D, Jones JL, Cantey PT, et al. Neglected parasitic infections: what every family physician needs to know. Am Fam Physician 2014;89(10): 803–11.
89. World Health Organization 2012. Accelerating work to overcome the global impact of neglected tropical diseases: a roadmap for implementation. Geneva, Switzerland. Available at: http://whqlibdoc.who.int/hq/2012/WHO_HTM_NTD_2012.1_eng.pdf. Accessed July 21, 2015.
90. Centers for Disease Control and Prevention (CDC). Congenital transmission of Chagas disease – Virginia, 2010. MMWR Recomm Rep 2012;61:26.
91. Bern C, Kjos S, Yabsley MJ, et al. Trypanosoma cruzi and Chagas' disease in the United States. Clin Microbiol Rev 2011;24(4):655–81.
92. Bern C, Montgomery SP. An estimate of the burden of Chagas disease in the United States. Clin Infect Dis 2009;49(5):e52–4.
93. Montgomery SP, Starr MC, Cantey PT, et al. Neglected parasitic infections in the United States: Chagas disease. Am J Trop Med Hyg 2014;90(5):814–8.
94. Bern C. Evaluation and treatment of Chagas disease in the United States: a systematic review. JAMA 2007;298:18.
95. Edwards MS, Rench MA, Todd CW, et al. Perinatal screening for Chagas disease in Southern Texas. J Pediatric Infect Dis Soc 2013;4(1):67–70.
96. Centers for Disease Control and Prevention (CDC). Blood donor screening for Chagas disease – United States, 2006-2007. MMWR Recomm Rep 2007; 56(7):141–3.
97. Mewara A, Goyal K, Sehgal R. Neurocysticercosis: a disease of neglect. Trop Parasitol 2013;3(2):106–13.
98. Cantey PT, Coyle CM, Sorvillo FJ, et al. Neglected parasitic infections in the United States: cysticercosis. Am J Trop Med Hyg 2014;90(5):805–9.
99. Garcia HH, Gonzalez AE, Gilman RH. Cysticercosis of the central nervous system: how should it be managed? Curr Opin Infect Dis 2011;24(5):423–7.

100. Garcia HH, Gilman RH, Gonzalez AE, et al. Hyperendemic human and porcine taenia solium infection in Peru. Am J Trop Med Hyg 2003;68(3):268–75.
101. Gilman RH, Gonzalez AE, Llanos-Zavalga F, et al. Prevention and control of Taenia solium taeniasis/cysticercosis in Peru. Pathog Glob Health 2012;106(5): 312–8.
102. Woodhall DM, Eberhard ML, Parise ME. Neglected parasitic infections in the United States: toxocariasis. Am J Trop Med Hyg 2014;90(5):810–3.
103. Ross AG, Bartley PB, Sleigh AC, et al. Schistosomiasis. N Engl J Med 2002; 346(16):1212–20.
104. Hotez PJ, Fenwick A. Schistosomiasis in Africa: an emerging tragedy in our new global health decade. PLoS Negl Trop Dis 2009;3(9):e485.
105. Mutapi F. Changing policy and practice in the control of pediatric schistosomiasis. Pediatrics 2015;135(3):536–44.
106. Gray DJ, Ross AG, Li YS, et al. Diagnosis and management of schistosomiasis. BMJ 2011;342:d2651.
107. Hermann LL, Gupta SB, Manoff SB, et al. Advances in the understanding, management, and prevention of Dengue. J Clin Virol 2015;64:153–9.
108. Bhatt S, Gething PW, Brady OJ, et al. The global distribution and burden of Dengue. Nature 2013;496(7446):504–7.
109. Verhagen LM, de Groot R. Dengue in children. J Infect 2014;69(Suppl 1): S77–86.
110. Villar L, Dayan GH, Arredondo-Garcia JL, et al. Efficacy of a tetravalent dengue vaccine in children in Latin America. N Engl J Med 2015;372(2):113–23.
111. Murray HW. Leishmaniasis in the United States: treatment in 2012. Am J Trop Med Hyg 2012;86(3):434–40.
112. Reithinger R, Dujardin J-C, Louzir H, et al. Cutaneous leishmaniasis. Lancet Infect Dis 2007;7(9):581–96.
113. Pace D. Leishmaniasis. J Infect 2014;69(Suppl 1):S10–8.
114. Fox TG, Manaloor JJ, Christenson JC. Travel-related infections in children. Pediatr Clin North Am 2013;60(2):507–27.
115. Practical guide for specimen collection and reference diagnosis of leishmaniasis. Available at: http://www.cdc.gov/parasites/leishmaniasis/resources/pdf/cdc_diagnosis_guide_leishmaniasis.pdf. Accessed May 31, 2015.
116. Bhutta ZA, Salam RA, Das JK, et al. Tackling the existing burden of infectious diseases in the developing world: existing gaps and the way forward. Infect Dis Poverty 2014;3:28.
117. Neglected tropical diseases: preventive chemotherapy and transmission control. Available at: http://whqlibdoc.who.int/hq/2006/WHO_CDS_NTD_2006.3a_eng.pdf. Accessed July 21, 2015.
118. Lassi ZS, Salam RA, Das JK, et al. The conceptual framework and assessment methodology for the systematic reviews of community-based interventions for the prevention and control of infectious diseases of poverty. Infect Dis Poverty 2014;3:22.
119. Bardosh K. Global aspirations, local realities: the role of social science research in controlling neglected tropical diseases. Infect Dis Poverty 2014;3(1):35.

# Prevention and Control of Childhood Pneumonia and Diarrhea

Daniel T. Leung, MD, MSc[a,b,]*,
Mohammod J. Chisti, MBBS, MMed, PhD[c], Andrew T. Pavia, MD[d]

KEYWORDS

- Pneumonia • Diarrhea • Vaccines • Global burden • Etiology

KEY POINTS

- Pneumonia and diarrhea are the 2 major preventable causes of childhood deaths in young children in low- and middle-income countries.
- Public health interventions, including nutritional rehabilitation, zinc supplementation, exclusive breastfeeding, and water-sanitation-and-hygiene strategies, have all contributed toward marked reductions in mortality; however, current coverage of these cost-effective interventions remains low.
- Respiratory syncytial virus, *Streptococcus pneumoniae*, and *Haemophilus influenza* are the leading causes of childhood pneumonia; the last two can be prevented through vaccination.
- Vaccines against diarrheal pathogens include that against cholera and rotavirus; development of vaccines against other leading causes of diarrhea, such as norovirus, *Cryptosporidium, Shigella, Campylobacter*, and enterotoxigenic *Escherichia coli*, are urgently needed.
- Successful implementation of the World Health Organization/United Nations Children's Fund's Integrated Global Action Plan for the Prevention and Control of Pneumonia and Diarrhea will need strong commitment from national governments, the private sector, and other stakeholders.

[a] Division of Infectious Diseases, Department of Medicine, University of Utah School of Medicine, 30 North 1900 East, SOM Room 4C416B, Salt Lake City, UT 84132, USA; [b] Division of Microbiology and Immunology, Department of Pathology, University of Utah School of Medicine, 15 North Medical Drive East, Salt Lake City, UT 84132, USA; [c] Centre for Nutrition and Food Security, ICU and Respiratory Wards, Dhaka Hospital, International Centre for Diarrhoeal Disease Research, GPO Box 128, Dhaka 1000, Bangladesh; [d] Division of Pediatric Infectious Diseases, Department of Pediatrics, University of Utah School of Medicine, 30 North 1900 East, Salt Lake City, UT 84132, USA
* Corresponding author. Division of Infectious Diseases, University of Utah School of Medicine, 30 North 1900 East, SOM Room 4C416B, Salt Lake City, UT 84132.
E-mail address: Daniel.leung@utah.edu

Pediatr Clin N Am 63 (2016) 67–79
http://dx.doi.org/10.1016/j.pcl.2015.08.003     **pediatric.theclinics.com**
0031-3955/16/$ – see front matter © 2016 Elsevier Inc. All rights reserved.

## INTRODUCTION

Pneumonia and diarrhea are the 2 leading infectious causes of death in children younger than 5 years worldwide, responsible for more than 1.5 million deaths annually. They accounted for 15% and 9%, respectively, of the 6.3 million deaths in children younger than 5 years that occurred globally in 2013.[1,2] There are an estimated 1.7 billion episodes annually of diarrhea and more than 150 million episodes of pneumonia. Marked decreases in mortality due to pneumonia and diarrhea over the past decade have been noted.[3] Between 2000 and 2013, there was an estimated 44% reduction in deaths due to pneumonia and 54% reduction in deaths due to diarrhea among children younger than 5 years.[2] Despite this, pneumonia and diarrhea continue to cause significant morbidity and mortality in young children worldwide, particularly those in Asia and Africa. Thus, efforts at optimizing prevention and control are needed. In this review, the authors describe strategies aimed at preventing and controlling childhood pneumonia and diarrhea.

## GLOBAL BURDEN

The World Health Organization (WHO) estimates that each year, there are greater than 150 million cases of pneumonia in children younger than 5 years, including 20 million cases that require hospitalization. Most of the morbidity and mortality worldwide due to pneumonia occur in low- and middle-income countries (LMICs). Using vital registration and verbal autopsy data, the Child Health Epidemiology Reference Group estimated the total number of pneumonia deaths in children younger than 5 years worldwide to be approximately 935,000.[3] Up to half of the deaths from pneumonia occurred in sub-Saharan Africa and approximately a third in Southern Asia. There were regional variations in the percentage of deaths attributable to pneumonia: from 5% of deaths in developed regions to 16% of deaths in sub-Saharan Africa. Most notably, 96% of episodes of pneumonia, and 99% of deaths from pneumonia, take place in LMICs.[4]

Although second to pneumonia in mortality burden, diarrheal illnesses occur more frequently. Children in LMICs who are younger than 5 years have an average of 2.9 episodes per year of diarrhea, accounting for nearly 1.7 billion episodes of diarrhea yearly,[5] resulting in more than 578,000 deaths per year.[3] The peak age of diarrheal disease incidence is during , from 6 to 11 months of age[5]; most of the deaths due to diarrhea occur in the first 2 years of life.[6]

## CAUSES OF PNEUMONIA

Because of logistical and ethical limitations, direct sampling of infected lung tissue is not commonly performed; our knowledge of the causes of pediatric pneumonia is based mostly on studies using various indirect sampling methods, such as nasopharyngeal swab, blood cultures, or induced sputum (**Box 1**). A large 10-country study conducted more than 25 years ago revealed respiratory viruses, especially respiratory syncytial virus (RSV), to be the leading cause of childhood pneumonia,[12] with the most common bacterial causes being *Streptococcus pneumoniae*, followed closely by *Haemophilus influenzae*. More contemporary studies have continued to identify RSV as the most common respiratory virus responsible for pneumonia worldwide, though improved molecular diagnostics have also implicated rhinovirus, influenza virus, human metapneumovirus, and adenovirus, with significant geographic variations.[7–9] Although viruses are detected in most cases of pneumonia, given the high frequency of copathogen isolation, their contribution to severe pneumonia is unclear. Notably,

---

**Box 1**
**Top pathogens causing childhood pneumonia and diarrhea**

*Pneumonia*[7–10]

Bacterial
  *Streptococcus pneumoniae*[a]
  *Haemophilus influenzae*[a]
  *Mycoplasma pneumonia*
  *Staphylococcus aureus*

Viral
  Respiratory syncytial virus
  Influenza A or B virus[a]
  Human rhinovirus
  Human metapneumovirus
  Adenovirus
  Parainfluenza virus

*Diarrhea*[6,11]

Bacterial
  *Shigella*
  Enterotoxigenic *Escherichia coli*
  *Campylobacter*
  *Aeromonas*
  *Vibrio cholerae*[a]

Viral
  Rotavirus[a]
  Norovirus
  Astrovirus
  Adenovirus

Protozoal
  *Cryptosporidium*

[a] Vaccine available.

---

a recent study from Gambia involving lung aspirates in children younger than 5 years with severe pneumonia demonstrated *S pneumoniae* to be present in 91% of lung aspirates, followed by *H influenzae* at 23%, and *Staphylococcus aureus* in 6%; in this small study, no viruses were present in greater than 5% of samples.[10] The authors have also shown that the causes of pneumonia in children with severe acute malnutrition differ from that of well-nourished children, with gram-negative bacteria being more common in those malnourished.[13] The Pneumonia Etiology Research for Child Health study, a 7-country case-control study of severe pneumonia in hospitalized children[14] and a similar study using the Global Approach to Biological Research, Infectious Diseases, and Epidemics in Low-Income Countries network in 9 countries[15] are both ongoing and are expected to provide more updated and comprehensive data regarding the causes of pneumonia in LMICs.

## CAUSES OF DIARRHEA

The etiologic determination of diarrheal disease and deaths are limited by the large number of pathogens present in the stool of children in LMICs, even during periods of relative health. For example, Bangladeshi infants without evidence of diarrhea had an average of 4.3 enteropathogens detected, compared with an average of 0.5 in infants from the United States.[16] The past decade saw the completion of 2 large multi-country studies using modern molecular diagnostic tools to provide insight into the cause and consequences of acute infectious diarrhea in children of LMICs (see **Box 1**).

The Global Enterics Multicenter Study, a 3-year cross-sectional case-control study, investigated the cause and incidence of moderate to severe diarrhea of more than 22,000 children at 7 sites in Africa and Asia.[6] It found that most cases were due to 4 pathogens: rotavirus, *Cryptosporidium*, *Shigella* spp, and heat-stable toxin-producing enterotoxigenic *Escherichia coli* (ST-ETEC). Rotavirus was the top attributable cause of diarrhea in children younger than 24 months of age, and *Shigella* was the top cause for those 2 to 5 years old. Other notable pathogens among the top causes included *Vibrio cholerae, Campylobacter jejuni,* adenovirus 40/41, and *Aeromonas spp*; but there was substantial geographic variation.

The Interactions of Malnutrition and Enteric Infections: Consequences for Child Health and Development project is a multi-site cohort that involved intensive surveillance for diarrhea and monthly asymptomatic stool collection from children, from birth to 24 months. Investigators found norovirus, rotavirus, *Campylobacter,* astrovirus, and *Cryptosporidium* to be the top causes of diarrhea in the first year of life, with the addition of *Shigella spp* in the second year.[11] These studies combine to demonstrate that bacterial, viral, and protozoal causes all play important roles in childhood diarrhea.

## PUBLIC HEALTH MEASURES FOR PREVENTION OF CHILDHOOD PNEUMONIA AND DIARRHEA

Pneumonia and diarrheal disease share several risk factors, including malnutrition, poor hygiene, poor socioeconomic status, lower education status, and lack of breastfeeding.[17] The authors have shown in a systematic review that young children with severe malnutrition are at an increased risk of death from pneumonia[13] and have high rates of death even after hospital discharge.[18] The authors have reported that severe acute malnutrition is associated with concurrent pneumonia and diarrhea; children with both illnesses have a greater than 80-fold increased risk of death compared with those with diarrhea alone.[19] Inpatient nutritional rehabilitation of malnourished children has been demonstrated to dramatically reduce case fatality rates, especially when implemented in units with standardized protocols and trained staff.[20,21] Interventions used in such units include appropriate rehydration therapy, targeted feeding, empiric antibiotics directed against gram-negative organisms, vitamin A supplementation, and management of hypoglycemia. Of the nutritional supplementation interventions studied, preventative zinc supplementation has been shown to reduce the incidence of diarrhea and pneumonia by more than 20% and all-cause mortality by 18% among children 12 to 59 months of age.[22] Additionally, exclusive breastfeeding of infants reduces deaths due to both pneumonia and diarrhea,[23] especially in the first 6 months of life.[24,25]

Diarrheal diseases have long been associated with ingestion of contaminated food and water. With the increasing recognition of viral causes of both pneumonia and diarrhea that may be transmitted person to person, efforts have also focused on strategies to improve water, sanitation, and hygiene (WASH) at the household level. Interventions, such as the encouragement of hand washing with soap, improving water quality, and proper disposal of excreta, have all been demonstrated to reduce diarrheal burden.[26] There are limited data behind the prevention of pneumonia through WASH interventions,[27] though a recent estimate suggested that hand washing with soap could prevent more than 600,000 deaths from diarrhea and pneumonia combined.[28]

The aforementioned preventive and protective measures form the backbone of public health efforts for children in LMICs. The marked reductions in mortality in the past decade have been in large part due to such nonspecific interventions. The remainder of this review focuses on the use of preventive vaccines for diarrheal and respiratory pathogens. Conjugate vaccines for *H influenza* type B and *S pneumoniae* and rotavirus vaccines have significantly decreased the burden of pneumonia and diarrhea in high-income countries (HICs). The uptake of these vaccines and the potential development of new vaccines are expected to further enhance the reductions in childhood mortality in LMICs.

## VACCINES TO PREVENT CHILDHOOD PNEUMONIA

Children younger than 2 years bear a large burden of bacterial respiratory infections, and polysaccharide antigens are poorly immunogenic in such children. The development of polysaccharide-protein conjugate vaccines has dramatically enhanced the prevention of pneumonia worldwide. Conjugate vaccines take advantage of a carrier protein to elicit a T cell–dependent antibody response to bacterial polysaccharide antigens. Conjugate vaccines against *S pneumoniae* and *H influenzae* type B, the top 2 causes of bacterial lower respiratory tract infections worldwide, are highly effective. Vaccines against the influenza virus are available but not widely used in LMICs; no vaccine is yet available against RSV, the most common cause of viral pneumonia.

## VACCINES AGAINST *STREPTOCOCCUS PNEUMONIAE* (PNEUMOCOCCUS)

The development of a pneumococcal vaccine that is effective in young children has been of great benefit to children worldwide. Available pneumococcal vaccines include 7-, 9-, 10-, 11-, 13-, and 15-valent conjugate vaccines and a 23-valent polysaccharide (nonconjugated) vaccine. Currently used conjugate vaccines worldwide include the 13-valent conjugate vaccines (pneumococcal conjugate vaccine 13 [PCV13]), which use CRM197 (diphtheria toxin mutant) as a carrier, and the 10-valent conjugate (PCV10), which uses 3 proteins: the diphtheria toxoid, the tetanus toxoid, and nontypeable *H influenzae* protein D.

PCVs prevent invasive pneumococcal disease (IPD), including meningitis, sepsis, and otitis media as well as pneumococcal pneumonia. In a meta-analysis that included 6 randomized controlled trials conducted in children younger than 2 years in Africa, the United States, Philippines, and Finland, the pooled efficacy of PCV7 was 80% for vaccine-serotype–associated IPD and 58% for all-serotype IPD. The effect of PCV7 on pneumonia was lower: the pooled efficacy for radiologically defined pneumonia was 27% and for clinical pneumonia 6%.[29] This finding likely reflects the importance of other pathogens in addition to *S pneumoniae* in childhood pneumonia. Several studies have suggested additional benefits of PCV beyond prevention of pneumococcal pneumonia in those vaccinated, including prevention of viral-attributed pneumonia,[30] reduction in IPD in older unvaccinated age groups due to herd immunity,[31] and serotype-associated IPD in younger unvaccinated age groups.[32]

The introduction of PCVs has had substantial impact on the burden of pneumococcal disease in every country where it has been widely adopted. The impact may be higher among young children in LMICs than those in HICs. A meta-analysis of serotypes causing IPD worldwide estimated that 49% to 88% of pneumococcal deaths in Africa and Asia are caused by serotypes covered in in PCV10 and PCV13.[33] Since 2006, the WHO has recommended that PCV be included in all routine immunization programs.

The uptake of PCV in LMICs has been limited, however, in large part because of the high cost of PCV. In response to this, the Global Alliance for Vaccines and

Immunization (GAVI) has worked to accelerate the introduction of PCVs in LMICs by working with manufacturers to commit supply and ensuring predictable vaccine pricing for the PCV10 and PCV13 vaccines. In total, more than 125 countries, including 50 GAVI-supported countries, have introduced universal PCV to their immunization programs, though greater than 50% of the world's infants still do not have access to PCV,[34] most notably many of those living in Asian LMICs.

Large randomized studies of 10- and 13-valent PCVs have not been conducted in LMICs, and their effectiveness is inferred from comparable immunogenicity as PCV7. With the use of PCV7, surveillance studies in HICs demonstrated a plateau in the reduction of pneumococcal infection rates in some populations due to serotype.[35] Notably, there are more than 90 pneumococcal serotypes. Although the factors that drive the epidemiology of *S pneumoniae* are complex and poorly understood, further serotype replacement seems likely. Vaccines aimed at inducing serotype-independent immunity are in early stages of development and hold promise of not being subject to serotype replacement.[36]

## VACCINES AGAINST *HAEMOPHILUS INFLUENZAE* TYPE B

As with pneumococcal vaccines, the first *Haemophilus influenzae* type b (Hib) vaccines were polysaccharide formulations that were poorly immunogenic in young children.[37] However, since 1987, several Hib conjugate vaccines (HibCVs) have become available, including ones conjugated to an outer membrane vesicle of *Neisseria meningitidis* and one conjugated to tetanus toxoid; HiBCVs have been combined with other childhood vaccines. Initial randomized controlled trials (RCTs) of HibCVs showed greater than 95% efficacy against invasive disease[38]; the introduction of HibCV has nearly eliminated invasive Hib disease from countries where the vaccine is widely used, including countries in sub-Saharan Africa.[39]

In 2006, the WHO issued a recommendation for the adoption of HibCVs in routine immunization programs worldwide. In response to the slow uptake of HibCV in LMICs, the Hib initiative was launched by GAVI to disseminate data regarding the burden of disease and provide advocacy for its introduction in low-income countries. Currently, more than 190 countries have introduced a Hib-containing vaccine into their national immunization program,[34] including all 73 GAVI countries. However, it is estimated that more than a third of infants worldwide are still not reached by the current immunization coverage.[34]

## VACCINES AGAINST INFLUENZA VIRUS

Despite the large burden of respiratory illness due to influenza virus infection among young children and the longstanding availability of the influenza vaccine in HICs, vaccines against influenza have not been widely implemented in any LMICs. The biggest reason is likely the cost and logistical resources needed to implement yearly immunizations. Inactivated influenza vaccines (IIVs) are produced to match influenza strains that circulate at the end of the last season. Efficacy depends on the degree of matching to actual circulating strains, and studies evaluating IIVs in children are limited. In a recent large multi-country RCT, a quadrivalent IIV had an efficacy of 60%.[40] On the other hand, the single-dose live attenuated influenza vaccine (LAIV) holds promise to be an effective and less costly option for LMICs. In contrast to IIVs, a large number of RCTs have shown that LAIVs are effective in preventing influenza illness in young children.[41] Furthermore, there is evidence that LAIVs may have activity against mismatched strains and possibly provide longer duration of protection than IIVs. A cost-effectiveness analysis conducted in Thailand showed vaccination with LAIV to be highly cost-effective, more than for IIV vaccine.[42] Current research efforts are focused on the feasibility of influenza vaccine implementation[43] as well as the protection of infants through vaccination during pregnancy.[44]

## VACCINES TO PREVENT CHILDHOOD DIARRHEA

Currently, there are few vaccines available for the prevention of childhood diarrhea. The rotavirus vaccine, highly efficacious and widely available in most HICs, has shown lower efficacy in some LMICs. Efforts to include it in national immunization programs have been slow. Recent enhancement and development of the oral cholera vaccine (OCV) has increased its availability, and the WHO now recommends it for use in both endemic and epidemic areas. The authors review these two available vaccines later. Vaccines against norovirus, *Shigella*, and ETEC are in advanced stages of development; given the surprisingly high burden of illness caused by *Cryptosporidium*, efforts are underway to increase our understanding of its host-pathogen relationship that could allow development of effective vaccines.

## VACCINES AGAINST ROTAVIRUS

Rotavirus is the most common cause of diarrhea in the first year of life,[6] which is the age with the highest incidence of, and deaths due to, diarrheal illness. The WHO has recommended that rotavirus vaccine for infants be included in national immunization programs. Two live attenuated oral rotavirus vaccines are available worldwide: a 3-dose pentavalent human-bovine reassortment vaccine containing serotypes G1, G2, G3, G4, and P1[8] (RV5) and a 2-dose monovalent vaccine derived from serotype combination G1P[8] (RV1), which likely has cross-protection against most other serotypes.

Several studies have shown that both rotavirus vaccines are effective in preventing gastroenteritis due to rotavirus in a variety of geographic settings. In large placebo-controlled studies of RV5 and RV1,[45,46] the vaccines were associated with approximately 90% efficacy against incidence of, hospitalization for, and emergency visits due to severe rotaviral gastroenteritis. The rotavirus vaccine has also been associated with a decrease in all-cause gastroenteritis and indirect protection of unvaccinated older siblings.[47] A total of 79 countries have introduced a rotavirus vaccine into their national immunization program, though an estimated three-quarter of the world's infants still do not have access to the rotavirus vaccine,[34] including most infants living in South and Southeast Asia.

Currently available rotavirus vaccines have lower immunogenicity and effectiveness in LMIC settings than seen in studies from North America, Europe, and South America. Large multi-country studies from sub-Saharan Africa[48,49] and Asia[50] showed vaccine efficacy estimates of 40% to 50%, a substantially lower number. Issues regarding immunogenicity, and the possible deleterious effect of environmental enteropathy, malnutrition, and alterations in gut microbiota, are currently being examined in the multi-site birth cohort Performance of Rotavirus and Oral Polio Vaccines in Developing Countries study.[51] Adjunctive interventions may be needed to optimize the delivery and efficacy of rotavirus and other oral vaccines in developing countries.

## VACCINES AGAINST *VIBRIO CHOLERAE*

Despite being available for several decades, vaccines against cholera have not been widely used in endemic countries because of concerns regarding efficacy, duration of protection, and costs. Recently, in efforts spearheaded by the International Vaccine

Initiative, an existing OCV produced and originally implemented in Vietnam was enhanced to meet WHO prequalification standards and licensed in India. This vaccine, Shanchol, is a bivalent (O1 and O139) heat- and formalin-killed whole-cell *V cholerae* vaccine, given as 2 doses 14 days apart. Unlike its precursor Dukoral, it does not contain a recombinant cholera toxin subunit. In a large double-blind cluster-randomized placebo-controlled trial in Kolkata, India, the vaccine was found to have a protective efficacy of 65% at 5 years of follow-up.[52]

In 2011, the WHO recommended that OCVs be used in both endemic and epidemic settings; in 2012, in response to recent epidemics, such as in Haiti and sub-Saharan Africa, the WHO established a global stockpile of OCV. Despite the high burden of cholera in young children,[53] OCVs have a lower protective efficacy and a shorter duration of protection in young children less than 5 years of age than in older persons.[54] The reasons for this are not fully understood. The authors have shown that children aged 24 to 59 months mount lower *V cholerae* polysaccharide-specific responses to OCV than older children and adults.[55] Given the logistical difficulties of completing a multiple-dose regimen in settings where cholera is present, efforts to study alternative dosing schedules of currently available OCVs are underway; several single-dose live-attenuated OCVs are under development.[56]

## INTEGRATED GLOBAL ACTION PLAN FOR THE PREVENTION AND CONTROL OF PNEUMONIA AND DIARRHEA

Despite the availability of effective cost-effective interventions to end preventable childhood deaths from diarrhea and pneumonia, access is low in many LMICs.[57] There are many barriers to the implementation and scale-up of interventions to end preventable deaths in children from pneumonia and diarrhea (**Box 2** and **Fig. 1**).[58,59] Following a series of regional and country workshops and subsequent follow-up and feedback from health care workers, the WHO conceptualized a "protect, prevent, and treat"

---

**Box 2**
**Barriers to the implementation and scale-up of pneumonia and diarrhea interventions**

- Lack of specific policy guidance for child health, CCM, or use of antibiotics and other essential health commodities by CHW
- Lack of harmonization, coordination, and collaboration between programs and sectors
- Insufficient involvement with the private sector
- Suboptimal vaccine coverage
- Financial constraints
- Scarcity of human resources
- Lack of adequate training for health care providers
- Lack of adequate health commodities and supplies (eg, antibiotics, zinc, vaccines)
- Health care access issues due to geographic and financial barriers
- Poor surveillance
- Inadequate monitoring and evaluation

*Abbreviations:* CCM, community case management; CHW, community health workers.
*Data from* Qazi S, Aboubaker S, MacLean R, et al. Ending preventable child deaths from pneumonia and diarrhea by 2025: the integrated global action plan for pneumonia and diarrhea. Arch Dis Child 2015;100(Suppl 1):s23–8.

Protect, Prevent and Treat framework

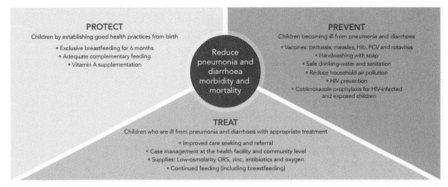

**Fig. 1.** WHO/UNICEF framework to protect, prevent, and treat pneumonia and diarrhea in children less than five years of age. (Used with permission from WHO/UNICEF. Ending preventable child deaths from pneumonia and diarrhea by 2025: the integrated global action plan for pneumonia and diarrhea. Geneva (Switzerland): WHO; 2013).

framework to reduce morbidity and mortality from pneumonia and diarrhea in LMICs.[59] In 2013, the WHO and The United Nations Children's Fund (UNICEF) launched the Integrated Global Action Plan for the Prevention and Control of Pneumonia and Diarrhea (GAPPD) with a goal to eliminate child deaths from pneumonia and diarrhea by 2025.[60] Community-based delivery platforms have been proposed to reach the poorest, hard-to-reach populations and reduce health care inequalities.[17]

Progress has been made in improving access to childhood vaccines to prevent pneumonia and diarrhea. Given the various challenges in modern vaccine development (eg, lack of investments, decreasing number of vaccine manufacturers), establishment of a global vaccine-development fund has been proposed.[61] Most experts in the field envision that GAPPD goals can be achieved, though successful implementation of the WHO/UNICEF Integrated GAPPD will need strong commitment from national governments, the private sector, and other stakeholders.[59]

## SUMMARY

Despite marked reductions in the past decade, pneumonia and diarrhea continue to be the leading killers of young children worldwide. There are now several effective and relatively low-cost interventions to control these diseases, and organizations such as GAVI have enabled many countries to implement pathogen-specific vaccines into their national immunization programs. Effective vaccines are needed against other major killers of children including RSV, ETEC, and norovirus. Further progress in this field will continue to depend on international commitment to fund, communicate, and advocate for the needs of these children.

## REFERENCES

1. Fischer-Walker CL, Rudan I, Liu L, et al. Global burden of childhood pneumonia and diarrhoea. Lancet 2013;381(9875):1405–16.
2. UNICEF committing to child survival: a promise renewed - progress report 2014. New York: UNICEF; 2014. Available at: http://files.unicef.org/publications/files/APR_2014_web_15Sept14.pdf.

3. Liu L, Oza S, Hogan D, et al. Global, regional, and national causes of child mortality in 2000-13, with projections to inform post-2015 priorities: an updated systematic analysis. Lancet 2015;385(9966):430–40.

4. Nair H, Simoes EA, Rudan I, et al. Global and regional burden of hospital admissions for severe acute lower respiratory infections in young children in 2010: a systematic analysis. Lancet 2013;381(9875):1380–90.

5. Fischer Walker CL, Perin J, Aryee MJ, et al. Diarrhea incidence in low- and middle-income countries in 1990 and 2010: a systematic review. BMC Public Health 2012;12:220.

6. Kotloff KL, Nataro JP, Blackwelder WC, et al. Burden and aetiology of diarrhoeal disease in infants and young children in developing countries (the Global Enteric Multicenter Study, GEMS): a prospective, case-control study. Lancet 2013; 382(9888):209–22.

7. Jain S, Williams DJ, Arnold SR, et al. Community-acquired pneumonia requiring hospitalization among U.S. children. N Engl J Med 2015;372(9):835–45.

8. Rudan I, O'Brien KL, Nair H, et al. Epidemiology and etiology of childhood pneumonia in 2010: estimates of incidence, severe morbidity, mortality, underlying risk factors and causative pathogens for 192 countries. J Glob Health 2013;3(1): 010401.

9. Mermond S, Zurawski V, D'Ortenzio E, et al. Lower respiratory infections among hospitalized children in New Caledonia: a pilot study for the Pneumonia Etiology Research for Child Health project. Clin Infect Dis 2012;54(Suppl 2):S180–9.

10. Howie SR, Morris GA, Tokarz R, et al. Etiology of severe childhood pneumonia in the Gambia, West Africa, determined by conventional and molecular microbiological analyses of lung and pleural aspirate samples. Clin Infect Dis 2014; 59(5):682–5.

11. Platts-Mills JA, Babji S, Bodhidatta L, et al. Pathogen-specific burdens of community diarrhoea in developing countries (MAL-ED): a multisite birth cohort study. Lancet Glob Health 2015;3(9):e564–75.

12. Selwyn BJ. The epidemiology of acute respiratory tract infection in young children: comparison of findings from several developing countries. Coordinated Data Group of BOSTID Researchers. Rev Infect Dis 1990;12(Suppl 8):S870–88.

13. Chisti MJ, Tebruegge M, La Vincente S, et al. Pneumonia in severely malnourished children in developing countries - mortality risk, aetiology and validity of WHO clinical signs: a systematic review. Trop Med Int Health 2009;14(10): 1173–89.

14. Levine OS, O'Brien KL, Deloria-Knoll M, et al. The Pneumonia Etiology Research for Child Health Project: a 21st century childhood pneumonia etiology study. Clin Infect Dis 2012;54(Suppl 2):S93–101.

15. Picot VS, Benet T, Messaoudi M, et al. Multicenter case-control study protocol of pneumonia etiology in children: Global Approach to Biological Research, Infectious diseases and Epidemics in Low-income countries (GABRIEL network). BMC Infect Dis 2014;14:635.

16. Taniuchi M, Sobuz SU, Begum S, et al. Etiology of diarrhea in Bangladeshi infants in the first year of life analyzed using molecular methods. J Infect Dis 2013; 208(11):1794–802.

17. Bhutta ZA, Das JK, Walker N, et al. Interventions to address deaths from childhood pneumonia and diarrhoea equitably: what works and at what cost? Lancet 2013;381(9875):1417–29.

18. Chisti MJ, Graham SM, Duke T, et al. Post-discharge mortality in children with severe malnutrition and pneumonia in Bangladesh. PLoS One 2014;9(9):e107663.

19. Leung DT, Das SK, Malek MA, et al. Concurrent pneumonia in children under 5 years of age presenting to a diarrheal hospital in Dhaka, Bangladesh. Am J Trop Med Hyg 2015. [Epub ahead of print].
20. Ahmed T, Ali M, Ullah MM, et al. Mortality in severely malnourished children with diarrhoea and use of a standardised management protocol. Lancet 1999; 353(9168):1919–22.
21. Ashworth A, Chopra M, McCoy D, et al. WHO guidelines for management of severe malnutrition in rural South African hospitals: effect on case fatality and the influence of operational factors. Lancet 2004;363(9415):1110–5.
22. Brown KH, Hess SY, Vosti SA, et al. Comparison of the estimated cost-effectiveness of preventive and therapeutic zinc supplementation strategies for reducing child morbidity and mortality in sub-Saharan Africa. Food Nutr Bull 2013;34(2):199–214.
23. Arifeen S, Black RE, Antelman G, et al. Exclusive breastfeeding reduces acute respiratory infection and diarrhea deaths among infants in Dhaka slums. Pediatrics 2001;108(4):E67.
24. Lamberti LM, Fischer Walker CL, Noiman A, et al. Breastfeeding and the risk for diarrhea morbidity and mortality. BMC Public Health 2011;11(Suppl 3):S15.
25. Lamberti LM, Zakarija-Grkovic I, Fischer Walker CL, et al. Breastfeeding for reducing the risk of pneumonia morbidity and mortality in children under two: a systematic literature review and meta-analysis. BMC Public Health 2013; 13(Suppl 3):S18.
26. Brown J, Cairncross S, Ensink JH. Water, sanitation, hygiene and enteric infections in children. Arch Dis Child 2013;98(8):629–34.
27. Aiello AE, Coulborn RM, Perez V, et al. Effect of hand hygiene on infectious disease risk in the community setting: a meta-analysis. Am J Public Health 2008; 98(8):1372–81.
28. Greenland K, Cairncross S, Cumming O, et al. Can we afford to overlook hand hygiene again? Trop Med Int Health 2013;18(3):246–9.
29. Lucero MG, Dulalia VE, Nillos LT, et al. Pneumococcal conjugate vaccines for preventing vaccine-type invasive pneumococcal disease and X-ray defined pneumonia in children less than two years of age. Cochrane Database Syst Rev 2009;(4):CD004977.
30. Simonsen L, Taylor RJ, Young-Xu Y, et al. Impact of pneumococcal conjugate vaccination of infants on pneumonia and influenza hospitalization and mortality in all age groups in the United States. MBio 2011;2(1):e00309–00310.
31. Whitney CG, Farley MM, Hadler J, et al. Decline in invasive pneumococcal disease after the introduction of protein-polysaccharide conjugate vaccine. N Engl J Med 2003;348(18):1737–46.
32. Olarte L, Ampofo K, Stockmann C, et al. Invasive pneumococcal disease in infants younger than 90 days before and after introduction of PCV7. Pediatrics 2013;132(1):e17–24.
33. Johnson HL, Deloria-Knoll M, Levine OS, et al. Systematic evaluation of serotypes causing invasive pneumococcal disease among children under five: the pneumococcal global serotype project. PLoS Med 2010;7(10):e1000348.
34. International Vaccine Access Center (IVAC) JHBSoPH. Vaccine information management system (VIMS) global vaccine introduction report. 2015. Available at: http://www.jhsph.edu/research/centers-and-institutes/ivac/vims. Accessed July 28, 2015.
35. Weinberger DM, Malley R, Lipsitch M. Serotype replacement in disease after pneumococcal vaccination. Lancet 2011;378(9807):1962–73.

36. Malley R, Anderson PW. Serotype-independent pneumococcal experimental vaccines that induce cellular as well as humoral immunity. Proc Natl Acad Sci U S A 2012;109(10):3623–7.

37. Ward JI, Broome CV, Harrison LH, et al. Haemophilus influenzae type b vaccines: lessons for the future. Pediatrics 1988;81(6):886–93.

38. Santosham M, Wolff M, Reid R, et al. The efficacy in Navajo infants of a conjugate vaccine consisting of Haemophilus influenzae type b polysaccharide and Neisseria meningitidis outer-membrane protein complex. N Engl J Med 1991;324(25): 1767–72.

39. Cowgill KD, Ndiritu M, Nyiro J, et al. Effectiveness of Haemophilus influenzae type b conjugate vaccine introduction into routine childhood immunization in Kenya. JAMA 2006;296(6):671–8.

40. Jain VK, Rivera L, Zaman K, et al. Vaccine for prevention of mild and moderate-to-severe influenza in children. N Engl J Med 2013;369(26):2481–91.

41. Osterholm MT, Kelley NS, Sommer A, et al. Efficacy and effectiveness of influenza vaccines: a systematic review and meta-analysis. Lancet Infect Dis 2012;12(1): 36–44.

42. Meeyai A, Praditsitthikorn N, Kotirum S, et al. Seasonal influenza vaccination for children in Thailand: a cost-effectiveness analysis. PLoS Med 2015;12(5): e1001829.

43. Ortiz JR, Goswami D, Lewis KD, et al. Safety of Russian-backbone seasonal trivalent, live-attenuated influenza vaccine in a phase II randomized placebo-controlled clinical trial among children in urban Bangladesh. Vaccine 2015; 33(29):3415–21.

44. Zaman K, Roy E, Arifeen SE, et al. Effectiveness of maternal influenza immunization in mothers and infants. N Engl J Med 2008;359(15):1555–64.

45. Ruiz-Palacios GM, Perez-Schael I, Velazquez FR, et al. Safety and efficacy of an attenuated vaccine against severe rotavirus gastroenteritis. N Engl J Med 2006; 354(1):11–22.

46. Vesikari T, Matson DO, Dennehy P, et al. Safety and efficacy of a pentavalent human-bovine (WC3) reassortant rotavirus vaccine. N Engl J Med 2006;354(1):23–33.

47. Cortese MM, Dahl RM, Curns AT, et al. Protection against gastroenteritis in US households with children who received rotavirus vaccine. J Infect Dis 2015; 211(4):558–62.

48. Madhi SA, Cunliffe NA, Steele D, et al. Effect of human rotavirus vaccine on severe diarrhea in African infants. N Engl J Med 2010;362(4):289–98.

49. Armah GE, Sow SO, Breiman RF, et al. Efficacy of pentavalent rotavirus vaccine against severe rotavirus gastroenteritis in infants in developing countries in sub-Saharan Africa: a randomised, double-blind, placebo-controlled trial. Lancet 2010;376(9741):606–14.

50. Zaman K, Dang DA, Victor JC, et al. Efficacy of pentavalent rotavirus vaccine against severe rotavirus gastroenteritis in infants in developing countries in Asia: a randomised, double-blind, placebo-controlled trial. Lancet 2010; 376(9741):615–23.

51. Kirkpatrick BD, Colgate ER, Mychaleckyj JC, et al. The "Performance of Rotavirus and Oral Polio Vaccines in Developing Countries" (PROVIDE) study: description of methods of an interventional study designed to explore complex biologic problems. Am J Trop Med Hyg 2015;92(4):744–51.

52. Bhattacharya SK, Sur D, Ali M, et al. 5 year efficacy of a bivalent killed whole-cell oral cholera vaccine in Kolkata, India: a cluster-randomised, double-blind, placebo-controlled trial. Lancet Infect Dis 2013;13(12):1050–6.

53. Deen JL, von Seidlein L, Sur D, et al. The high burden of cholera in children: comparison of incidence from endemic areas in Asia and Africa. PLoS Negl Trop Dis 2008;2(2):e173.
54. Sinclair D, Abba K, Zaman K, et al. Oral vaccines for preventing cholera. Cochrane Database Syst Rev 2011;(3):CD008603.
55. Leung DT, Uddin T, Xu P, et al. Immune responses to the O-specific polysaccharide antigen in children who received a killed oral cholera vaccine compared to responses following natural cholera infection in Bangladesh. Clin Vaccine Immunol 2013;20(6):780–8.
56. Desai SN, Cravioto A, Sur D, et al. Maximizing protection from use of oral cholera vaccines in developing country settings: an immunological review of oral cholera vaccines. Hum Vaccin Immunother 2014;10(6):1457–65.
57. WHO/UNICEF. Countdown to 2015. Building a future for women and children: the 2012 report. Washington, DC. 2012. Available at: who.int/pmnch/topics/part_publications/introduction.pdf. Accessed July 28, 2015.
58. Gill CJ, Young M, Schroder K, et al. Bottlenecks, barriers, and solutions: results from multi-country consultations focused on reduction of childhood pneumonia and diarrhea deaths. Lancet 2013;381:1487–98.
59. Qazi S, Aboubaker S, MacLean R, et al. Ending preventable child deaths from pneumonia and diarrhea by 2025: the integrated global action plan for pneumonia and diarrhea. Arch Dis Child 2015;100(Suppl 1):s23–8.
60. WHO/UNICEF. Ending preventable child deaths from pneumonia and diarrhea by 2025: the integrated global action plan for pneumonia and diarrhea. Geneva (Switzerland): WHO; 2013.
61. Plotkin SA, Mahmoud AF, Farrar J. Establishing a global vaccine-development fund. N Engl J Med 2015;373(4):297–300.

# Global Delivery of Human Papillomavirus Vaccines

Jannah Wigle, MSc[a], Holly B. Fontenot, PhD, RN[b], Gregory D. Zimet, PhD[c],*

## KEYWORDS

- Human papillomavirus • HPV • Vaccine • Immunization • Global • Progress

## KEY POINTS

- As of 2012, more than 100 countries had licensed human papillomavirus (HPV) vaccines. As of February, 2015, there were an estimated 80 national HPV vaccination programs and 37 pilot programs.
- Financing mechanisms through GAVI, the Vaccine Alliance, and the Pan American Health Organization have helped many low-income and middle-income countries (LMICs) implement HPV vaccination programs, though funding challenges continue to represent a significant barrier in many countries.
- School-based approaches to HPV vaccine delivery have generally been very successful in both LMICs and high-income countries.
- Clinic-based or office-based delivery strategies have been evaluated, with some countries showing limited success (eg, the United States) and others having greater success (eg, Denmark).
- Community outreach approaches have shown some success in HPV vaccine uptake, particularly in reaching children who are not in school.

## INTRODUCTION

Worldwide, genital human papillomavirus (HPV) is very common. In most cases, HPV infections are symptomless and do not progress to disease; however, persistent HPV infection can progress to cause genital warts (via nononcogenic or low-risk types), as well as cancers of the anogenital area and head and neck (via oncogenic or high-risk types).[1] Worldwide, HPV types 16 and 18 are causally implicated in the development

Disclosures: J. Wigle and H.B. Fontenot report no relevant disclosures. G.D. Zimet is an investigator on investigator-initiated research funded by Merck & Co, Inc and has served within the past year as a consultant to Merck & Co, Inc.
[a] Division of Social and Behavioural Health Sciences, Dalla Lana School of Public Health, University of Toronto, 155 College Street, 6th Floor, Toronto, Ontario, M5T 3M7, Canada; [b] W.F. Connell School of Nursing, Boston College, 140 Commonwealth Avenue, Chestnut Hill, MA 02467, USA; [c] Department of Pediatrics, Indiana University School of Medicine, 410 West 10th Street, HS 1001, Indianapolis, IN 46202, USA
* Corresponding author.
E-mail address: gzimet@iu.edu

of approximately 70% of cervical cancers, whereas HPV types 6 and 11 cause about 90% of genital warts.[1] Globally, cervical cancer is the fourth most common cancer among women. In 2012, an estimated 527,624 women were diagnosed with cervical cancer and more than 85% of the 265,653 deaths occurred in developing countries (**Fig. 1**).[2,3] In the United States it is estimated that more than 17,000 women and more than 9000 men are diagnosed with HPV-related cancers each year (**Table 1**).[4]

There are currently 3 vaccines that prevent HPV infections and diseases: a bivalent vaccine (HPV2) that protects against types 16 and 18[5]; a quadrivalent vaccine (HPV4) that protects against types 16, 18, as well as 6 and 11[6,7]; and a 9-valent vaccine (HPV9) that protects against the 4 types covered in HPV4, plus 5 additional oncogenic types (31, 33, 45, 52, and 58).[8] HPV vaccine efficacy, effectiveness, and safety are well-established.[9–12]

Key points on HPV vaccines include
- As of 2012, more than 100 countries had licensed HPV vaccines[13]
- As of February, 2015, there were an estimated 80 national HPV vaccination programs and 37 pilot programs, with many of these implemented in low-income and middle-income countries (LMICs; **Fig. 2**)[14]
- The HPV9 vaccine was licensed by the US Food and Drug Administration in December, 2014[15]
- The World Health Organization (WHO) recommends a 2-dose vaccination schedule for patients younger than 15 years of age[16]
- The United States continues, for now, to recommend a 3-dose schedule, regardless of age.[8]

In the United States, the national goal for HPV vaccination 3-dose series completion is 80% of all children by age 13 to 15 years.[17] However, the 2013 National Immunization Survey-Teen found that only 37.6% of females and 13.9% of males, ages 13 to 17 years, had received 3 or more doses of the vaccine.[18] In contrast, other high-income countries (HICs), such as Canada, the United Kingdom, Denmark, and Australia, have achieved very high HPV vaccination rates, as have several LMICs (see **Fig. 2**).[19–25] The relative success or failure of HPV vaccination programs is likely due to many factors, including vaccine funding, implementation approaches, logistical and resource barriers, and cultural and political issues related to vaccination. See later sections for discussion of these factors.

## HUMAN PAPILLOMAVIRUS VACCINE FUNDING

HPV vaccine cost is a central factor in successful implementation of vaccination programs. High out-of-pocket costs for individuals decrease HPV vaccine acceptability[26–28] and high costs for LMICs may limit the ability to provide vaccine for citizens. The cost for the vaccine in the public sector ranges by country and region, from US $4.50 to more than $100 per dose,[29] representing a potential barrier to its implementation in many countries worldwide.

Significant progress has been made to improve the affordability of HPV vaccine to LMICs through financing mechanisms, including GAVI, the Vaccine Alliance, and the Pan American Health Organization (PAHO) Revolving Fund. In June, 2011, Merck & Co (West Point, PA, USA), announced that HPV4 would be offered to GAVI for $5 per dose for GAVI-eligible countries.[30] In 2013, a further record-low price of $4.50 per dose was announced.[31] Many GAVI-eligible countries are able to procure the vaccine for a small copayment of $0.20 per dose,[32] increasing affordability. However, this low cost is only available to the 49 LMICs that are currently eligible for GAVI

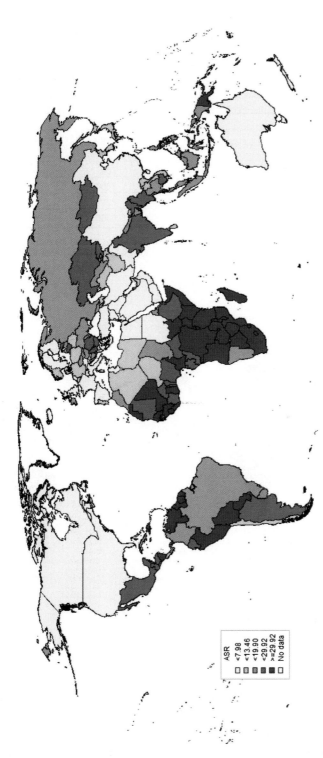

**Fig. 1.** Age-standardized incidence rates per 100,000 of cervical cancer in the world (estimations for 2012). (*From* Ferlay J, Soerjomataram I, Ervik M, et al. GLOBOCAN 2012 v1.0, Cancer Incidence and Mortality Worldwide: IARC CancerBase No. 11. Lyon (France): International Agency for Research on Cancer; 2013. Available at: http://globocan.iarc.fr. Accessed May 19, 2015; with permission.)

ASR
<7.98
<13.46
<19.90
<29.92
>=29.92
No data

**Table 1**
**United States burden of human papillomavirus–related cancers in men and women**

| Type of Cancer | Average Annual Number of Cases | Cases Probably Caused by HPV |
|---|---|---|
| Cervix | 11,422 | 10,400 |
| Vagina | 735 | 600 |
| Vulva | 3168 | 2200 |
| Anus (W) | 2821 | 2600 |
| Oropharynx (W) | 2443 | 1800 |
| Total Women | 20,589 | 17,600 |
| Penis | 1048 | 700 |
| Anus (M) | 1549 | 1400 |
| Oropharynx (M) | 9974 | 7200 |
| Total Men | 12,571 | 9300 |

*Data from* Centers for Disease Control and Prevention, United States Cancer Statistics (USCS), 2006-2010. Available at: http://www.cdc.gov/cancer/hpv/statistics/cases.htm. Accessed July 27, 2015.

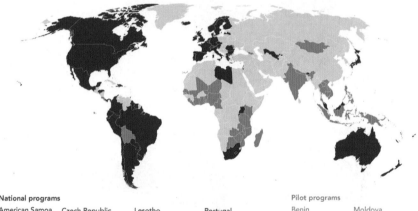

**National programs**

| | | | | |
|---|---|---|---|---|
| American Samoa | Czech Republic | Lesotho | Portugal | |
| Argentina | Denmark | Libya | Romania | |
| Aruba | Dominican Republic | Luxembourg | Rwanda | |
| Australia | Ecuador | Macedonia | San Marino | |
| Austria | Fiji | Malaysia | Seychelles | |
| Bahamas | Finland | Malta | Singapore | |
| Barbados | France | Marshall Islands | Slovenia | |
| Belgium | French Polynesia | Mexico | South Africa | |
| Belize | Germany | Micronesia | Spain | |
| Bermuda | Greece | Monaco | St. Eustatius | |
| Bhutan | Guam | Netherlands | Suriname | |
| Brazil | Guyana | New Caledonia | Sweden | |
| Brunei | Honduras | New Zealand | Switzerland | |
| Bulgaria | Iceland | Niue | Trinidad and Tobago | |
| Canada | Ireland | Northern Marianas | Uganda | |
| Cayman Islands | Israel | Norway | United Kingdom | |
| Chile | Italy | Palau | United States | |
| Colombia | Japan | Panama | Uruguay | |
| Cook Islands | Kiribati | Paraguay | Uzbekistan | |
| Curacao | Latvia | Peru | Vanuatu | |

**Pilot programs**

| | |
|---|---|
| Benin | Moldova |
| Bolivia | Mongolia |
| Botswana | Mozambique |
| Burundi | Nepal |
| Cambodia | Niger |
| Cameroon | Nigeria |
| Costa Rica | Papua New |
| Cote d'Ivoire | Guinea |
| Gambia | Philippines |
| Georgia | Senegal |
| Ghana | Sierra Leone |
| Haiti | Solomon |
| India | Islands |
| Indonesia | Tanzania |
| Kenya | Thailand |
| Lao PDR | Togo |
| Liberia | Vietnam |
| Madagascar | Zambia |
| Malawi | Zimbabwe |
| Mali | |

**Fig. 2.** Global progress in HPV vaccine introduction (February, 2015). (*From* Cervical Cancer Action. Global maps: global progress in HPV vaccination. 2015. Available at: http://www.cervicalcanceraction.org/comments/comments3.php. Accessed May 27, 2015.)

support, which have a gross national income per capita in 2015 less than $1580.[33] Countries that have successful experiences delivering HPV vaccines to adolescents are eligible to apply to GAVI for financial support for national implementation or, if additional experience is required, can apply for support to implement demonstration projects.[29,34] The cost to procure the HPV vaccine for LMICs in Latin America and the Caribbean through the PAHO Revolving Fund is approximately $10 to $15.[32,35] The PAHO Revolving Fund was established in 1978 as a mechanism for procurement of supplies and equipment necessary for sustained delivery of vaccines.[36]

The cost for the vaccine and delivery approach of HPV vaccine programs has been found to vary by country and program.[32,35,37,38] Reasons for variation in cost between pilot projects included scope and scale, delivery strategy, national income levels and public health cost, infrastructure and the compensation structure for health staff, and health system policies. A recent study comparing the costs of HPV pilot, demonstration, or national programs in Peru, Uganda, Vietnam, India, Bhutan, and Tanzania found that introduction costs per fully immunized girl ranged from $1.49 to $18.94, with recurring costs from $1.00 to $15.69.[37] Despite subsidization of the HPV vaccine for many LMICs, costs to deliver and sustain HPV vaccination programs remain a significant ongoing investment and potential financial barrier. In addition, although significant progress has been made to achieve lower prices for the vaccine, many middle-income countries are ineligible for the low prices and copayment systems offered through GAVI, or may have graduated from GAVI-eligibility. These countries may continue to experience barriers to fund and sustain HPV vaccination programs and opportunities to support these countries should be investigated.[39]

In HICs, vaccine financing varies greatly from a patchwork combination of private and public funding in the United States to publically funded programs in, for example, Canada, Australia, the United Kingdom, and several European countries.[12] Not all European countries provide public financing for HPV vaccine, however, and several require self-pay.[40]

## HUMAN PAPILLOMAVIRUS VACCINATION IMPLEMENTATION APPROACHES
### School-Based Approaches

School-based delivery methods have been an effective approach to achieve high coverage in several LMICs through demonstration projects, donation programs, and national vaccination programs.[23,25,38,41–43] Demonstration programs through the international nongovernmental organization PATH have achieved high coverage through school-based delivery in Peru (82.6%), Uganda (88.9%), and Vietnam (96.1%).[42] High coverage has also been seen in school-based demonstration projects in South Africa,[44] Brazil,[45] and Nepal.[24] The Gardasil Access Program (GAP) was implemented by Axios Healthcare Development, and received small donations of vaccine by Merck & Co, to support countries to gain experience in the design and implementation of HPV vaccination programs.[38,46] Between 2009 and 2012, 21 vaccination programs were implemented in 14 LMICs around the world.[38] The GAPs achieved an average vaccine uptake rate of 88.7% through 3 delivery strategies, including school-based, facility-based, and mixed approaches. The school-based strategy was specifically identified as a factor that positively influenced vaccine uptake rates.[38] In 2011, national implementation of the HPV vaccine in Rwanda achieved 93.2% coverage for girls in grade 6 through school-based vaccination and community sensitization and involvement.[23]

School-based HPV vaccination programs have also been implemented successfully in several HICs, including the United Kingdom, Australia, and Canada.[19–21] Of the European countries that report an organized HPV vaccination program, more than 50% use a school-based delivery approach.[40] In the United States, there has been very limited implementation of school-based HPV vaccination, though this approach has been identified as an ideal way to reach the largest number of adolescents.[47] A pilot school-based adolescent vaccination initiative evaluated in Chicago, IL, was only modestly successful in delivering HPV vaccination. Obstacles included difficulty getting informed consent forms returned from parents and inconsistent participation by schools over time.[48] In some areas of the United States, vaccines, including HPV vaccine, can be delivered via school-based health centers (SBHCs). However, while this approach eliminates some barriers to vaccination, vaccines are delivered on an individual patient basis and, therefore, SBHC-delivery is not as efficient as an approach that involves administration of vaccines on a single day to groups of youth.[49] Attitudes of key stakeholders in the United States (eg, parents, school nurses, school administrators) about the feasibility of school-based HPV vaccination implementation are mixed, with some research showing relatively little concern among parents and administrators[48] and other research indicating uncertain support and doubts about program implementation.[50]

### Clinic-Based or Office-Based Approaches

The principal approach to HPV vaccine delivery in the United States and several European countries is via medical clinics and doctors' offices. Office-based vaccination is standard practice for most childhood vaccines in the United States. For vaccines required for school-entry, this approach has generally been quite successful, with high levels of vaccination coverage achieved.[51] However, with the exception of the state of Virginia and the District of Columbia, HPV vaccination is not required for school entry.[52] Moreover, Virginia has a relatively weak HPV vaccine school entry law, which has not proven particularly effective.[18,53] Without a clear public health policy supporting HPV vaccination, the burden of decision-making and recommendations largely falls to health care providers (HCPs) and parents. As a result, despite the licensure of HPV4 in 2006 and public and private financing for vaccination, HPV vaccination rates in the United States remain at lower than desired levels.[18]

Reasons for nonvaccination seem to be related to unwarranted parental concerns about safety; failure of HCPs to make strong, routine recommendations for vaccination at the targeted ages of 11 to 12 years; lack of knowledge; and access issues (particularly for follow-up doses).[54–57] **Box 1** contains a list of factors that have been identified as barriers to HCPs making a strong recommendation for HPV vaccination.

A variety of intervention approaches have been explored, including the use of electronic health message prompts directed to HCPs,[58,59] reminder messages sent to parents and adolescents,[60–63] communication messaging targeting parents and youth,[64] and practice-based interventions.[65–68] Results of these interventions have been mixed, with some showing modest improvements in vaccination rates and others showing no significant effects.[64,69]

In contrast to the United States experience, Denmark, which also uses an office-based approach to HPV vaccination, has had remarkable success. In 2009, Denmark began providing free HPV vaccine for all 12-year-old girls. After just 1 year, 80% of eligible girls had initiated vaccination and 62% had received all 3 doses of vaccine.[22] Over time, even greater success was achieved in Denmark, with more than 90% of girls receiving 1 or more dose of vaccine and more than 80% completing the 3-dose series.[70] Interestingly, even with this impressive level of success, HPV

---

**Box 1**
**Health care provider barriers to recommendation of HPV vaccine for adolescents**

- Limited knowledge and understanding of HPV-related disease, particularly in male patients
- Concerns of the vaccine's safety and efficacy
- Uncomfortable discussing sexual behavior with young adolescents
- Preference for vaccinating older adolescents (potentially linked to discomfort on discussing sexual behavior)
- Apprehension of parental resistance
- Insufficient time available to discuss vaccines
- Inadequate systems to remind HCPs to recommend vaccines to age-appropriate patients

*Adapted from* National Foundation for Infectious Diseases. Call to action: HPV vaccination as a public health priority. 2014. Available at: http://www.adolescentvaccination.org/hpv-cta. Accessed July 27, 2015.

---

vaccination rates in Denmark are significantly lower among girls from immigrant families and those from families with fewer socioeconomic resources.[70]

### Community Outreach Approaches

Community outreach delivery strategies, which have principally been implemented in LMICs, have demonstrated some success reaching out-of-school girls or providing opportunities for vaccine catch-up services, particularly in countries with low school enrollment and poor attendance.[25,42,43] Community approaches are also generally paired with other strategies for a mixed approach to achieve vaccination. A school-based vaccination program in combination with existing community-based child-focused public health campaign was used in Uganda to reach out-of-school girls.[42] Coverage through this approach only achieved 52.6% for their population during the first year.[42] In Vietnam, both community health center and school-based strategies were tested over 2 years and both approaches achieved high HPV vaccination coverage.[71] Achievement of high coverage in Rwanda's national HPV vaccine program has also been attributed to the combination of a school-based vaccination program, high levels of community involvement to identify absent or out-of-school girls, as well as strong national sensitization efforts and outreach before the initiation of the campaign.[23]

The PATH demonstration project in India achieved high coverage through a mixed approach using school-based and health center–based delivery with existing immunization programs (68% urban, 83% rural coverage), as well as special public health campaigns at 3 fixed time points (77%–88% coverage).[41,42] Despite these achievements in India, adverse events were falsely linked to the vaccine and the demonstration project was incorrectly characterized as an experimental clinical trial.[72,73] These claims were refuted, citing that appropriate review and approvals were obtained, that extensive research on the safety found no deaths related to the HPV vaccine, and that demonstration projects are not clinical trials.[74,75] Nonetheless, the PATH program was suspended by the Ministry of Health and Family Welfare,[72,76] a decision highlighting potential inadequate recognition of public distrust and a history in India of justifiable suspicion of the motives of outside organizations.[77,78] Findings from demonstration and national programs highlight the importance of incorporating community outreach and sensitization to the successful implementation of the HPV vaccine in LMICs.

## CHALLENGES AND FUTURE DIRECTIONS

Understanding and addressing the potential logistical and sociocultural challenges has been, and continues to be critical to ensuring the acceptability and effectiveness of HPV vaccine programs worldwide.

Logistical and resource barriers with vaccine delivery

- Health system capacity and infrastructure, including cold chain systems to transport and store the vaccine, as well as the availability of human resources for cold chain and logistics management[41,79];
- Financial costs to introduce and sustain HPV programs[37];
- Girls (including pre-adolescents and adolescents) represent a new population that has not been regularly targeted for routine immunization by the Expanded Program on Immunization[25];
- School-based programs may experience challenges including: absenteeism, determining eligibility for vaccination (eg, grade vs age-based criteria), capturing out-of-school girls, coordination of diverse immunization and education stakeholders, as well as scheduling 3 doses during the academic year[25,42,80];
- Delays or lags in delivery of vaccination programs, caused by supply shortages may decrease interest among girls and parents to complete all doses[38];
- Straining health systems and human resources by introducing new vaccines, including the HPV vaccine.[71,81]

### Cultural and Political Barriers

Sociocultural challenges to implementation and delivery of the HPV vaccine highlight the importance of improving attitudes and knowledge of HPV, HPV related diseases, and awareness of the vaccine and vaccination programs. For example, as discussed previously the PATH demonstration project in India demonstrates problems that may occur related to not fully understanding the cultural constructs when implementing vaccine programs.

Other potential cultural and political challenges to HPV vaccine delivery may include

- Stigma and controversy, targeting female adolescents ages 9 to 13 years for a sexually transmitted infection[79,82];
- Parental concerns over the vaccine's safety and its potential side effects, including unjustified fears of future infertility, early sexual debut, and potential for increased sexual activity[83–85];
- Differences in acceptable communication strategies and dissemination of health information, as well as parental consent preferences (eg, opt-in vs opt-out)[86];
- Skepticism and concerns related to research and introducing new vaccines and medicines[86];
- Political will and commitment of decision makers to prioritize demonstration projects and/or national implementation of the HPV vaccine[87]

In order to influence the acceptability and uptake of the vaccine in all countries it is critical to provide information and improve knowledge of the intervention. In Africa, despite low levels of knowledge or awareness of HPV (on average 26%), and the HPV vaccine (15%), high levels of acceptability were achieved across 10 countries (59%–100%) due to the vaccine's accessibility, costs and cues to action by health workers and decision makers.[85] Another systematic review supported findings that high levels of willingness to vaccinate and acceptability of the HPV vaccine can be achieved, despite low levels of knowledge and awareness of HPV, the vaccine or cervical cancer.[88] Early experiences from demonstration projects in Peru, Vietnam, Uganda, and India also found limited initial awareness and inadequate information of cervical cancer, HPV, the HPV vaccine and the vaccination program before community sensitization efforts.[42] Adequate community engagement and sensitization are key factors in successful implementation and overcoming sociocultural barriers.[23,38,42,83,89]

## Future Directions

With progress in HPV science and continued work toward global herd immunity, challenges will continue to transform and change as countries both achieve greater vaccination rates and encounter new barriers toward adopting a comprehensive approach. In 2014, the US CDC and the President's Cancer Panel identified adolescent HPV vaccine uptake as a public health priority to prevent HPV-related cancers and recommended key strategies to HCPs (**Box 2**).[57] The National Foundation for Infectious Diseases in collaboration with multiple stakeholders have developed a comprehensive online educational resources related to HPV and HPV vaccines for HCP (adolescentvaccination.org/hpv-resource-center)

Future challenges to, and directions for, HPV vaccine implementation in LMIC may include

- Meeting the WHO 2014 guidelines on cervical cancer, and introducing the HPV vaccine within a comprehensive cervical cancer prevention and control strategy and program[90];
- Delivering the HPV vaccine in conjunction with other nonvaccine interventions targeting adolescents, for example, iron supplementation[91];
- Potential risks for health disparities with unequal distribution of HPV vaccination globally, particularly with the introduction of the 9-valent vaccine;

---

**Box 2**
**Recommendations and key strategies for health care providers to improve HPV vaccination rates**

- Recommend the HPV vaccine with the same strength and conviction used to recommend other adolescent vaccines. A recommendation by an HCP is the most important reason that adolescents get the HPV vaccine.

- Health care providers should recommend the vaccine with a presumptive, rather than participatory style to improve parental acceptance of the vaccine

- Emphasize that the HPV vaccine prevents cancer

- Health care providers should educate themselves on HPV and HPV vaccines

- Address potential barriers through key elements of HPV education including: (1) provide sufficient information to parents on the disease and cancer prevention, (2) outline the rationale for vaccinating ages 11 to 12, (3) discuss safety and efficacy of the vaccine, (4) remind parents/patients of the 3-shot series, (5) address system barriers (eg, cost), and (6) highlight the benefit of male vaccination.

- Inform colleagues and staff to ensure that everyone delivers the same messages on HPV

- Communicate vaccination benefits to parents and adolescents at every opportunity

- Make vaccination procedures routine and focus on ways to reduce missed opportunities

*Adapted from* National Foundation for Infectious Diseases. Call to action: HPV vaccination as a public health priority. 2014. Available at: http://www.adolescentvaccination.org/hpv-cta. Accessed July 27, 2015.

- Potential changes to cervical cancer screening programs and protocols in the post vaccination era;
- Changes to vaccine administration programs related to 2-dose HPV vaccination, which is now recommended by the WHO for youth ages 9 to 13 years[17];
- Potential risk for lower public acceptance due to changes in vaccine composition and dosing schedules.

## SUMMARY

Pilot, demonstration and national HPV vaccination programs have successfully achieved high coverage and vaccine uptake among many countries worldwide. Financing mechanisms have improved the affordability of the vaccine in these settings and drastically contributed to overcoming this barrier to implementation in many countries. LMICs have achieved success through the introduction of diverse delivery strategies, including school-based approaches and community engagement and sensitization. Among many HICs success has also been achieved with diverse delivery strategies, including school-based and clinic/office-based approaches, as evidence by the success in Australia, Denmark, and the United Kingdom among others. The United States continues to have a slow but steady rise in vaccination rates with primarily a clinic/office based approach. Nearly a decade after the first HPV vaccine was made available, considerable progress to global delivery has been achieved, however, continued efforts to address challenges and share successes will be critical to ensure equitable and universal access to the HPV vaccine globally.

## REFERENCES

1. Forman D, de Martel C, Lacey CJ, et al. Global burden of human papillomavirus and related diseases. Vaccine 2012;30(Suppl 5):F12–23.
2. Bruni L, Barrionuevo-Rosas L, Albero G, et al. ICO Information Centre on HPV and Cancer (HPV Information Centre). Human Papillomavirus and Related Diseases in the World. Summary Report 2015-04-08;2015. Available at: http://www.hpvcentre.net/summaryreport.php. Accessed September 27, 2015.
3. Ferlay J, Soerjomataram I, Ervik M, et al. GLOBOCAN 2012 v1.0, Cancer Incidence and Mortality Worldwide: IARC CancerBase No. 11. Lyon (France): International Agency for Research on Cancer; 2013. Available at: http://globocan.iarc.fr. Accessed May 19, 2015.
4. Centers for Disease Control and Prevention, United States Cancer Statistics (USCS). Available at: http://www.cdc.gov/cancer/hpv/statistics/cases.htm. Accessed July 27, 2015.
5. Centers for Disease Control & Prevention. FDA licensure of bivalent human papillomavirus vaccine (HPV2, Cervarix) for use in females and updated HPV vaccination recommendations from the Advisory Committee on Immunization Practices. MMWR Morb Mortal Wkly Rep 2010;59:626–7.
6. Centers for Disease Control & Prevention. Quadrivalent human papillomavirus vaccine: recommendations of the Advisory Committee on Immunization Practices (ACIP). MMWR Morb Mortal Wkly Rep 2007;56(No. RR-2):1–26.
7. Centers for Disease Control & Prevention. FDA licensure of quadrivalent human papillomavirus vaccine (HPV4, Gardasil) for use in males and guidance from the advisory committee on immunization practices (ACIP). MMWR Morb Mortal Wkly Rep 2010;59:630–2.
8. Petrosky E, Bocchini JA Jr, Hariri S, et al. Use of 9-Valent Human Papillomavirus (HPV) vaccine: updated HPV vaccination recommendations of the advisory

committee on immunization practices. MMWR Morb Mortal Wkly Rep 2015;64: 300–4.

9. La Torre G, de Waure C, Chiaradia G, et al. HPV vaccine efficacy in preventing persistent cervical HPV infection: a systematic review and meta-analysis. Vaccine 2007;25:8352–8.

10. Joura EA, Giuliano AR, Iversen OE, et al. A 9-valent HPV vaccine against infection and intraepithelial neoplasia in women. N Engl J Med 2015;372:711–23.

11. Drolet M, Benard E, Boily MC, et al. Population-level impact and herd effects following human papillomavirus vaccination programmes: a systematic review and meta-analysis. Lancet Infect Dis 2015;15:565–80.

12. Scheller NM, Svanstrom H, Pasternak B, et al. Quadrivalent HPV vaccination and risk of multiple sclerosis and other demyelinating diseases of the central nervous system. JAMA 2015;313:54–61.

13. Markowitz LE, Tsu V, Deeks SL, et al. Human papillomavirus vaccine introduction – the first five years. Vaccine 2012;30:F139–48.

14. Cervical Cancer Action. Global maps: global progress in HPV vaccination. 2015. Available at: http://www.cervicalcanceraction.org/comments/comments3.php. Accessed May 27, 2015.

15. U.S. Food & Drug Administration. FDA approves Gardasil 9 for prevention of certain cancers caused by 5 additional types of HPV. 2014. Available at: http://www.fda.gov/NewsEvents/Newsroom/PressAnnouncements/ucm426485.htm. Accessed May 31, 2015.

16. World Health Organization. Human papillomavirus vaccines: WHO position paper, October 2014-Recommendations. Vaccine 2015;33(36):4383–4.

17. U.S. Department of Health & Human Services. Healthy People 2020. 2015. Available at: http://www.healthypeople.gov/2020/topics-objectives/topic/immunization-and-infectious-diseases/objectives. Accessed May 31, 2015.

18. Elam-Evans LD, Yankey D, Jeyarajah J, et al. National, regional, state, and selected local area vaccination coverage among adolescents aged 13-17 Years—United States, 2013. MMWR Morb Mortal Wkly Rep 2014;63:625–33.

19. Shearer BD. HPV vaccination: understanding the impact on HPV disease. Purple Paper 2011;34:1–18.

20. Brotherton JM, Murray S, Hall M, et al. Human papillomavirus vaccine coverage among female Australian adolescents: success of the school-based approach. Med J Aust 2013;199:614–7.

21. Franceschi S. Monitoring HPV 16/18 immunisation in England and elsewhere. Br J Cancer 2010;103:157–8.

22. Widgren K, Simonsen J, Valentiner-Branth P, et al. Uptake of the human papillomavirus-vaccination within the free-of-charge childhood vaccination programme in Denmark. Vaccine 2011;29:9663–7.

23. Binagwaho A, Wagner CM, Gatera M, et al. Achieving high coverage in Rwanda's national human papillomavirus vaccination programme. Bull World Health Organ 2012;90:623–8.

24. Singh Y, Shah A, Singh M, et al. Human papilloma virus vaccination in Nepal: an initial experience in Nepal. Asian Pac J Cancer Prev 2010;11:615–7.

25. Watson-Jones D, Baisley K, Ponsiano R, et al. Human papillomavirus vaccination in Tanzanian schoolgirls: cluster-randomized trial comparing 2 vaccine-delivery strategies. J Infect Dis 2012;206:678–86.

26. Sauvageau C, Duval B, Gilca V, et al. Human papilloma virus vaccine and cervical cancer screening acceptability among adults in Quebec, Canada. BMC Public Health 2007;7:304.

27. Lenehan JG, Leonard KC, Nandra S, et al. Women's knowledge, attitudes, and intentions concerning human papillomavirus vaccination: findings of a waiting room survey of obstetrics-gynaecology outpatients. J Obstet Gynaecol Can 2008;30:489–99.
28. Liau A, Stupiansky NW, Rosenthal SL, et al. Health beliefs and vaccine costs regarding human papillomavirus (HPV) vaccination among a U.S. national sample of adult women. Prev Med 2012;54:277–9.
29. GAVI. Human papillomavirus vaccine support. 2015. Available at: http://www.gavi.org/support/nvs/human-papillomavirus-vaccine-support. Accessed April 20, 2015.
30. GAVI. Gavi welcomes lower prices for life-saving vaccines. 2011. Available at: http://www.gavi.org/library/news/press-releases/2011/gavi-welcomes-lower-prices-for-life-saving-vaccines. Accessed May 27, 2015.
31. GAVI. Millions of girls in developing countries to be protected against cervical cancer thanks to new HPV vaccine deals. 2013. Available at: http://www.gavi.org/library/news/press-releases/2013/hpv-price-announcement. Accessed May 27, 2015.
32. Levin CE, Van Minh H, Odaga J, et al. Delivery cost of human papillomavirus vaccination of young adolescent girls in Peru, Uganda and Viet Nam. Bull World Health Organ 2013;91:585–92.
33. GAVI. Countries eligible for support. 2015. Available at: http://www.gavi.org/support/apply/countries-eligible-for-support. Accessed April 20, 2015.
34. Hanson CM, Eckert L, Bloem P, et al. Gavi HPV programs: application to implementation. Vaccine 2015;3:408–19.
35. Portnoy A, Ozawa S, Grewal S, et al. Costs of vaccine programs across 94 low- and middle-income countries. Vaccine 2015;33(Suppl 1):A99–108.
36. Andrus JK, Sherris J, Fitzsimmons JW, et al. Introduction of human papillomavirus vaccines into developing countries - international strategies for funding and procurement. Vaccine 2008;26S:K87–92.
37. Levin A, Wang SA, Levin C, et al. Costs of introducing and delivering HPV vaccines in low and lower middle income countries: inputs for GAVI policy on introduction grant support to countries. PLoS One 2014;9:e101114.
38. Ladner J, Besson MH, Rodrigues M, et al. Performance of 21 HPV vaccination programs implemented in low and middle-income countries, 2009-2013. BMC Public Health 2014;14:670.
39. Kaddar M, Schmitt S, Makinen M, et al. Global support for new vaccine implementation in middle-income countries. Vaccine 2013;31(Suppl 2):B81–96.
40. Elfstrom KM, Dillner J, Arnheim-Dahlstrom L. Organization and quality of HPV vaccination programs in Europe. Vaccine 2015;33:1673–81.
41. Paul P, Fabio A. Literature review of HPV vaccine delivery strategies: considerations for school- and non-school based immunization program. Vaccine 2014;32:320–6.
42. LaMontagne DS, Barge S, Le NT, et al. Human papillomavirus vaccine delivery strategies that achieved high coverage in low- and middle-income countries. Bull World Health Organ 2011;89:821–30B.
43. Penny M, Bartolini R, Mosqueira NR, et al. Strategies to vaccinate against cancer of the cervix: feasibility of a school-based HPV vaccination program in Peru. Vaccine 2011;29:5022–30.
44. Moodley I, Tathiah N, Mubaiwa V, et al. High uptake of Gardasil vaccine among 9-12-year-old schoolgirls participating in an HPV vaccination demonstration project in KwaZulu-Natal, South Africa. S Afr Med J 2013;103:318–21.

45. Fregnani JH, Carvalho AL, Eluf-Neto J, et al. A school-based human papilloma-virus vaccination program in Barretos, Brazil: final results of a demonstrative study. PLoS One 2013;8:e62647.
46. Ladner J, Besson MH, Hampshire R, et al. Assessment of eight HPV vaccination programs implemented in lowest income countries. BMC Public Health 2012;12:370.
47. Limper HM, Burns JL, Lloyd LM, et al. Challenges to school-located vaccination: lessons learned. Pediatrics 2014;134:803–8.
48. Caskey RN, Macario E, Johnson DC, et al. A school-located vaccination adolescent pilot initiative in Chicago: lessons learned. J Pediatr Infect Dis Soc 2013;2: 198–204.
49. Rickert VI, Auslander BA, Cox DS, et al. School-based HPV immunization of young adolescents: effects of two brief health interventions. Hum Vaccin Immunother 2015;11:315–21.
50. Nodulman JA, Starling R, Kong AS, et al. Investigating stakeholder attitudes and opinions on school-based human papillomavirus vaccination programs. J Sch Health 2015;85:289–98.
51. Orenstein WA, Hinman AR. The immunization system in the United States - the role of school immunization laws. Vaccine 1999;17(Suppl):S19–24.
52. Laugesen MJ, Mistry R, Carameli KA, et al. Early policy responses to the human papillomavirus vaccine in the United States, 2006-2010. J Adolesc Health 2014; 55:659–64.
53. Pitts MJ, Adams Tufts K. Implications of the Virginia human papillomavirus vaccine mandate for parental vaccine acceptance. Qual Health Res 2013;23: 605–17.
54. Stokley S, Jeyarajah J, Yankey D, et al. Human papillomavirus vaccination coverage among adolescents, 2007-2013, and postlicensure vaccine safety monitoring, 2006-2014-United States. MMWR Morb Mortal Wkly Rep 2014;63: 620–4.
55. Kester LM, Zimet GD, Fortenberry JD, et al. A national study of HPV vaccination of adolescent girls: rates, predictors, and reasons for non-vaccination. Matern Child Health J 2013;17:879–85.
56. Donahue KL, Stupiansky NW, Alexander AB, et al. Acceptability of the human papillomavirus vaccine and reasons for non-vaccination among parents of adolescent sons. Vaccine 2014;32:3883–5.
57. National Foundation for Infectious Diseases. Call to Action: HPV Vaccination as a Public Health Priority. 2014. Available at: http://www.adolescentvaccination.org/hpv-cta. Accessed July 27, 2015.
58. Szilagyi PG, Serwint JR, Humiston SG, et al. Effect of provider prompts on adolescent immunization rates: a randomized trial. Acad Pediatr 2015;15:149–57.
59. Ruffin MT, Plegue MA, Rockwell PG, et al. Impact of an electronic health record (EHR) reminder on human papillomavirus (HPV) vaccine initiation and timely completion. J Am Board Fam Med 2015;28:324–33.
60. Kharbanda EO, Stockwell MS, Fox HW, et al. Text message reminders to promote human papillomavirus vaccination. Vaccine 2011;29:2537–41.
61. Matheson EC, Derouin A, Gagliano M, et al. Increasing HPV vaccination series completion rates via text message reminders. J Pediatr Health Care 2014;28: e35–9.
62. Rand CM, Brill H, Albertin C, et al. Effectiveness of centralized text message reminders on human papillomavirus immunization coverage for publicly insured adolescents. J Adolesc Health 2015;56(5 Suppl):S17–20.

63. Bar-Shain DS, Stager MM, Runkle AP, et al. Direct messaging to parents/guardians to improve adolescent immunizations. J Adolesc Health 2015;56(5 Suppl): S21–6.
64. Fu LY, Bonhomme LA, Cooper SC, et al. Educational interventions to increase HPV vaccination acceptance: a systematic review. Vaccine 2014;32:1901–20.
65. Mayne S, Karavite D, Grundmeier RW, et al. The implementation and acceptability of an HPV vaccination decision support system directed at both clinicians and families. AMIA Annu Symp Proc 2012;2012:616–24.
66. Fiks AG, Grundmeier RW, Mayne S, et al. Effectiveness of decision support for families, clinicians, or both on HPV vaccine receipt. Pediatrics 2013;131: 1114–24.
67. Perkins RB, Zisblatt L, Legler A, et al. Effectiveness of a provider-focused intervention to improve HPV vaccination rates in boys and girls. Vaccine 2015;33: 1223–9.
68. Gilkey MB, Moss JL, Roberts AJ, et al. Comparing in-person and webinar delivery of an immunization quality improvement program: a process evaluation of the adolescent AFIX trial. Implement Sci 2014;9:21.
69. Dempsey AF, Zimet GD. Interventions to improve adolescent vaccination: what may work and what still needs to be tested. Am J Prev Med 2015. [Epub ahead of print].
70. Slattelid Schreiber SM, Juul KE, Dehlendorff C, et al. Socioeconomic predictors of human papillomavirus vaccination among girls in the Danish childhood immunization program. J Adolesc Health 2015;56:402–7.
71. LaMontagne DS, Nghi NQ, Nga le T, et al. Qualitative study of the feasibility of HPV vaccine delivery to young adolescent girls in Vietnam: evidence from a government-implemented demonstration program. BMC Public Health 2014; 14:556.
72. Sharma DC. Rights violation found in HPV vaccine studies in India. Lancet Oncol 2013;14:e443.
73. Sengupta A, Shenoi A, Sarojini NB, et al. Human papillomavirus vaccine trials in India. Lancet 2011;377:719.
74. Tsu VD. Indian vaccine study clarified. Nature 2011;475:296.
75. Lamontagne DS, Sherris JD. Addressing questions about the HPV vaccine project in India. Lancet Oncol 2013;14:e492.
76. Sarojini N, Deepa V. Trials and tribulations: an expose of the HPV vaccine trials by the 72nd Parliamentary Standing Committee Report. Indian J Med Ethics 2013; 10:220–2.
77. Larson HJ, Brocard P, Garnett G. The India HPV-vaccine suspension. Lancet 2010;376:572–3.
78. Towghi F. The biopolitics of reproductive technologies beyond the clinic: localizing HPV vaccines in India. Med Anthropol 2013;32:325–42.
79. Biellik R, Levin C, Mugisha E, et al. Health systems and immunization financing for human papillomavirus vaccine introduction in low-resource settings. Vaccine 2009;27:6203–9.
80. Kane MA, Serrano B, de Sanjosé S, et al. Implementation of human papillomavirus immunization in the developing world. Vaccine 2012;30:F192–200.
81. Burchett HE, Mounier-Jack S, Torres-Rueda S, et al. The impact of introducing new vaccines on the health system: case studies from six low- and middle-income countries. Vaccine 2014;32:6505–12.
82. Tsu VD. Overcoming barriers and ensuring access to HPV vaccines in low-income countries. Am J Law Med 2009;35:401–13.

83. Bingham A, Drake K, LaMontagne S. Sociocultural issues in the introduction of human papillomavirus vaccine in low-resource settings. Arch Pediatr Adolesc Med 2009;163:455–61.
84. Vermandere H, Naanyu V, Mabeya H, et al. Determinants of acceptance and subsequent uptake of the HPV vaccine in a cohort in Eldoret, Kenya. PLoS One 2014; 9:e109353.
85. Cunningham MS, Davison C, Aronson KJ. HPV vaccine acceptability in Africa: a systematic review. Prev Med 2014;69:274–9.
86. Bartolini RM, Winkler JL, Penny ME, et al. Parental acceptance of HPV vaccine in Peru: a decision framework. PLoS One 2012;7:e48017.
87. Wigle J, Coast E, Watson-Jones D. Human papillomavirus (HPV) vaccine implementation in low- and middle-income countries (LMICs): health system experiences and prospects. Vaccine 2013;31:3811–7.
88. Perlman S, Wamai RG, Bain PA, et al. Knowledge and awareness of HPV vaccine and acceptability to vaccine in sub-Saharan Africa: a systematic review. PLoS One 2014;9:e90912.
89. Mugisha E, LaMontagne DS, Katahoire AR, et al. Feasibility of delivering HPV vaccine to girls aged 10 to 15 years in Uganda. Afr Health Sci 2015;15:33–41.
90. World Health Organization. Comprehensive cervical cancer control: a guide to essential practice. 2nd edition. Geneva (Switzerland): WHO; 2014.
91. Hindin M, Bloem P, Ferguson J. Effective nonvaccine interventions to be considered alongside human papilloma virus vaccine delivery. J Adolesc Health 2015; 56:10–8.

# Integrating Children's Mental Health into Primary Care

Lawrence S. Wissow, MD, MPH[a],*, Nadja van Ginneken, MRCGP, PhD[b],
Jaya Chandna, MSc[b], Atif Rahman, MB BS, PhD[b]

## KEYWORDS

• Mental health • Children/youth • Prevention • Primary care

## KEY POINTS

• Mental health problems in children and adolescents are common and begin early in life.
• Mental health promotion and early intervention during childhood are global public health priorities.
• Primary care can help meet this need through collaboration with specialists and by recognizing the centrality of mental health to physical health.
• Mental health interventions can be re-designed to fit the work flow and staffing of primary care sites.
• Taking on mental health promotion and care is a "whole office" task that includes families in its design and execution.

## UNMET NEED FOR CHILD MENTAL HEALTH SERVICES

Children's mental health problems are among global health advocates' highest priorities[1] because they are among the leading causes of disability for children and youth and often go untreated for years, significantly disrupting healthy development.[2,3] In addition, advocates increasingly see mental health promotion in childhood as the only viable short-term path to reducing the burden of adult mental disorders.[4,5] Nearly three-quarters of adult disorders have their onset or origins during childhood, becoming harder to treat and incurring ever-greater social, educational, and economic consequences over time. In contrast, there is good evidence that commonly occurring problems such as anxiety and depression can be prevented or ameliorated through intervention in childhood and adolescence.[6–10]

---

[a] Center for Mental Health in Pediatric Primary Care, Department of Health, Behavior, and Society, Johns Hopkins School of Public Health, 703 Hampton House, 624 North Broadway, Baltimore, MD 21205, USA; [b] Departments of Psychological Sciences and Health Services, Institute of Psychology, Health & Society, University of Liverpool, Waterhouse Building, 2nd Floor Block B, 1-5 Brownlow Street, Liverpool L69 3GL, UK
* Corresponding author.
E-mail address: lwissow@jhmi.edu

Pediatr Clin N Am 63 (2016) 97–113
http://dx.doi.org/10.1016/j.pcl.2015.08.005       pediatric.theclinics.com
0031-3955/16/$ – see front matter © 2016 Elsevier Inc. All rights reserved.

Designing an expanded program to address mental health in childhood presents many challenges. Even in the most highly resourced countries, child mental health professionals are in short supply and their optimal use is hampered by fragmented systems and competition for limited public funding. In much of the world, specialized care is virtually unavailable except to the most privileged.[11] In the United States, the 2003 National Health Interview Survey found that 56% of children aged 4 to 17 years with definite or severe functional difficulties attributable to mental health problems had not seen a mental health professional in the past year.[12] A decade later, a study in Massachusetts, after the start of mandatory child mental health screening in primary care, found that 40% of screen-positive children had no previous history of mental health service use.[13]

## A ROLE FOR PRIMARY CARE

Strategies for improving children's access to mental health care focus largely on increasing the number and kinds of providers who can deliver preventive and treatment services. This includes engaging family members, improving the mental health promotion and treatment capacity of schools and community programs, and increasing the capacity of primary care.[14]

Around the world, primary care is delivered in many different ways and by professionals and paraprofessionals with differing skill sets. The extent to which child mental health care integrates with primary care thus varies, and also depends on opportunities to expand services in schools and from community-based organizations. For example, in the United States, primary care providers (family physicians, primary care pediatricians, nurse practitioners, physicians' assistants, and the others who work with them) are tasked with a variety of health maintenance and monitoring functions that, in other systems, are carried out by public health workers. Thus, integration efforts in the United States focus mostly on primary care sites themselves, whereas in other countries (such as the United Kingdom) they involve work with a combination of primary care, school-based, and public health services.

Whether in primary care predominantly, or in a combination of primary care and public health, the philosophy of promoting and tracking children's healthy development creates the benefit of integration, forming a natural base from which to promote mental health and detect emerging problems. Mental health care can then be delivered in the context of care for co-occurring medical conditions, and with a focus on periods of individual and family vulnerability. Ongoing relationships can build willingness to share sensitive information and trust in the appropriateness of diagnosis and treatment.

Developing primary care as a resource for mental health has involved 2 strategies (collaborative care and task shifting), which in fact are inseparable. Collaborative care emphasizes effective partnerships between primary and specialty care, allowing patients to receive treatments that take advantage of specialty expertise, while benefiting from the comprehensiveness and longitudinal aspects of primary care.[15] However, collaborative care cannot function without some degree of task shifting, the delivery of some specialized services by primary care providers themselves.[16] Task shifting is needed for several reasons: early detection and intervention (as well as efforts at health promotion) may identify situations that do not qualify for specialty care; waiting times for specialty care may be too long; many patients may prefer to be treated in primary care and opt for no care at all rather than accepting a referral. Task shifting may be the only alternative in settings where specialty care is available only at great expense or in extraordinary circumstances.

## BARRIERS TO TASK SHIFTING

The biggest barrier to task shifting, and even to the co-location of mental health providers in primary care offices, is that most current mental health treatment does not fit with how primary care is practiced by clinicians or used by families. Primary care practice is characterized by the need to conduct many visits in a short time and accommodate unscheduled visits for acute illness. In contrast, mental health treatments are usually delivered in sessions lasting from 30 to 60 minutes.[17] Primary care continuity is defined as longitudinal access and monitoring over an indefinite time frame, while mental health treatments are delivered in a series of closely spaced visits, often for a finite time. These differences may apply both to primary care providers themselves and to co-located practitioners. Business models supporting co-located providers may not allow for extended visits, and families may find it just as hard to return for serial visits to a primary care site as they do for mental health service sites.[18,19]

Other difficulties with currently available treatments lie in their therapeutic targets. A recent analysis of child-youth treatments supported by randomized trials found that, even if a full set of those targets recommended by the Substance Abuse and Mental Health Services Administration were to be available, nearly 50% of youth in need of services would technically not be considered appropriate candidates because their age, gender, or disorder did not match the characteristics of children among whom the intervention had been studied.[20] The situation in primary care is even worse: up to 20% to 30% of children seen in primary care have behavioral or emotional problems that impair their function but do not meet criteria for any disorder; thus, the range of available evidence-based treatments is even smaller.[21]

Many evidence-based treatments fail to take an ecologic perspective. Children's problems may stem from difficulties within their family or community and include parental mental health problems, food and housing insecurity, or exposure to dangerous neighborhoods or challenging schools.[22] The child may be the "identified patient" in these situations, but intervention may be more effectively directed to the underlying issues rather than the child's resulting behavioral or emotional state. The links between these so-called social determinants and mental health are becoming increasingly clear. In the United States, an estimated 7% of infants and young children live with severely depressed mothers, a recognized and treatable cause of child mental health problems.[23] The prevalence increases to 11% for children living in poverty, and to 41% and 55% for all children and those in poverty, respectively, if mild and moderate depression are included. Poverty itself affects parental functioning in ways that have an impact on children's mood and behavior; the daily hassles of poverty, even when not experienced as stress, reduce cognitive "bandwidth," making it harder for parents to reason through problems and sustain goal-directed attention.[24]

Another shortcoming of current mental health services is that they are separate from or lacking interventions that promote mental wellness. The "dual continuum model"[25] posits that mental illness and mental wellness are 2 separate although related concepts. Both mental illness and mental wellness predict lifetime medical problems and mortality, with mental illness markedly reducing lifespan and mental wellness increasing it.[26] Importantly, promoting wellness can prevent illness, but treating illness may not necessarily promote wellness. Promoting mental wellness has long been an aspiration of primary care in the United States,[27] but there are no widely disseminated practical interventions beyond infancy and toddlerhood. The "Triple P" program shows promise as a primary care and community-based approach based on parenting training, but evidence for its effectiveness remains limited.[28]

Finally, despite the demand and need for mental health services, current treatments are far from widely embraced by families. In 1 US study, more than half of parents with emotional, behavioral, or developmental concerns about their children did not discuss them with their child's doctor,[29] and even in highly integrated health care systems anywhere from a significant minority to a majority of referrals from primary care to mental health are never completed.[30] Patient preferences are important; in 1 primary care study of medication for adult depression, treatment was highly cost-effective for patients with favorable attitudes toward medication but showed no advantage over usual care for patients with negative attitudes.[31] In pediatrics, parents vary considerably in their attitudes toward therapeutic options for common childhood mental health problems.[32]

## DESIGNING MENTAL HEALTH INTERVENTIONS FOR PRIMARY CARE

In this article, we focus on what types of mental health treatment and promotion interventions might be practical, engaging to families, and effective for use by primary care providers and primary care–based mental health professionals. The goals of providing these services include

- Being an effective gateway to specialty services
- Being part of a safety net: identifying and helping families who fall out of the specialized mental health system for one reason or another
- Providing early intervention: catching things before they get worse
- Promoting positive mental health: the attributes that help children "flourish"

We divide the remaining sections of the paper into 3 groups: what primary care providers might do, how they might be supported to learn how to do it, and what could make it sustainable and become part of routine.

## WHAT MIGHT PROVIDERS DO?
### A Holistic Framework for Care

Much of the reasoning in this section flows from the concept that the brain is the principle organ of human adaptation.[33] The brain's processing of, and responses to, the environment determine both mental and physical health. Appraisal of the environment drives autonomic, endocrine, and immunologic responses, with long-term implications for health; emotional responses to the environment drive behaviors that have profound implications for physical health as well as social connectedness, cognitive development, and ultimately reproductive success. Thus, thinking about mental health is integral to good medical care; it is not an add-on. If mental health care is then integral to all of pediatric care, it needs to begin with interventions that permeate all care but are particularly put into play when working with families in which a child may have a mental health problem.

There are several possibilities for universal interventions that mesh seamlessly with day-to-day medical practice (**Table 1**). First, the "common factors" literature from psychotherapy demonstrates that there are aspects of the client-therapist interaction predicting outcomes across conditions and treatments.[34] This parallels observations of how patient-provider interactions and organizational culture influence outcomes in medical and agency-based services.[35,36] Second, studies of "single session" psychotherapy demonstrate the effectiveness of providing problem (rather than diagnostic) targeted treatment in brief pulses across extended periods, similar to patterns of medical care.[37] Third, "stepped care" models suggest that generalists can provide first-contact mental health treatment based on brief problem-oriented assessments if they follow patients to ascertain need for further diagnosis or intervention.[38]

| Table 1 Promising adaptations of mental health treatment for primary care ||
| --- | --- |
| **Community and General Medical Settings** | **Parallels in Mental Health Services** |
| Emphasis on patient-centered care and joint decision making building trust and activation | "Common factors" in psychotherapeutic processes promoting engagement, optimism, alliance |
| Treatment delivered in pulses with follow-up for monitoring or as needed | "Single session" treatment models |
| Initial treatment often presumptive or relatively nonspecific | Stepped care models with increasing specificity of diagnosis and intensity of treatment |
| Treatment based on brief counseling focused on patient-identified problems | "Common elements" |
| Links with community services, advice addressing family and social determinants | Peer/family navigators |

### Targeted Brief Interventions

The major gap in our ability to provide mental health services in primary care is the need for brief interventions more specifically targeting particular common problems. To reach a large number of children, these interventions need to be relatively few in number (crossing current diagnostic categories), easy to implement, and broadly address early intervention, family and social influences, and wellness promotion.

These brief interventions can be developed from more complex evidence-based treatments. In 2004, Hawaii's Evidence Based Services Committee pioneered the technique of identifying "practice elements" used repeatedly across multiple evidence-based therapies for specific conditions.[39] Since then, the process of identifying elements has been refined,[40] and trials in outpatient child mental health programs have found that using treatment where problems are matched to elements (as opposed to diagnoses being matched to evidence-based interventions) was effective and well received by families.[41,42]

Although there have yet to be similar trials in primary care, a pilot study that trained pediatricians to use an elements-based approach for children with anxiety found evidence of effectiveness and feasibility within the structure of primary care practice.[43] **Table 2** shows elements extracted from evidence-based treatments by the Hawaii Evidence Based Services Committee for 4 major child behavioral and emotional problems encountered by pediatricians. There are a relatively small number of discrete interventions, most of which are already suggested for use in primary care.[44]

### Beyond Diagnosis to Promoting Core Components of Mental Health

Whereas the conditions in **Table 2** are readily recognizable, they still are "problems" rather than qualities related to positive mental health. Ideally, we want to be able to address issues that are at the root of healthy functioning, and we want to be able to acknowledge that children's behavior and emotional problems are closely linked to developmental, family, school, and community issues that might be important primary or simultaneous targets of intervention.

Over the last several years, the US National Institute of Mental Health has developed what it calls the Research Domain Criteria (RDoC) framework as a way identifying core brain circuits identified with mental illness and wellness independently of current diagnostic categories.[45] Although not suggesting that there is a neurologic correlate to all behaviors and mental states, RDoC follows a line of inquiry in developmental

**Table 2**
Most frequently appearing "common elements" in evidence-based practices, grouped by common presenting problems in pediatric primary care

| Presenting Problem Area | Most Common Elements of Related Evidence-Based Practices |
|---|---|
| Anxiety | Graded exposure, modeling |
| ADHD and oppositional problems | Tangible rewards, praise for child and parent, help with monitoring, time out, effective commands and limit setting, response cost |
| Low mood | Cognitive/coping methods, problem-solving strategies, activity scheduling, behavioral rehearsal, social skills building |

*Abbreviation:* ADHD, attention deficit hyperactive disorder.

psychology that tries to identify processes underlying the frequently comorbid and variable conditions seen in children's mental health problems.[46] Multidisciplinary panels identified 5 major domains: negative and positive valence systems, cognitive systems, social processes, and arousal systems. Within each domain, particular constructs represent feelings and behaviors associated with both successful adaptation and difficulty functioning. Although the domains have evidence for their independent existence and functioning, they clearly work together to promote positive mental health or influence states of emotional distress or behavioral dysfunction.

Although the RDoC framework is new, it has shown promise as a clinical as well as a research tool, helping clinicians consider patients' strengths and difficulties in ways that open additional avenues for treatment.[47] It offers the promise of grouping treatments in ways that are more intuitive to clinicians, using fewer categories than current schemes, thus increasing ease of dissemination.

**Table 3** maps key circuits identified by RDoC with mental states associated with positive mental health[26,48] and then with a tentative selection of interventions for promoting mental health or intervening early with potential difficulties. The entries in the intervention columns of the table can be thought of as involving treatments aimed at children or parent-child dyads. Interventions in the bottom row of the table target the family overall or a parent in particular.

As an example of how treatments and mental health promotion interventions might be mapped onto RDoC, we can take the case of a school-age child with trouble paying attention in school. Exercise might be associated with promoting overall brain states that favor effortful control, which is believed to be important in child anxiety, oppositional behavior, and attention deficit hyperactive disorder (ADHD). Helping parents promote children's organizational and emotion regulating abilities might be associated with more specific training that accomplishes the same end.[46] Thinking through the child's problems using RDoC constructs might lead to exploration of problems the child might have with chronic worry (about poor performance or related to trauma) and poor self-image (from feeling inferior to peers or being singled out as a problem in school). This is in contrast to current approaches based on diagnosis, which might elicit symptoms suggestive of ADHD and move to an evidence-based treatment such as stimulant medication.

Supporting parents or the family environment might also be considered, and likely fall within or not far from existing pediatric practice. Self-care is already an established part of counseling for parents of infants,[44] as is smoking cessation advice for parents of children with asthma and family dietary counseling for children with weight problems.[49,50] Larger pediatric practices may work with social workers and other peer and professional staff capable of linking families to community services or advocating for them

**Table 3**
Research Domain Criteria constructs, related mental states, and strategies for promotion/prevention and early intervention

| RDoC Domain/Construct | States Related to Positive Mental Health | Promotion/Prevention | Early Intervention |
|---|---|---|---|
| Cognitive systems<br>• Effortful control<br>• Working memory | Reasonable ability to sustain attention, engage in problem solving | Parent-child joint attention activities, play involving concentration and memory, learning to structure work<br>Whole-school interventions | Task monitoring, organizational support, rewards for sustained attention |
| Positive valence systems | Reasonable ability to derive satisfaction from constructive social and intellectual activity | Early cognitive and social stimulation, early exposure to role models intellectually stimulating peer activities | Identification and intervention for learning disorders and other impediments to school success |
| Negative valence, low mood | Reasonable ability to regulate emotions and moderate responses to perceived threats | Contingent responsiveness, parental warmth, cognitive coping skills, promotion of self-esteem, self-efficacy (via social processes domain), skills and activities that build social capital | Behavioral activation, solution-focused problem solving |
| Negative valence<br>• Acute, potential, and sustained threat | | | Differentiation of sustained vs acute or potential fears: cognitive coping, behavioral rehearsal, modeling, graded exposure |
| Tolerance of negative valence states | | | Relaxation, distraction, mindfulness, controlled avoidance |
| Social processes<br>• Attachment<br>• Social communications<br>• Self-representation | Positive sense of self, ability to form bonds with others, ability to read and express emotions | Parenting guidance<br>Whole-classroom programs<br>Community-based group activities for children | Social skills groups<br>Parent-child bibliotherapy |
| Arousal<br>• Sleep cycles | Evolving ability to match sleep needs with cultural norms | Monitoring of electronic activities, sufficient physical activity, limiting intake of substances interfering with sleep and arousal | Sleep hygiene, problem solving around schedules, substance intake, increasing physical activity |
| Parent/family interventions | | Support for parent to maintain these interactions over time, promotion of parental self-efficacy, mentalization, developmental knowledge<br>Support for the family in the community: social support of various kinds, promotion of financial stability; attention to mental health promotion and prevention across the lifespan | Support from across formal and informal community agencies to provide these interventions; treatment of parental mental health problems |

with schools or government agencies. Brief counseling models for adult substance use and depression might readily be incorporated into pediatric practice and are even more readily used by family practitioners providing care for both parents and children.[38,51]

## HOW CAN PROVIDERS LEARN NEW SKILLS?

In some countries, primary care providers already have a strong toolkit of early interventions targeting mental health promotion and treatment, but may need help building confidence,[52] or need more than brief refreshers to build particular skills.[35] In other countries, community health workers, health officers, and peer counselors have or can develop skills for both case finding and brief counseling.[53] Especially in communities where mental health problems are especially stigmatized, building a mental health component into interventions for other conditions may be the most effective avenue of dissemination. Doing this can leverage counseling skills that providers have learned for other purposes, including HIV-related counseling or the promotion of breast feeding.[54,55]

Many of the basic "common factors" skills and attitudes are developed in clinicians' basic training; using them may be more dependent on shifts in office priorities and routines than learning new methods. However, other skills, such as those derived from motivational interviewing or solution-focused therapy, may require additional learning and practice. They can be learned at workshops (in the United States by the Institute for Healthcare Communication and others), and via online training, including new resources being developed by the American Academy of Pediatrics (AAP; www.aap.org/mentalhealth).

Although continuing medical education activities have traditionally focused on 1-time educational sessions, it has long been recognized that knowledge and skills related to psychosocial concerns are best learned over time through collaborative relationships with specialists and exchange of experience with colleagues. In the 1950s, British psychoanalyst Michael Balint initiated group meetings with general practitioners to discuss difficult patients and ways to try to better understand and address their concerns.[56] The Balint movement continues in North America and the United Kingdom, including the possibility of obtaining training and forming a group oneself (www.americainbalintsociety.org). Since 1989, the Maternal and Child Health Training Program, part of the US federal Maternal and Child Health Bureau, has funded several centers to organize "Collaborative Office Rounds," community meetings based on the Balint concept but specifically addressing mental health aspects of pediatric care.[57] The groups are jointly led by pediatricians and child psychiatrists and may target trainees or established practitioners. A list of current grantees is available at http://www.mchb.hrsa.gov/training/projects.asp?program=3.

Most recently, several states have implemented programs that provide free, informal child mental health consultations to primary care providers caring for children and youth (and in some cases pregnant women). Based on a model originally developed in Massachusetts,[58] the programs typically offer some form of optional training, assistance with finding mental health referrals, and a telephone "warm line" through which primary care providers can connect with a child mental health specialist to discuss diagnostic, treatment, or referral dilemmas. Initial evaluations of state programs suggest that they are effective in increasing primary care providers' willingness and ability to manage child mental health problems.[52,59] The newly formed National Network of Child Psychiatry Access Programs (www.nncpap.org) provides a directory of existing programs and can link providers with advice on program development and functioning.

## IMPLEMENTING AND SUSTAINING A MENTAL HEALTH PROGRAM IN PRIMARY CARE
### The Chronic Care Model as a Blueprint

Mental health brings into sharp focus the reality that health care is distinct from many other public services in that it depends on human interactions at multiple levels.[60] Communities must develop goals for well-being and embrace services as being legitimate and effective. Individuals within communities need trusting relationships with health care providers and confidence in the relevance of the providers' knowledge. Providers may need new roles and relationships; community agencies may need to work more closely with each other and with medical services. Many cultural, structural, and financial barriers stand in the way of these collaborations. Collaboration across staff levels and disciplines, involvement of families, and a willingness to rethink processes have proved to be necessary elements of integrating psychosocial concerns with the more medical model of primary care.[61,62]

Elaborations on Wagner's Chronic Care Model (CCM)[15] have been the basis of most programs to integrate mental health with adult and pediatric primary care and with community services (**Table 4**). Several CCM interventions with positive outcomes have been reported for adult depression; 2 positive trials have been reported for adolescent depression and 1 for disruptive behaviors among younger children, both using co-located personnel.[63–65]

The CCM sets out some key structural elements for specialist-generalist collaboration and task shifting.

- Generalists should systematically be looking for certain kinds of problems faced by their patients so that they can intervene early or try to prevent problems altogether. This process usually involves some combination of formal screening and a variety of changes to pre- and intra-visit interactions to promote discussion of patients' concerns.
- Generalists should have the tools and back-up to provide immediate first-line care for the problems, usually through a combination of training, reference materials, and ready access to consultation and collaboration.
- Office systems and routines may need small but important modifications to be able to accommodate families with mental health concerns. These include some flexibility in assignment of visit slots when a slightly longer visit would be helpful, "huddles" or brief team meetings at the start of the day to identify families who will likely need more support, and review of protocols for helping those who are acutely distressed.
- Systems should be in place to follow up first-line treatment and decide if it has been successful. Medical home models, for example, call for tracking referrals and creating registries of patients or families with particular needs.
- When more treatment is needed, generalists should be able to work closely with specialists (ideally with whom they have a personal relationship) to assure that patients get the added care they need, and that the added care fits with the patient's other medical needs (often referred to as "stepped care").

The CCM is also a model of both patient and provider behavior change.[66] It posits that patient engagement is central to outcomes in conditions (like mental health) that rely heavily on self-management.[60] Engagement is supported at the interpersonal level through patients' interactions with providers, at the social level through involvement with formal and informal community-based services, and at the systems level through the organization and financing of care. Within this engagement-promoting structure, clinical sites are organized to detect problems early and deliver evidence-informed treatments in collaboration with specialists.

**Table 4**
Core elements of the collaborative Chronic Care Model and related interventions

| Element | Focus | Potential Practice Components |
|---|---|---|
| Patient self-management support | Practice able to provide coaching, problem solving, skills-focused psychotherapy and psychoeducation to promote self-management and engagement in care | Primary care provider training in use of common factors skills during routine visits; universal brief advice for parent-child interactions, stress reduction, problem solving; brief advice for specific clusters of symptoms |
| Clinical information systems use | Facilitation of information flow from relevant clinical sources to treating clinicians | Data systems for tracking progress and referrals |
| Delivery system re-design | Re-definition of work roles of physicians and staff to facilitate anticipatory or preventive care rather than reactive care | All staff oriented and helped to develop common factors skills; scheduling to accommodate families with greater needs, team huddles to share information and anticipate family needs; integration of co-located services; consideration of processes for systematizing prevention and case finding |
| Provider decision support | Facilitated provision of expert-level input to generalists to reduce need for consultation separated in time and space from clinical needs | Primary care staff training, development of collaborative and consulting linkages including warm lines, co-located services |
| Community resource linkage | Support for clinical and nonclinical needs from resources outside the health care organization | Development of guides for referral to community services and family support programs |
| Health care organization support | Organization leadership and tangible resources to support goals and practices | Articulating the case for providing mental health care; developing markers for key goals |

Adapted from Woltmann E, Grogan-Kaylor A, Perron B, et al. Comparative effectiveness of collaborative chronic care models for mental health conditions across primary, specialty, and behavioral health care settings: systematic review and meta-analysis. Am J Psychiatry 2012;169:792; with permission.

## Getting Started

The AAP's Task Force on Mental Health "Toolkit" (www.aap.org/mentalhealth) provides a comprehensive blueprint for practices contemplating a full-fledged effort to take on mental health care, and largely follows the CCM. It addresses steps in planning, office readiness, universal interventions, condition-specific treatments, and collaboration with specialists. To conclude, we highlight 2 areas that have emerged as particularly important to beginning and sustaining mental health work: screening and team involvement.

## Screening for Problems and Hooks for Engagement

The CCM emphasizes the need for systematic assessment, and screening is often where practices begin when thinking about taking on mental health care. Screening has many appealing aspects, but it is much more complicated than it seems. There are clinical issues (how it will be presented to families, integrated with developmental screening or other pre-visit questionnaires, how the results will be used as a part of care) and logistic issues (how screens will be systematically given out, scored, entered into the medical record, and their results made available for use during the visit). A full discussion of screening is beyond the scope of this article, and many models and details can be found in the AAP Toolkit.

A concept that can guide screening implementation is to think of it as only 1 step in a process designed to initiate discussions about families' most pressing concerns. Screening can signal the acceptability of discussing topics that families may have assumed were out of scope for the visit, give time for family members to formulate and prioritize their questions, and give providers an indication, at the start of the visit, about a likely agenda. Framing screening as "routine" helps bring up sensitive issues without families feeling targeted or stigmatized.[67]

A critical component of the process is the conversation between the clinician and family about the screening results. Not discussing the results diminishes their importance in the eyes of families and risks sending a message that the screen is just 1 more piece of paperwork that serves the system but not the patient. Both "negative" and "positive" screens need follow-up. Screens may be negative because the family truly senses that there are no difficulties to discuss, because they are not comfortable disclosing difficulties, because they do not understand the questions being asked, or because they have problems but do not believe that they are reflected in the questions on the screen. A negative screen offers a chance to confirm that there are no problems and to ask if there might be something related that the family would like to discuss. Screens can be positive because the family in fact has difficulties to discuss, or because they misinterpret questions or the directions for completing the form. Verifying that the responses truly reflect a concern offers the chance to get a better understanding of what the family might want to discuss. The conversations between provider and patient that emerge from the use of the screener are more important than the positive/negative results of the screening tool itself. Although clinicians often fear that screening will uncover more issues than can be dealt with in a single visit, the overlapping nature of family mental health problems, and their often common roots, create a situation in which complexity is a good thing; it offers multiple possible "hooks" by which a family might be engaged. Any issue that a family sees as a priority is likely to eventually lead to exploring the others that have been uncovered.

It is also important to remember that the positive/negative cut-points, even in "validated" screening tools, may not be applicable to the population that is being cared for, or have limited predictive value in a generally well population. For example, the Pediatric Symptom Checklist, the Strengths and Difficulties Questionnaire, and the Patient Health Questionnaire have positive predictive values of 50% or less at the prevalence rates found in well-child visits.[68–70]

### Mental Health Visits Start at the Front Desk

Patients coming to medical and medical health sites develop therapeutic relationships with a variety of staff members, not just the clinician who conducts the formal "visit."[71,72] Impressions made at the front desk and during the process of getting to an examining room or having vital signs measured can carry over into willingness to discuss sensitive information once the formal visit starts.[73] Thus, getting ready to provide mental health care involves the entire office team, and a consideration of how the office environment promotes a sense of safety and respect. The best way to involve and gain the collaboration (and wisdom) of team members is to involve them in planning the start-up or expansion of mental health care. Family representatives in particular are essential to developing effective plans and making the case for change, and increasingly are taking on a formal role as part of treatment teams.[74]

## SUMMARY

Mental health problems in children remain a major public health challenge in both high-income countries and low- and middle-income countries. Promising models exist to address this challenge but there remain gaps in knowledge.[75] Two studies of primary care–based treatment of adolescent depression[63,64] found that use of a collaborative/integrated care model (some degree of task shifting to primary care providers themselves, use of a "care-manager" to deliver treatment, and an algorithm for seeking more intensive care) improved outcomes and was feasible in a variety of settings (although neither study included stand-alone private practices). Another study focusing only on child behavior problems[65] had similar findings, again with a co-located therapist, in academic-affiliated practices. These studies show that collaborative care can be effective, but they involve single conditions and leave unanswered the question of how the additional clinical resources can be financed in the long term.

Although not yet evaluated with regard to outcomes, advanced "child psychiatry access programs," such as Massachusetts' "MCPAP,"[59] have used a model promoting primary care services for a range of conditions (via regional hubs providing direct care, training, and support for primary care management). These programs, now in operation in some form in more than 20 states, have garnered strong acceptance from policymakers and the primary care community. They offer potential economies of scale, and the potential for impact across a broad range of conditions. However, again, in addition to uncertainty about their clinical impact, how they will be financed in the long term remains a question.

Solutions may come from 2 directions warranting active research agendas. First, refining and determining the impact of trans-diagnostic and combined illness/wellness approaches to treatment offers the promise of designing interventions that address a broad range of problems, are more readily adapted to use by primary care and other community-based providers, and are also potentially more potent. Second, technology may offer ways of promoting task shifting and collaborative care that preserve the strengths of one-to-one mentoring that seem most effective but that are practical at scale, especially in settings where specialist consultants are in short supply.[76] In the meantime, there are many steps that individual practitioners, health systems, and educational and social welfare agencies can take that are sufficiently well developed to warrant thoughtful implementation.

## ACKNOWLEDGMENTS

The authors are grateful to Dr Jane Foy, whose encouragement and insights have been central to the themes developed in this paper. This work was supported in part by NIMH grant P20MH086048 and by a visiting professorship from the University of Liverpool.

## REFERENCES

1. Collins PY, Patel V, Joestl SS. Grand challenges in global mental health. Nature 2011;475:27–30.
2. World Health Organization (WHO). Caring for children and adolescents with mental disorders: setting WHO directions. Geneva (Switzerland): World Health Organization; 2003.
3. World Health Organization (WHO). Adolescent mental health: mapping actions of nongovernmental organizations and other international development organizations. Geneva (Switzerland): World Health Organization; 2012.
4. Insel TR, Scolnick EM. Cure therapeutics and strategic prevention: raising the bar for mental health research. Mol Psychiatry 2006;11:11–7.
5. Wong EH, Yocca F, Smith MA, et al. Challenges and opportunities for drug discovery in psychiatric disorders: the drug hunters' perspective. Int J Neuropsychopharmacol 2010;13:1269–84.
6. Bayer J, Hiscock H, Scalzo K, et al. Systematic review of preventive interventions for children's mental health. Aust NZ J Psychiatry 2009;43:695–710.
7. Cuijpers P, Van Straten A, Smit F. Preventing the incidence of new cases of mental disorders: a meta-analytic review. J Nerv Ment Dis 2005;193:119–25.
8. Cuijpers P, van Straten A, Smit F, et al. Preventing the onset of depressive disorders: a meta-analytic review of psychological interventions. Am J Psychiatry 2008;165:1272–80.
9. Durlak JA, Wells AM. Primary prevention programs for children and adolescents: a meta-analytic review. Am J Community Psychol 1997;25:115–53.
10. Merry S, McDowell H, Hetrick S, et al. Psychological and/or educational interventions for the prevention of depression in children and adolescents. Cochrane Database Syst Rev 2004;(2):CD003380.
11. Kim WJ, American Academy of Child and Adolescent Psychiatry Task Force on Workforce Needs. Child and adolescent psychiatry workforce: a critical shortage and national challenge. Acad Psychiatry 2006;27:277–82.
12. Simpson GA, Bloom B, Cohen RA, et al. U.S. children with emotional and behavioral difficulties: Data from the 2001, 2002, and 2003 National Health Interview Surveys. Adv Data 2005;23:1–13.
13. Hacker KA, Penfold R, Arsenault L, et al. Screening for behavioral health issues in children enrolled in Massachusetts Medicaid. Pediatrics 2014;133:46–54.
14. World Health Organization (WHO). Atlas: child and adolescent mental health resources: global concerns, implications for the future. Geneva (Switzerland): World Health Organization; 2005.
15. Wagner EH, Austin BT, Von Korff M. Organizing care for patients with chronic illness. Milbank Q 1996;74:511–44.
16. World Health Organization (WHO). Task shifting to tackle health worker shortages. Geneva (Switzerland): World Health Organization; 2007.
17. American Academy of Pediatrics Committee on Coding and Nomenclature. Application of the resource-based relative value scale system to pediatrics. Pediatrics 2004;113:1437–40.

18. Areán PA, Ayalon L, Jin C, et al. Integrated specialty mental health care among older minorities improves access but not outcomes: results of the PRISMe study. Int J Geriatr Psychiatry 2008;23:1086–92.
19. Williams J, Shore SE, Foy JM. Co-location of mental health professionals in primary care settings: three North Carolina models. Clin Pediatr (Phila) 2006; 45:537–43.
20. Bernstein A, Chorpita BF, Daleiden EL, et al. Building an evidence-informed service array: considering evidence-based programs as well as their practice elements. J Consult Clin Psychol 2015. [Epub ahead of print].
21. Briggs-Gowan MJ, Horwitz SM, Schwab-Stone ME, et al. Mental health in pediatric settings: distribution of disorders and factors related to service use. J Am Acad Child Adolesc Psychiatry 2000;39:841–9.
22. Odgers CL, Caspi A, Russell MA, et al. Supportive parenting mediates neighborhood socioeconomic disparities in children's antisocial behavior from ages 5 to 12. Dev Psychopathol 2012;24:705–21.
23. Vericker T, Macober J, Golden O. Infants of depressed mothers living in poverty: opportunities to identify and serve. Washington, DC: Urban Institute; 2010.
24. Mani A, Mullainathan S, Shafir E, et al. Poverty impedes cognitive function. Science 2013;341:976–80.
25. Keyes CL. Promoting and protecting mental health as flourishing: a complementary strategy for improving national mental health. Am Psychol 2007;62:95–108.
26. Keyes CL, Simoes EJ. To flourish or not: positive mental health and all-cause mortality. Am J Public Health 2012;102:2164–72.
27. Brazelton TB. Working with families. Opportunities for early intervention. Pediatr Clin North Am 1995;42:1–9.
28. Wilson P, Rush R, Hussey S, et al. How evidence-based is an 'evidence-based parenting program'? A PRISMA systematic review and meta-analysis of Triple P. BMC Med 2012;10:130.
29. Horwitz SM, Leaf PJ, Leventhal JM. Identification of psychosocial problems in pediatric primary care: do family attitudes make a difference? Arch Pediatr Adolesc Med 1998;152:367–71.
30. Hacker K, Myagmarjav E, Harris V, et al. Mental health screening in pediatric practice: factors related to positive screens and the contribution of parental/ personal concern. Pediatrics 2006;126:1896.
31. Pyne JM, Rost KM, Farahati F, et al. One size fits some: the impact of patient treatment attitudes on the cost-effectiveness of a depression primary care intervention. Psychol Med 2005;35:839–54.
32. Bussing R, Koro-Ljungberg ME, Gary F, et al. Exploring help-seeking for ADHD symptoms: a mixed-methods approach. Harv Rev Psychiatry 2005;13: 85–101.
33. McEwen BS. Brain on stress: how the social environment gets under the skin. Proc Natl Acad Sci U S A 2012;109(Suppl 2):17180–5.
34. Karver MS, Handelsman JB, Fields S, et al. A theoretical model of common process factors in youth and family therapy. Ment Health Serv Res 2005;7:35–51.
35. Wissow L, Gadomski A, Roter D, et al. Aspects of mental health communication skills training that predict parent and child outcomes in pediatric primary care. Patient Educ Couns 2011;82:226–32.
36. Glisson C, Green P. Organizational climate, services, and outcomes in child welfare systems. Child Abuse Negl 2011;35:582–91.

37. Perkins R, Scarlett G. The effectiveness of single session therapy in child and adolescent mental health. Part 2: an 18-month follow-up study. Psychol Psychother 2008;81(Pt 2):143–56.
38. Katon W, Ünützer J, Wells K, et al. Collaborative depression care: history, evolution and ways to enhance dissemination and sustainability. Gen Hosp Psychiatry 2010;32:456–64.
39. Evidence Based Services Committee. Summary of effective interventions for youth with behavioral and emotional needs. Honolulu (HI): Child and Adolescent Mental Health Division, Hawaii Department of Health; 2004.
40. Chorpita BF, Daleiden EL, Weisz JR. Identifying and selecting the common elements of evidence based interventions: a distillation and matching model. Ment Health Serv Res 2005;7:5–20.
41. McGarry J, McNicholas F, Buckley H, et al. The clinical effectiveness of a brief consultation and advisory approach compared to treatment as usual in child and adolescent mental health services. Clin Child Psychol Psychiatry 2008;13: 365–76.
42. Weisz JR, Chorpita B, Palinkas LA, et al. Testing standard and modular designs for psychotherapy treating depression, anxiety, and conduct problems in youth: A randomized effectiveness trial. Arch Gen Psychiatry 2012;69:274–82.
43. Ginsburg G, Drake K, Winegrad H, et al. An open trial of the *Anxiety Action Plan (AxAP)*: a brief pediatrician-delivered intervention for anxious youth. Child and Youth Care Forum, in press.
44. Jellinek M, Patel BP, Froehle MC, editors. Bright futures in practice: mental health, volume I, practice guide. Arlington (VA): National Center for Education in Maternal and Child Health; 2002.
45. Franklin JC, Jamieson JP, Glenn CR, et al. How developmental psychopathology theory and research can inform the Research Domain Criteria (RDoC) project. J Clin Child Adolesc Psychol 2015;44:280–90.
46. Steinberg EA, Drabick DA. A developmental psychopathology perspective on ADHD and comorbid conditions: the role of emotion regulation. Child Psychiatry Hum Dev 2015. [Epub ahead of print].
47. Etkin A, Cuthbert B. Beyond the DSM: development of a transdiagnostic psychiatric neuroscience course. Acad Psychiatry 2014;38:145–50.
48. Heckman JJ, Stixrud J, Urzua S. The effects of cognitive and non-cognitive abilities on labor market outcomes and social behavior. J Labor Econ 2006;24: 411–82.
49. Pérez-Stable EJ, Juarez-Reyes M, Kaplan C, et al. Counseling smoking parents of young children: comparison of pediatricians and family physicians. Arch Pediatr Adolesc Med 2001;155:25–31.
50. Resnicow K, McMaster F, Bocian A, et al. Motivational interviewing and dietary counseling for obesity in primary care: an RCT. Pediatrics 2015;135: 649–57.
51. Madras BK, Compton WM, Avula D, et al. Screening, brief interventions, referral to treatment (SBIRT) for illicit drug and alcohol use at multiple healthcare sites: comparison at intake and six months. Drug Alcohol Depend 2010; 99:280–95.
52. Gadomski AM, Wissow LS, Palinkas L, et al. Encouraging and sustaining integration of child mental health into primary care. Gen Hosp Psychiatry 2014;36: 555–62.

53. Zafar S, Sikander S, Haq Z, et al. Integrating maternal psychosocial well-being into a child-development intervention: the five-pillars approach. Ann N Y Acad Sci 2014;1308:107–17.
54. Sikander S, Maselko J, Zafar S, et al. Cognitive-behavioral counseling for exclusive breastfeeding in rural pediatrics: A cluster RCT. Pediatrics 2015;135:e424–31.
55. Wissow LS, Tegegn T, Legesse H, et al. Collaboratively re-framing mental health for integration with HIV care in Ethiopia. Health Policy Plan 2015;30(6):791–803.
56. Kjeldmand D, Holmström I. Balint groups as a means to increase job satisfaction and prevent burnout among general practitioners. Ann Fam Med 2008;6: 138–45.
57. Fishman ME, Kessel W, Heppel DE, et al. Collaborative office rounds: continuing education in the psychosocial/developmental aspects of child health. Pediatrics 1997;99:E5.
58. Connor DF, McLaughlin TJ, Jeffers-Terry M, et al. Targeted child psychiatric services: a new model of pediatric primary clinician–child psychiatry collaborative care. Clin Pediatr (Phila) 2006;45:423–34.
59. Sarvet B, Gold J, Straus JH. Bridging the divide between child psychiatry and primary care: the use of telephone consultation within a population-based collaborative system. Child Adolesc Psychiatr Clin North Am 2011;20:41–53.
60. Leykum LK, Lanham HJ, Pugh JA, et al. Manifestations and implications of uncertainty for improving healthcare systems: an analysis of observational and interventional studies grounded in complexity science. Implement Sci 2014;9:165.
61. Nutting PA, Crabtree BF, Miller WL, et al. Transforming physician practices to patient-centered medical homes: lessons from the National Demonstration Project. Health Aff 2011;30:439–45.
62. Stange KC, Etz RS, Gullett H, et al. Metrics for assessing improvements in primary health care. Annu Rev Public Health 2014;35:423–42.
63. Asarnow JR, Jaycox LH, Duan N, et al. Effectiveness of a quality improvement intervention for adolescent depression in primary care clinics: a randomized controlled trial. JAMA 2005;293:311–9.
64. Richardson LP, Ludman E, McCauley E, et al. Collaborative care for adolescents with depression in primary care: a randomized clinical trial. JAMA 2014;312: 809–16.
65. Kolko DJ, Campo J, Kilbourne AM, et al. Collaborative care outcomes for pediatric behavioral health problems: a cluster randomized trial. Pediatrics 2014;133: e981–92.
66. Woltmann E, Grogan-Kaylor A, Perron B, et al. Comparative effectiveness of collaborative chronic care models for mental health conditions across primary, specialty, and behavioral health care settings: systematic review and meta-analysis. Am J Psychiatry 2012;169:790–804.
67. Fothergill K, Gadomski A, Olson A, et al. Assessing the impact of a web-based comprehensive somatic and mental health screening tool in pediatric primary care. Acad Pediatr 2013;13:340–7.
68. Gardner W, Klima J, Chisolm D, et al. Screening, triage, and referral of patients who report suicidal thought during a primary care visit. Pediatrics 2010;125: 945–52.
69. Goodman R. Psychometric properties of the strengths and difficulties questionnaire. J Am Acad Child Adolesc Psychiatry 2001;40:1337–45.
70. Richardson LP, McCauley E, Grossman DC, et al. Evaluation of the patient health questionnaire-9 item for detecting major depression among adolescents. Pediatr 2010;126:1117.

71. Ware NC, Tugenberg T, Dickey B, et al. An ethnographic study of the meaning of continuity of care in mental health services. Psychiatr Serv 1999;50:395–400.
72. Pulido R, Monari M, Rossi N. Institutional therapeutic alliance and its relationship with outcomes in a psychiatric day hospital program. Arch Psychiatr Nurs 2008; 22:277–87.
73. Christensen A, Brown J, Wissow LS, et al. Spillover of ratings of patient- and family-centered care: an example for physicians and medical assistants in a Federally Qualified Health Center. J Ambul Care Manage, in press.
74. Young MH, McMenamy JM, Perrin EC. Parent advisory groups in pediatric practices: parents' and professionals' perceptions. Arch Pediatr Adolesc Med 2001; 155:692–8.
75. Campo JV, Bridge JA, Fontanella CA. Access to mental health services: implementing an integrated solution. JAMA Pediatr 2015;169:299–300.
76. Hamdani SU, Atif N, Tariq M, et al. Family networks to improve outcomes in children with intellectual and developmental disorders: a qualitative study. Int J Ment Health Syst 2014;8(1):7.

# Caring for Children in Immigrant Families

## Vulnerabilities, Resilience, and Opportunities

Julie M. Linton, MD[a],*, Ricky Choi, MD, MPH[b],
Fernando Mendoza, MD, MPH[c]

### KEYWORDS

- Immigrant children • Children in immigrant families • Health disparities
- Cultural and linguistic disparities • Toxic stress • Resilience • Advocacy

### KEY POINTS

- Pediatricians will increasingly care for children in immigrant families (CIF) as part of routine practice.
- A large proportion of CIF are at risk for health disparities relating to socioeconomic disadvantage and cultural and/or linguistic challenges.
- CIF and their families often have strengths that can offer a positive contribution to their health (immigrant paradox).
- Changes in global communication, including cultural media, can have a particular impact on immigrant children and families that may modify acculturation process.
- Pediatricians have a professional responsibility to address the medical, mental health, and social needs of immigrant children and families to optimize the potential of this growing sector of the population.

## INTRODUCTION

Children in immigrant families (CIF) represent the fastest growing segment of the US population and will soon represent 1 out of every 3 US children.[1,2] Although CIF are a heterogeneous group with respect to culture, language, social class, and residential status, there are common health-related issues related to provider-patient differences

---

Disclosures: None.
[a] Department of Pediatrics, Wake Forest School of Medicine, Medical Center Boulevard, Winston-Salem, NC 27157, USA; [b] Pediatrics, Asian Health Services Community Health Center, 818 Webster Street, Oakland, CA 94607, USA; [c] Department of Pediatrics, Stanford University School of Medicine, Medical School Office Building, X240, 1265 Welch Road, Stanford, CA 94305-5459, USA
* Corresponding author.
E-mail address: jlinton@wakehealth.edu

Pediatr Clin N Am 63 (2016) 115–130
http://dx.doi.org/10.1016/j.pcl.2015.08.006           **pediatric.theclinics.com**

in language and culture. This article highlights the current demographic trends of CIF and reviews the risk for health disparities relating to socioeconomic disadvantage and cultural and/or linguistic challenges, with an emphasis on those CIF who are most at risk for adversity, primarily Latino and some Asian subgroups. Health care providers have a critical role to play to address access to care, address unique health risks and needs, and cultivate resiliency in these new Americans.

## DEMOGRAPHICS

CIF are defined as children who are either born outside the United States (immigrant children) or are US citizens and have at least 1 parent born outside the United States. First-generation immigrant children are defined as those born outside the United States, whereas second-generation immigrant children represent US-born children with at least 1 immigrant parent (**Table 1**). Between 1994 and 2014, the percentage of first-generation or second-generation immigrant children in the United States has risen by 45% (to 18.7 million). Currently, they represent one-quarter of the 75 million children in the US.[2,3] It is predicted that by 2050, CIF will comprise one-third of more than 100 million US children.[1,3] It is estimated that during the next 40 years, immigrants and their US-born children will generate almost all growth in the young adult population[2] and nearly all growth of the nation's labor force.[1]

Although just 10 states (Arizona, California, Florida, Georgia, Illinois, Massachusetts, New Jersey, New York, Texas, and Washington) house nearly three-fourths of these children,[3] there has been significant growth in immigrant populations in other states in recent years. Between 1990 and 2009, the number of CIF increased by more than fivefold in North Carolina, Georgia, Nevada, and Arkansas.[4] State-level data in 2013 indicate that California (48%), Nevada (37%), and New Jersey (36%) have the highest populations of CIF among children living in these states; West Virginia (3%), Montana (4%), and Mississippi (4%) have the lowest[5] (**Fig. 1**). These data underscore the need for pediatricians to realize the health needs of CIF as part of routine training, practice, and continuing education.

As pediatricians prepare to care for more CIF, demographic shift and linguistic diversity of immigrant populations must be considered. Most CIF are of Latin American origin (including 40% of CIF with parents from Mexico), followed by 20% with parents from Asia[6] (predominantly China, India, and the Philippines).[2] Besides race and Hispanic origin, major differences have been noted among first-generation and second-generation immigrant children by generation, country of origin, poverty status, and family structure.[2] A non-English language is spoken in the homes of 20.3% of the US population.[7] Among CIF, 56% of parents have difficulty speaking English, and 22% of CIF live in linguistically isolated households where no person at least 14 years old speaks English "very well,"[5] However, arrival in the United States before adolescence, living in the United States for a longer period of time, and having a higher level of education are associated with English proficiency.[7] Time in the United States affects immigrant children and their US-born siblings, particularly with respect to language and culture.

Legal status is a complex issue for many CIF. Of CIF, 88% to 89% are US citizens.[5,8] The remainder include refugees, asylees, those with temporary protected status, and unauthorized children (see **Table 1**). Unauthorized children, or those who are foreign-born without legal status, represent 4% to 6% of the CIF population.[8–10] The number of US-born children of unauthorized immigrants has been growing and represents about 8% of all US births.[9,10] It is estimated that 5.5 million children live with 1 unauthorized parent, and 4.5 million of these children are born in the United States[11] Most

| Table 1 | |
|---|---|
| **Definitions and legal statuses of immigrant children** | |
| **Generational Status** | **Definition** |
| First-generation | Children born outside of the United States |
| Second-generation | US-born children with at least 1 immigrant parent |
| Third-generation (and higher) | Children born to US-born parents |
| **Immigration Status** | **Definition as Defined by the United States Citizenship and Immigration Services (USCIS), an Agency of the Department of Homeland Security** |
| US Citizen | Children born in the United States or children who are residing as green card holders in the United States and both parents are naturalized before the child's turns 18 y old |
| Lawful permanent resident (Green Card holder) | Any person not a citizen of the United States who is residing the in the United States under legally recognized and lawfully recorded permanent residence as an immigrant. |
| Refugee | A person outside his or her country of nationality who is unable or unwilling to return to that country because of persecution or a well-founded fear of persecution (and is granted refugee status by USCIS) |
| Asylee | An alien in the United States or at a port of entry who is found to be unable or unwilling to return to his or her country of nationality, or to seek the protection of that country, because of persecution or a well-founded fear of persecution |
| Temporary protected status | Conditions in the country temporarily prevent the country's nationals from returning safely or, in certain circumstances, in which the country is unable to handle the return of its nationals adequately |
| Special Immigrant Juvenile Status (SIJS) | Humanitarian form of relief available to noncitizen minors who enter the child welfare system due to abuse, neglect, or abandonment by 1 or both parents<br>To be eligible for SIJS, a child must be under 21, unmarried, and the subject of certain dependency orders issued by a juvenile court |
| T Nonimmigrant Status (T visa) | Visa that protects victims of human trafficking and allows victims to remain in the United States to assist in an investigation or prosecution of human trafficking |
| U Nonimmigrant Status (U visa) | Visa for victims of certain crimes who have suffered mental or physical abuse and are helpful to law enforcement or government officials in the investigation or prosecution of criminal activity |
| Mixed-status families | More than 1 US-citizen child and at least 1 undocumented parent |

*Data from* Passel JS. Demography of immigrant youth: past, present, and future. Future Child 2011;21:19–1; and USCIS. Available at: http://www.uscis.gov/tools/glossary. Accessed July 25, 2015.

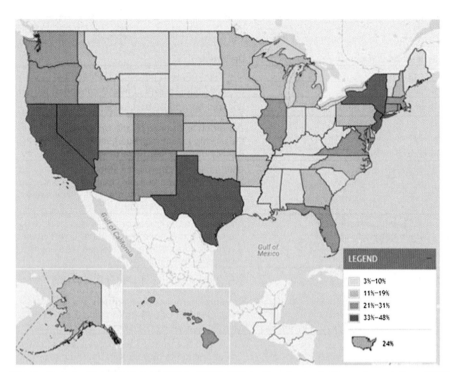

**Fig. 1.** State-level estimates of CIF in 2013. (*From* The Annie E. Casey Foundation, KIDS COUNT Data Center. Available at: http://datacenter.kidscount.org/data/Map/115-children-in-immigrant-families?loc=1&loct=1#national. Accessed June 9, 2015.)

children of unauthorized immigrants are Latino, with the largest percentage from Mexico.[9] Although 79% of the children of undocumented immigrants are US citizens,[10] mixed-resident status families may include undocumented children. Among undocumented children, unaccompanied minors and children who have been separated from their families are the most vulnerable. Beginning in October 2011, the US government recorded a dramatic rise in the number of unaccompanied and separated children arriving to the United States from El Salvador, Guatemala, and Honduras, as well as children continuing to arrive from Mexico.[12]

Although the United States is a country founded by immigrants, immigration policy is a topic historically marked by confusion and conflict. Immigration policy debate often ensues following increased migration due to war, armed conflict, or political unrest that incites larger flows of immigrants. Several key historical changes (**Table 2**) in US immigration policy have affected the current state of CIF, particularly the Immigrant Act of 1965, which focused on family reunification. The impact of immigration policy is 2-pronged: the effect on the child and on the parent. Adult deportation policy is a topic of importance for pediatricians because of the profound impact of parental deportation on children's health. Total deportations more than doubled during the past decade.[9] Yet, recent executive orders, including Deferred Action for Childhood Arrivals (DACA) and the Deferred Action for Parents of Americans and Lawful Permanent Residents (DAPA) program, have aimed to promote safety and well-being of children and families who reside in the United States by deferring deportation and allowing work for select undocumented immigrants.

**Table 2**
**A select timeline of immigration policy in the United States**

| Unrestricted Immigration | → 1875 | → 1882 | → 1921 | → 1965 | → 1980 | → 1990 | → 2000 | → 2008 |
|---|---|---|---|---|---|---|---|---|
| | Immigration restriction for criminals, prostitutes, and Chinese contract laborers | Chinese Exclusion Act of 1882 specifically prohibits naturalization of Chinese workers | The first numerical immigration quotas provoked a shift in U.S. immigration from Europe to Latin America and Asia | Previous national origin quota systems were abolished, and a new visa system focused on family reunification and skills | Following the Vietnam War, Congress enacted refugee and asylum provisions that brought the United States into compliance with international standards of refugee protection | Temporary Protected Status offers legal status to individuals unable to return to their home countries because of a political or environmental catastrophe | Trafficking Victims Protection Act, addresses human trafficking concerns | All unaccompanied alien children must be screened as potential victims of human trafficking; children from non-contiguous states must be transferred to ORR[a] within 72 h and simultaneously placed in removal proceedings with EOIR[b] within the Department of Justice |

[a] Office of Refugee and Resettlement.
[b] Executive Office for Immigration Review.
*Data from* Refs.[13-16]

## RISK FROM SOCIAL DETERMINANTS OF HEALTH

A myriad of issues are faced by CIF at an individual, family, and societal level (**Table 3**). Because the health and safety of children depend on the people and environment around them, social determinants of health, briefly defined as "the economic and social conditions that shape the health of individuals and communities,"[17] deserve particular consideration in pediatric practice. US immigrant populations have a broad range of health risks from social determinants, and not all CIF share comparable risks for health disparities. For many immigrant children, however, poverty, low educational level, poor access to health care, legal status, language barriers, and discrimination can have health impacts. Although data exist for some racial and ethnic groups, many health disparities are obscured by the lack of disaggregated data for smaller ethnic populations. Yet, some themes are common across populations, particularly those at greatest risk for health disparities such as Latinos and some Asian subgroups.

Among CIF, 54% live at or below 200% of the poverty line and 12% of parents have less than a ninth-grade education.[5] In the setting of poverty, exposure to violence,[18] and family separation due to migration patterns or deportation,[6] some immigrant children may be predisposed to the impact of toxic stress. When stressful events are long-term, overwhelming, and/or lacking the buffer of stable, responsive support from adults, toxic stress can affect children's health and even brain architecture.[19,20] Given that toxic stress can affect children's health,[19] toxic stress must be considered when evaluating the well-being of CIF. The early identification of CIF who are at risk for toxic stress remains a challenge. Use of validated screening tools for social determinants of health[21,22] may offer an opportunity to screen CIF for risk factors associated with toxic stress.

Resilience is characterized by successful adaptation to adversity, such as "transforms potentially toxic stress into tolerable stress."[23] The most important way to build resilience in a child is through a stable, supportive relationship with at least 1 parent or other caring adult.[23] Despite the potential risks for toxic stress, immigrants often demonstrate resilience as observed in several psychological, behavioral, and educational outcomes.[18] In particular, strong social support systems may enhance resilience among CIF, such as being raised in 2-parent families, of which there are a

**Table 3**
**Issues for immigrant children**

| Individual | Family | Society |
|---|---|---|
| Individual health (infectious, congenital, etc) | Intergenerational conflict | Poverty |
| Nutrition and obesity | Acculturation | Health disparities |
| Oral health | Linguistic isolation | Language barriers |
| School readiness | Parental education | Educational opportunity |
| Mental health | Immigration status | Immigration policy |
| Medications (home country, alternative therapies) | Traditional parenting practices | Transportation (access, driver's license) |
| Fear of parental deportation | Deportation | Unemployment |
| Abuse | Domestic violence | Fear and stigma |
| Health insurance status | Mobility or migration | Health policy |
| Federal benefit eligibility | Food or housing insecurity | Federal benefit eligibility |

higher proportion in immigrant families,[5] and using extended familial and/or social networks as a way to increase social support and resiliency to toxic stress environments.

## The Immigrant Paradox and Health

The immigrant paradox is a phenomenon that highlights the success of children of immigrants beyond expectation based on the key social determinants. Despite higher poverty rates, lower educational levels, and lower access to health care among Hispanic immigrants compared with non-Hispanic whites and US-born Hispanics, they demonstrate similar or better outcomes in several key indicators, including low birth weight and infant mortality.[24] Immigrant women are more likely to initiate and sustain breastfeeding than native women,[25] and immigrants seem to have lower risk of smoke exposure and several chronic physical and mental health conditions when compared with racially and ethnically matched peers.[26] Furthermore, despite a higher prevalence of obesity, physical inactivity, and parental reports of fair or poor child health among immigrant children versus US-born members of the same racial or ethnic groups, ultimate life expectancy is higher among immigrants compared with matched peers.[26] Theories to explain this paradox include the "healthy immigrant effect" (the concept that immigrants may be healthier than those staying in their native countries), lower health-risk behaviors, and higher family and social support.[26] Specifically, CIF are markedly more likely to live in 2-parent households than are children of native-born US citizens.[6] Thus, supporting cultural behaviors may significantly benefit CIF and their families, a role that pediatricians should play in practicing family pediatrics as recommended by the American Academy of Pediatrics (AAP).[27]

## The Immigrant Paradox and Education

Immigrant children face learning and education challenges. As early as infancy, immigrant children demonstrate smaller gains in cognitive proficiencies between 9 and 24 months compared with middle-class populations.[28] Children of undocumented parents may face particular risk for lower levels of cognitive development.[11]

Low parental literacy is linked to a limited cognitive home environment.[29] As immigrant toddlers approach early childhood, they are less likely than children of US-born parents to be enrolled in school or center-based preschool programs.[30] Limited school readiness confers academic risk, particularly among children of Latino origin.[31] Due to language barriers and limited functional literacy, many immigrant parents have limited access to early educational opportunities or may struggle to communicate concerns with the school system.[32] Access to early childhood education and care may be particularly exacerbated among smaller minority groups and speakers of languages other than Spanish.[32] At home, parents in immigrant families are less likely to share books with children during early childhood, which can translate into delays in language skills and literacy.[33]

However, older immigrant children show unanticipated educational success. Another aspect of the immigrant paradox, children of immigrant parents have better high school completion, grade point average, and standardized test scores than peers of the same racial, ethnic, or national background who have US-born parents.[34] This phenomenon is stronger for boys than girls and for children of Asian and African immigrants than other groups.[31] Although CIF show this paradox, early childhood development still needs to be a critical focus for these children.

## Identity Formation and Health Behaviors in a Changing World

Immigration to a new country is a transformational event in the life of a child and family. It means learning to live, work, and attend school in a new culture with different rules and expectations. Acculturation is defined as "the process of cultural and psychological change in cultural groups, families, and individuals following intercultural contact."[35] Immigrant children and adolescents may struggle with their identities as Americans because the process of immigration no longer entails complete severance of ties to a native culture. Media (television, print, and Internet) allows immigrant families to live in the United States while maintaining a virtual connection with their home countries. Therefore, mass media and social media may help children and their families develop a hybrid identity as new Americans by offering a connection to their home country while introducing them to the norms of their new home country.[36] This connection is a resource for cultural and identity grounding for children during acculturation.

The process of acculturation varies among CIF based on immigrant parents' sociocultural, economic, and educational levels with differing impact on physical health, mental health, and behavior. For example, when compared with whites, first-generation Asian adolescents' preventive health behaviors are reported to be worse but to improve over subsequent generations. Latino adolescents' behaviors are in some areas similar to whites, and in others worse, with limited change across generations.[37] Among Latino children and adults, acculturation has a mixed impact. It has been associated with poorer health and nutritional outcomes; however, with improved access to and satisfaction with health care come reports of better health.[38] Social activities may reflect different approaches to acculturation, such as participation in traditional dance versus engaging in ballet, and may promote identity formation and resilience. Pediatricians should discuss issues of acculturation with parents and children to evaluate the impact it has on the child's health and well being.

As immigrant children reach adolescence, sexual health becomes a crucial cultural issue. Nationally, teen birth rates are highest among Hispanic and Latino teens and lowest among Asians and Pacific Islanders.[5] However, teen pregnancy rates vary markedly between and within ethnic groups and must be evaluated in the context of cultural and generational status. Among Hispanic youth, although first-generation youth and those who prefer speaking Spanish are less likely than second-generation and third-generation youth to engage in sexual intercourse before age 18, they are also less likely to consistently use contraception.[39] As sexual behavior may be a taboo topic in some communities, pediatricians should address these issues within a confidential setting and build trust with families while remaining mindful of their cultural values in this important area of adolescent development.

### Physical Health Among Immigrant Children

On entry into the health care system, immigrant children and families may be at risk for particular conditions affecting physical health related to disease prevalence in their country of origin or the process of immigration. Infectious diseases are among the most common medical risks for immigrant children. The most commonly encountered infectious diseases include tuberculosis, hepatitis B, parasitic infectious, and sexually transmitted infections; prevalence for these conditions varies significantly based on country of origin, age of child, and individual risk factors. Nutritional issues, impaired vision, and hearing are also important. Children's health and safety is contingent on a comprehensive medical evaluation that includes screening for and management of commonly encountered medical conditions. Additionally, immigrants visiting their country of origin have disproportionate travel-related infections due to factors such as travel to high-risk destinations, belief that they are immune to disease, and last minute travel planning.[40] The AAP Immigrant Health Toolkit[41] (http://bit.ly/1y6HR1D)

offers recommendations regarding particular risk factors and screening for immigrant children (**Box 1**).

## *Mental Health in Families*

Complex factors, including social determinants of health, identify formation, past experiences, and family circumstances, may place CIF at risk for mental health problems. Data on mental health of immigrant children are limited. However, as part of an increasingly transnational lifestyle, immigrant parents and children may be separated for sustained periods of time.[42] This separation can disrupt attachment relationships important for healthy development.[42]

Immigrant children can be exposed to trauma, before immigration, during transit, and after settlement in the United States. Children at high risk for traumatic exposures, such as border children,[43] refugees,[44] and unaccompanied minors,[12] may be particularly vulnerable to related mental health conditions. It is estimated that more than half of the unaccompanied and separated children who arrive in the United States from Mexico, Guatemala, El Salvador, and Honduras could qualify for refugee status based on violence exposures in their countries of origin.[12] Refugees who resettle in developed nations have about a 10-times increased likelihood of suffering from posttraumatic stress disorder (PTSD) than the general population, and approximately 11% of refugee children have been found to have PTSD.[44] After relocation, continued exposure to violence and fear can perpetuate traumatic experiences. Living in unsafe neighborhoods and concerns for physical safety after relocation can be associated with an increased risk of PTSD.[45] Because immigrant children and families may not routinely volunteer experiences of neighborhood violence and school bullying with pediatricians, these topics should be explicitly addressed in routine pediatric care.

Like immigrant children, immigrant parents may face stress in countries of origin, during migration, and when adjusting to life in the United States. Immigrant and minority families demonstrate significantly higher levels of parenting aggravation, defined as stress experienced by parents associated with caring for children.[46] Among immigrant children, supervision neglect (being left home alone without adult supervision), physical neglect, and physical assault are more common. However, risk for physical neglect and assault are mitigated by other sociodemographic factors such as income level, parent's education, and race or ethnicity.[47] These risks place a critical responsibility on pediatricians to not only screen for adverse childhood experiences but also

---

**Box 1**
**Components of the Academy of Pediatrics immigrant child health toolkit**

- Key facts
- Clinical care, including medical screening and treatment recommendations for newly arrived immigrant children
- Access to health care and public benefits
- Mental and emotional health
- Immigration status and related concerns
- State legal resources for immigrant children and families
- AAP Advocacy

*Data from* AAP Immigrant Child Health Toolkit, AAP Council on Community Pediatrics. Available at: http://bit.ly/1y6HR1D. Accessed July 26, 2015.

to help families to cope with these experiences, to prevent further exposure, and optimize positive outcomes.

### Access to Health Care

For CIF, the parent or guardian enrolling in health insurance mediates access to health care. However, Medicaid-eligible CIF have high rates of noninsurance, reaching more than 20% in some states.[48] Medicaid-eligible children with immigrant parents are significantly more likely than children with native-born parents to be uninsured.[48] The enrollment gap varies substantially between states. Although some states, such as New York and Massachusetts, boast an enrollment differential approaching zero, other states approach 20% differences in enrollment between CIF and children with native-born parents.[48] Children without health insurance and those who speak a primary language other than English at home are much less likely to have access to a medical home.[49] Low health literacy, particularly for those with limited English proficiency, is common among immigrant parents and has been associated with lack of health insurance and difficulty understanding health information such as medication labels.[50] Finally, fear associated with immigration enforcement policies can translate into reduced use of services such as prenatal care.[51]

Language barriers limit health care access and have been associated with increased risk for serious medical events, including medical errors.[52,53] Use of professional interpreters is associated with lower likelihood of errors than not using an interpreter or using an ad hoc interpreter.[54] National Standards for Culturally and Linguistically Appropriate Services (CLAS) in Health and Health Care[55] are endorsed by health care organizations across the country and advocate for universal standards in care for increasingly diverse populations. However, more than half of pediatricians use family members to communicate with patients and families with limited English proficiency.[56] CIF may serve as cultural, linguistic, and technological brokers for parents, working to schedule, appointments, translate for their parents during doctor visits, or link families to access services and benefits.[57] Children may ultimately place the family's needs above their own, placing them at risk for school absenteeism and failure to complete homework.[57] Protecting CIF through culturally and linguistically appropriate care is essential to providing optimal pediatric care in all settings.

## CLINICAL CARE, RESEARCH, AND ADVOCACY FOR CHILDREN IN IMMIGRANT FAMILIES

Pediatricians have a unique opportunity to make a powerful difference in the lives of immigrant children and their families. Key research agenda for CIF include improving their access to health care, enhancing their quality of health care, and evaluating cultural factors that promote positive health and improve developmental outcomes.[24] Advocacy, or speaking out on behalf of patients and families, is a fundamental role of pediatricians.[58] Advocacy can occur at the level of the practice, community, state, nation, or beyond. The strategies listed in **Box 2** offer examples of opportunities to enhance clinical care, scholarship, and advocacy on behalf of CIF.

## SUMMARY

In a changing progressively transnational world, pediatricians will increasingly care for immigrant children and families as part of routine practice. Because immigrant children represent the foundation of the nation's future, it is essential to develop strategies to address persistent health disparities among CIF. In the context of multiple risk factors, pediatricians must pay particular attention to the social determinants of health when caring for CIF. Paradoxic strengths offer incredible opportunities to build

**Box 2**
**Clinical care, research, and advocacy on behalf of children in immigrant families**

*Optimal care and advocacy at the practice level*

1. Identify CIF in the practice and follow recommended medical, developmental, and psychosocial screening for immigrant children[40,59]

2. Develop a new patient orientation that includes a basic introduction to the US health care system, including the role of primary care and ways to access urgent care

3. Appreciate cultural practices and concerns. The process of listen, explain, acknowledge and discuss differences and similarities, recommend treatment, and negotiate agreement (LEARN) offers providers strategies to manage interactions with diverse patient populations.[60]

4. Promote CLAS Standards in your organization.[55] Providers and staff should be trained in cultural competence.[61] Interpretation using trained staff is key, and children should never be used as interpreters. Consider adding alerts for CIF whose families prefer interpretation for visits.[62] Offer translated patient education information at an appropriate reading level.[63]

5. Screen CIF regarding social determinants of health. Use validated mnemonic-based screening questions such as IHELLP[22] and WE CARE[21]; and then connect patients with positive responses to relevant local, state, or national resources.

6. Support enrollment in public programs for qualifying children such as Medicaid, State Children's Health Insurance Program (SCHIP) and Women, Infants, and Children (WIC), and encourage preschool and early child development programs.

7. Emphasize literacy from early infancy through book sharing and story telling,[33] book distribution programs such as Reach Out and Read, and enrollment in Head Start and preschool programs.

*Research and Data at the Practice Level*

1. Optimize use of the electronic health record (EHR) to improve understanding of population health for CIF. The EHR can not only incorporate routine medical information, such as disease prevalence and treatment, but can also integrate essential social determinants of health, such as living situation, parental literacy, household numbers, and social support networks, which can be analyzed to better understand health of CIF.

2. Engage in community-based research on topics with limited available data specific to CIF, including screening tools for toxic stress, the potential impact of Internet access, capacity to navigate resources such as social services, and inclusion of smaller immigrant populations.

3. Support interdisciplinary collaboration research, particularly with educators and child development specialists. Collaboration across disciplines has the potential to develop a more comprehensive and systematic way for this population of children and youth to get what they need to be healthy and successful.

*Advocacy in the community*

1. Establish partnerships with other professional organizations. Medical-legal partnerships can address common legal and social issues with significant health implications, including housing, educational issues, and eligibility for federal benefits such as WIC, SNAP, and Temporary Assistance for Needy Families (TANF). Specifically, low-income immigrants may be eligible for Special Supplement Nutrition Program for WIC. Close proximity or colocation with WIC services would facilitate patient access to services.

2. Connect with local health departments and the public health sector. Health departments often emphasize surveillance for infectious disease, vaccination, and family planning and may offer treatment or vaccination for infectious disease not typically managed in the outpatient clinic or as well as related educational materials. Health departments may also be the entry point to the health system for many immigrant communities. A partnership between health departments and medical homes may improve access to medical homes for all immigrant children.

3. Engage local schools to open lines of communication and to understand programs and services available to new English learners. Learning disabilities and delays may go unrecognized when the child is not a proficient English speaker.

4. Get involved with community groups. Partnering with cultural centers offers opportunities to learn about other resources in the area, educate the community about a health issue, or to help a patient find a community.[61] Cultural centers may be potential partners for grant funding to address community health concerns or can assist with training peer educators or patient navigators.

5. Identify opportunities to engage with local and ethnic media. Ethnic media plays a powerful role in many immigrant communities. In public health emergencies (ie, H1N1) or changes in health policy (ie, Affordable Care Act), ethnic media becomes a valuable outlet to educate the broader ethnic community. Pediatricians can offer to serve as consultants for ethnic media.

6. Shape medical education. Offer training on interpreter use, promote additional language training in medical school,[63] and include community-based experiences in caring for CIF in routine medical education.

*Advocacy at the state and national levels*

1. Engage professional societies. Professional societies can be an important network to share information on community resources and practice experiences. For instance, in 2011, the AAP formed the Immigrant Child Health Special Interest Group. Through this group, the AAP has developed an agenda to educate pediatricians on the care of this growing population as well as advocate nationally on behalf of immigrant children.

2. Participate in legislative advocacy. Immigration-related policy and legislation have been historically controversial in the United States. As a nation of immigrants, it would behoove the United States to embrace a forward-looking policy that supports success for all residents, beginning with meeting the needs of immigrant children. Pediatricians have a charge to elevate patient stories to elected officials to support inclusion into safety net programs and to address health disparities.

resilience and support children and families to contribute positively to the changing world. Advocacy offers an opportunity for pediatricians to not only affect the health of individual children and families but to incite systems-level change to improve the health of potentially vulnerable but resilient populations.

## ACKNOWLEDGMENTS

We would like to thank Dr Daniel Krowchuk for critical review of this article.

## REFERENCES

1. Passel JS, Cohn D. U.S. population projections: 2005-2050. Washington, DC: Pew Hispanic Center; 2008. Available at: http://pewhispanic.org/files/reports/85.pdf. Accessed June 10, 2015.

2. Child Trends Data Bank. Immigrant Children. Indicators on Children and Youth. October 2014. Available at: http://www.childtrends.org/?indicators=immigrant-children. Accessed July 21, 2015.

3. Passel JS. Demography of immigrant youth: past, present, and future. Future Child 2011;21:19–41.

4. Fortuny K, Chaudry A. Children of immigrants: growing national and state diversity. Washington, D.C: Children of Immigrants Research. Urban Institute, Brief No. 5; 2011.

5. Annie E. Casey Foundation. Kids Count Data Center. The Annie E. Casey Foundation, KIDS COUNT Data Center, Available at: http://datacenter.kidscount.org. Accessed June 9, 2015.

6. Landale NS, Thomas KJA, Van Hook J. The living arrangements of children of immigrants. Future Child 2011;21:43–70.

7. Rumbaut RG, Massey DS. Immigration & language diversity in the United States (2013). Daedalus 2013;142(3):141–54. Available at: http://ssrn.com/abstract=2293262. Accessed June 10, 2015.

8. Hernandez D, Cervantes W. Children in immigrant families: ensuring opportunity for every child in America. Washington, D.C: First Focus and Foundation for Child Development; 2011. Available at: http://fcd-us.org/resources/children-immigrant-families-ensuring-opportunity-every-child-america. Accessed June 2, 2015.

9. Passel JS, Cohn D. Unauthorized immigrant population: national and state trends, 2010. Washington, DC: Pew Hispanic Center; 2011.

10. Passel JS, Taylor P. Unauthorized immigrants and their U.S.-born children. Washington, DC: Pew Hispanic Center; 2010. Available at: http://pewhispanic.org/files/reports/125.pdf. Accessed July 15, 2015.

11. Yoshikawa H, Kholoptseva J. Unauthorized immigrant parents and their children's development: a summary of the evidence. Washington, DC: Migration Policy Institute; 2013.

12. UNHCR (United Nations High Commissioner for Refugees). Children on the run. Washington, DC. 2014. Available at: http://www.unhcrwashington.org/children/reports. Accessed March 6, 2015.

13. American Immigration Council. Children in danger: a guide to the humanitarian challenge at the border. 2014. Available at: http://www.immigrationpolicy.org/sites/default/files/docs/children_in_danger_a_guide_to_the_humanitarian_challenge_at_the_border_final.pdfPublished. Accessed March 2, 2014.

14. Ewing WA. Opportunity and exclusion: a brief history of U.S. immigration policy. Washington, D.C: Immigration Policy Center; 2012. Available at: http://www.immigrationpolicy.org/sites/default/files/docs/opportunity_exclusion_011312.pdf. Accessed June 6, 2015.

15. Giovagnoli M. Overhauling immigration law: a brief history and basic principles of reform. Washington, D.C: American Immigration Council, Immigration Policy Center; 2013. Available at: http://www.immigrationpolicy.org/. Accessed March 2, 2015.

16. Messick M, Bergeron C. Temporary protected status in the United States: a grant of humanitarian relief that is less than permanent. Washington, D.C.: Migration Policy Institute; 2014. Available at: http://www.migrationpolicy.org/article/temporary-protected-status-united-states-grant-humanitarian-relief-less-permanent. Accessed March 2, 2015.

17. AAP Council on Community Pediatrics. Policy statement: community pediatrics: navigating the intersection of medicine, public health, and social determinants of children's health. Pediatrics 2012;131:623–8.

18. American Psychological Association, Presidential Task Force on Immigration. 2012. Crossroads: The psychology of immigration in the new century. Available at: http://www.apa.org/topics/immigration/report.aspx. Accessed June 6, 2015.

19. National Scientific Council on the Developing Child. 2005/2014. Excessive stress disrupts the architecture of the developing brain: working paper 3. Updated Edition. Available at: http://developingchild.harvard.edu/index.php/resources/reports_and_working_papers/working_papers/wp3/. Accessed June 6, 2015.

20. AAP Committee on Psychosocial Aspects of Child and Family Health, Committee on Early Childhood, Adoption, and Dependent Care, Section on Developmental

and Behavioral Pediatrics. The lifelong effects of early childhood adversity and toxic stress. Pediatrics 2012;129:e232–46.

21. Garg A, Butz AM, Dworkin PH, et al. Improving the management of family psychosocial problems at low-income children's well-child care visits: the WE CARE Project. Pediatrics 2007;120:547–58.

22. Kenyon C, Sandel M, Silverstein M, et al. Revisiting the social history for child health. Pediatrics 2007;120:e734–8.

23. National Scientific Council on the Developing Child. (2015). Supportive relationships and active skill-building strengthen the foundations of resilience: working paper 13. Available at: http://developingchild.harvard.edu/resources/reports_and_working_papers/working_papers/wp13/. Accessed June 6, 2015.

24. Mendoza FS. Health disparities and children in immigrant families: a research agenda. Pediatrics 2009;124(S3):S187–95.

25. Singh GK, Kogan MD, Dee DL. Nativity/immigrant status, race/ethnicity, and socioeconomic determinants of breastfeeding initiation and duration in the United States, 2003. Pediatrics 2007;119(S1):S38–46.

26. Singh GK, Rodriguez-Lainz A, Kogan MD. Immigrant health inequalities in the US: use of eight major national data systems. ScientificWorldJournal 2013;2013: 512313.

27. AAP Task Force on the Family. Family pediatrics: report of the Task Force on the Family. Pediatrics 2003;111(6 pt 2):1541–71.

28. Fuller B, Bridges M, Bein E, et al. The health and cognitive growth of Latino toddlers: at risk or immigrant paradox? Matern Child Health J 2009;13:755–68.

29. Green CM, Berkule SM, Dreyer BP, et al. Maternal literacy and associations between education and the cognitive home environment in low-income families. Arch Pediatr Adolesc Med 2009;163(9):832–7.

30. Magnuson K, Lahaie C, Waldfogel J. Preschool and school readiness of children of immigrants. Soc Sci Q 2006;87(5):1241–62.

31. Crosnoe R, Lopez Turley RN. K-12 educational outcomes of immigrant youth. Future Child 2011;21:129–52.

32. Park M, McHugh M. Immigrant parents and early childhood programs: addressing barriers of literacy, culture, and systems knowledge. Washington, DC: Migration Policy Institute; 2014.

33. Festa N, Loftus PD, Cullen MR, et al. Disparities in early exposure to book sharing within immigrant families. Pediatrics 2014;134(1):e162–8.

34. Crosnoe R. Preparing the children of immigrants for early academic success. Washington, DC: Migration Policy Institute; 2013.

35. Berry JW. Acculturation strategies and adaptation. In: Lansford JE, Deater-Deckard K, Bornstein MH, editors. Immigrant families in contemporary society. New York: Guildford Press; 1999. p. 69–82.

36. Elias N. Media and immigrant children. In: Lemish D, editor. The Routledge International Handbook of Children, Adolescents, and Media. Oxfordshire (UK): Routledge; 2013. p. 336–43. Available at: http://www.academia.edu/5100215/Media_and_immigrant_children. Accessed June 6, 2015.

37. Allen ML, Elliot MN, Morales LS, et al. Adolescent participation in preventive health behaviors, physical activity, and nutrition: differences across immigrant generations for Asians and Latinos compared with Whites. Am J Public Health 2007;97(2):337–43.

38. Lara M, Gamboa C, Kahramanian M, et al. Acculturation and Latino health in the United States: a review of the literature and its sociopolitical context. Annu Rev Public Health 2005;26:367–97.

39. McDonald JA, Manlove J, Ikramulla EN. Immigration measures and reproductive health among Hispanic youth: findings from the national longitudinal survey of youth, 1997-2003. J Adolesc Health 2009;44:14–24.
40. Centers for Disease Control and Prevention. CDC health information for international travel 2014. New York: Oxford University Press; 2014. Available at: http://wwwnc.cdc.gov/travel/yellowbook/2014/chapter-8-advising-travelers-with-specific-needs/immigrants-returning-home-to-visit-friends-and-relatives-vfrs. Accessed June 6, 2015.
41. AAP Council on Community Pediatrics. Immigrant Health Toolkit, Available at: http://bit.ly/1y6HR1D. Accessed July 26, 2015.
42. Bohr Y, Tse C. Satellite babies in transnational families: a study of parents' decision to separate from their infants. Infant Ment Health J 2009;30:203–19.
43. Griffin M, Son M, Shapleigh E. Children's lives on the border. Pediatrics 2013;133: e1117–9.
44. Fazel M, Wheeler J, Danesh J. Prevalence of serious mental disorder in 7000 refugees resettled in western countries: a systematic review. Lancet 2005;365: 1390–414.
45. Fawzi MCS, Betancourt TS, Marcelin L, et al. Depression and post-traumatic stress disorder among Haitian immigrant students: implications for access to mental health services and educational programming. BMC Public Health 2009;9:482.
46. Yu SM, Singh GK. High parenting aggravation among US immigrant families. Am J Public Health 2012;102:2102–18.
47. Hussey JM, Chang JJ, Kotch JB. Child maltreatment in the United States: prevalence, risk factors, and adolescent health consequences. Pediatrics 2006;118: 993–1042.
48. Seiber EE. Which states enroll their Medicaid eligible, citizen children with immigrant parents? Health Serv Res 2013;48:519–38.
49. Strickland BB, Jones JR, Ghandour RM, et al. The medical home: health care access and impact for children and youth in the United States. Pediatrics 2011;127: 604–11.
50. Yin HS, Johnson M, Mendelsohn AL, et al. The health literacy of parents in the United States: a nationally representative study. Pediatrics 2009;124(S3): S289–98.
51. Rhodes SD, Mann L, Siman FM, et al. The impact of local immigration enforcement policies on the health of immigrant Hispanics/Latinos in the United States. Am J Public Health 2015;105:329–37.
52. Cohen AL, Rivara F, Marcuse EK, et al. Are language barriers associated with serious medical events in hospitalized pediatric patients? Pediatrics 2005; 116(3):575–9.
53. Flores G, Laws MB, Mayo SJ, et al. Errors in medical interpretation and their potential clinical consequences in pediatric encounters. Pediatrics 2003;111:6–14.
54. Flores G, Abreu M, Barone CP, et al. Errors of medical interpretation and their potential clinical consequences: a comparison of professional versus ad hoc versus no interpreters. Ann Emerg Med 2012;60(5):545–53.
55. National standards for culturally and linguistically appropriate services in health and health care: a blueprint for advancing and sustaining CLAS policy and practice. Washington, DC: Office of Minority Health, U.S. Department of Health and Human Services; 2013.
56. DeCamp LR, Kuo DZ, Flores G, et al. Changes in language services use by US Pediatricians. Pediatrics 2013;132:e396–406.

57. Katz VS. Kids in the middle: how children of immigrants negotiate community interactions for their families. New Brunswick (Canada): Rutgers University Press; 2014.
58. AAP Advocacy Guide. 2009. Available at: www.aap.org/moc/advocacyguide. Accessed June 9, 2015.
59. AAP Council on Community Pediatrics. Policy statement: providing care for immigrant, migrant, and border children. Pediatrics 2013;131:e2028-34.
60. Berlin EA, Fowkes WC Jr. A teaching framework for cross-cultural health care—application in family practice. In cross-cultural medicine. West J Med 1983; 139:934-8.
61. Bustamante AV, Van der Wees PJ. Integrating immigrants into the U.S. health system. AMA J Ethics 2012;14:318-23.
62. RWJF. Electronic health records alerts to increase utilization of interpreter services. Available at: http://www.rwjf.org/en/library/articles-and-news/2013/02/ehr-_alerts_-increase-use-of-interpreters.html. Accessed May 13, 2015.
63. Tucker JD, Chen AH, Glass RI. Foreign language assessment and training in U.S. medical education is a must. Acad Med 2012;87(3):257.

# Orphans and Vulnerable Children Affected by Human Immunodeficiency Virus in Sub-Saharan Africa

CrossMark

Malcolm Bryant, MBBS, MPH*, Jennifer Beard, PhD, MA, MPH

## KEYWORDS

- Child • Orphaned • Vulnerable populations • HIV • Sub-Saharan Africa

## KEY POINTS

- Sub-Saharan Africa has the greatest human immunodeficiency virus (HIV) and acquired immunodeficiency syndrome (AIDS) burden in the world, with children disproportionately affected by HIV compared with any other region of the world.
- Affected children face significant challenges to their education, mental health, physical health, social wellbeing, and are more likely to live in poverty than unaffected children.
- Global investments in achieving an AIDS-free generation focus on prevention of mother-to-child transmission and treatment of children infected with HIV, whereas the social, emotional, and developmental health of children orphaned or otherwise affected are less well-addressed.
- Children orphaned and otherwise affected by HIV are largely supported by external donor assistance, leaving children made vulnerable by poverty with few or no supports. Because poverty is a stronger predictor of negative outcomes for children than HIV status alone, this can result in the neediest being passed over for services and support.

## INTRODUCTION

Globally, 39 million people have died since the beginning of the human immunodeficiency virus (HIV) pandemic.[1] An estimated 17.8 million children have lost 1 or both parents to acquired immunodeficiency syndrome (AIDS) and countless more have had to leave school to take care of ill parents and been propelled into a state of economic and emotional insecurity. Yet these data do little to communicate the extent of HIV's impact on children, families, and communities.[2] Considerably more is known

Disclosure Statement: The authors have nothing to disclose.
Department of Global Health, Boston University School of Public Health, 801 Massachusetts Avenue, Boston, MA 02118, USA
* Corresponding author.
E-mail address: bryatm@bu.edu

Pediatr Clin N Am 63 (2016) 131–147
http://dx.doi.org/10.1016/j.pcl.2015.08.007
0031-3955/16/$ – see front matter © 2016 Elsevier Inc. All rights reserved.

about the number of children infected with HIV, than about the number of children who are uninfected but whose lives have been affected by HIV. In 2013, more than 3 million children were living with the virus and 250,000 new pediatric infections were detected.[3] Every day, approximately 660 children become infected with HIV and 530 die of an AIDS-related illness. Gender inequity results in disproportionately high infection rates in girls, who represent two-thirds of HIV-infected adolescents.[4] In addition to the 15 million children orphaned by HIV in Sub-Saharan Africa (SSA), the United Nations Children's Fund (UNICEF) has estimated that as many as 1 million children are made vulnerable each year when a parent becomes sick.[5]

Preventing and treating pediatric HIV is well-understood and the global community has seen a measure of success with 58% fewer pediatric infections between 2001 and 2013, and the number of children receiving antiretroviral therapy (ART) more than doubling from 255,000 in 2009 to 740,000 in 2013.[6] These improvements are largely due to the Global Plan to Establish an AIDS-Free Generation by 2015.[2] The major components of the plan include prevention of mother-to-child transmission (PMTCT), treatment of children living with HIV, and mitigation of the social and economic impact faced by children.

During the last 15 years, children orphaned and made otherwise vulnerable by HIV have been a major focus of international policy and donor funding. On a continent where millions of children are living in poverty, undernourished, or struggling to stay in school and achieve their full potential, differential vulnerability between children affected by HIV and those who are not is largely determined by global donor assistance. Affected children being reached by services targeting their needs may, as a result, be no more vulnerable than their unaffected peers.[7] However, in the absence of this assistance, the social impact of HIV on children in many African countries continues to overwhelm families and communities.

A child affected by HIV faces the emotional trauma of losing a parent and the stigma associated with an incurable sexually transmitted infection. Families caring for an ill adult or grieving a death caused by AIDS are frequently catapulted into poverty, with the ensuing problems of maintaining food, shelter, and a safe environment for children. In the absence of effective treatment of adult HIV, parents become ill and are forced to stop working. Children in these households are often required to leave school to work or care for parents and siblings. Even if HIV were eliminated in the near future, the devastating social and emotional impacts will continue to affect multiple generations of children. Prolonged conflict, political instability, and extreme poverty also contribute to child orphaning and vulnerability in some settings in SSA. The global community must continue to place high priority on mitigating the impacts of HIV on children for many years to come.

This article synthesizes background information and evidence from a wide variety of sources to provide an overview of the burden HIV has placed on children and families in SSA. Relevant policy developments at global and national levels are reviewed, key program innovations attempting to reduce disparities faced by orphans and vulnerable children (OVC) are summarized, and the core human rights challenges faced by OVC are examined. A glossary of terms commonly used when referring to children affected by HIV can be found in **Table 1**.

### Orphans and Vulnerable Children in Sub-Saharan Africa

The 920 million people living in SSA represent only 12% of the world's population yet carry 75% of the total HIV burden. This burden falls disproportionately on children because 90% of the world's HIV-positive (HIV +) children under the age of 15 years and 84% of AIDS-orphaned children live in SSA. Overall, 15.1 million children in

**Table 1**
**Definition of terms in common usage when working children affected by HIV**

| Term | Definition |
|------|------------|
| Orphan | Child who has lost 1 or both parents. Children who have been orphaned are often referred to as single (1 parent dead) or double (both parents dead) or maternal (mother dead) and paternal (father dead). Children living without their parents are sometimes referred to as social or de facto orphans because their parents may be alive but uninvolved in their lives. |
| Vulnerable Child | Child who is at risk of or currently lacking adequate care and protection. Can include children who are infected with HIV as well as those who are not. The World Bank describes child vulnerability as a "downward spiral where each shock leads to a new level of vulnerability, and each new level opens up for a host of new risks. In other words, the probability of a child experiencing a negative outcome rises with each shock."[8] |
| Generalized Epidemic | Context in which HIV infection is sustained through heterosexual transmission. HIV prevalence usually exceeds 1% among pregnant women attending antenatal clinics.[9] |
| Concentrated Epidemic | Context in which HIV prevalence is relatively low in the general population but high in 1 or more subpopulations, such as men who have sex with men, people who inject drugs, or sex workers and their clients. In these key populations, HIV has multiple modes of transmission, including unprotected anal and vaginal sex, unsafe injection, exchanging sex for money or favors, and multiple concurrent partners. |
| Sex Work | The exchange of sex for money. Sex worker is the term applied to women, men, and transgender individuals who professionally self-identify as such. |
| Transactional & Survival Sex | The exchange of sex for money, favors, or gifts. Women and men who engage in transactional sex (known in some contexts as survival sex) often do not identify their actions as sex work. Rather, they see it as a temporary means to a needed or desired end. |
| Stigma & Discrimination | Stigma is a negative stereotype about a person rooted in social perceptions of shameful or taboo behavior. Discrimination is unfair treatment of others who are perceived to be different. Stigma can also be internalized by those who are stereotyped and excluded, causing them to accept negative actions inflicted on them as justified. |

*Data from* World Bank. OVC Toolkit. Available at: http://info.worldbank.org/etools/docs/library/138974/toolkit/howknow/definitions.htm. Accessed May 18, 2015; and UNAIDS. UNAIDS Terminology Guidelines. 2011. Available at: http://www.unaids.org/sites/default/files/media_asset/JC2118_terminology-guidelines_en_0.pdf. Accessed July 27, 2016.

SSA have lost 1 or both parents to HIV.[10] The number of children affected by HIV is much larger, though difficult to estimate. **Table 2** presents information on the impact of HIV on children and adults both globally and in SSA.

These numbers hide significant regional and national variation. Ten countries (South Africa, Nigeria, Kenya, Mozambique, Uganda, Tanzania, Zimbabwe, Zambia, Malawi, and Ethiopia) account for 80% of the continent's HIV burden.[11] Similarly, 40% of HIV + children in East and Southern Africa have access to ART, compared with 15% in West and Central Africa.[2] Adult access to ART is an important proxy for

**Table 2**
**Impact of human immunodeficiency virus on children**

| Key Indicators | Global | Sub-Saharan Africa |
|---|---|---|
| Number of PLHIV[1] (all ages) | 35 million | 26 million |
| Number of Children Orphaned by HIV | 17.8 million | 15.1 million |
| Number of HIV + Children (0–14) | 3.2 million | 2.9 million |
| Number of HIV-infected Adolescents and Young Adults (15–24) | 4.9 million | 4 million |
| Number of AIDS-related deaths | 1.5 million | 1.1 million |
| Proportion of HIV + Adults with Access to ART | 64% | 36% |
| Proportion of HIV + Children with Access to ART | 34% | 33% |
| Proportion of HIV + Pregnant Women Receiving PMTCT | 67% | 52% |

*Abbreviation:* PLHIV, people living with HIV.
   *Data from* Refs.[1,2,8,10]

estimating vulnerability of affected children to orphaning and the array of challenges created by living in a household where 1 or more adults cannot work due to a terminal illness.

## VULNERABILITIES FACED BY CHILDREN AFFECTED BY HUMAN IMMUNODEFICIENCY VIRUS
### Poverty

During the last 10 years, Africa has had one of the fastest growing economies in the world. The World Bank now ranks 7 SSA countries as high middle income and 15 are ranked as lower middle income. Despite these advances, 47% of Africans live on less than $1.25 per day.[12] The links between poverty and HIV are well-documented, providing strong evidence that HIV drives families into poverty, which in turn creates vulnerability to HIV.[13–16] Families affected by HIV begin to founder when parents become so ill that they can no longer work, causing a chain of events that push them, their children, and others who rely on them for support more deeply into poverty and food insecurity.[16] Similarly, poverty also drives decisions to engage in sex work or survival sex, which often brings a higher financial benefit without a condom,[17] along with increased risk for HIV.

  Children living in households affected by HIV or who have been orphaned are particularly vulnerable to deepening poverty (**Table 3** presents data from 5 SSA countries on

**Table 3**
**Prevalence of orphans and poverty in countries with a generalized adult epidemic**

| Country | Adult HIV Prevalence | Orphans Prevalence | Orphans Living in Households in the 2 Lowest Wealth Quintiles |
|---|---|---|---|
| Swaziland | 26.5% | 24.3% | 12% |
| Zambia | 12.7% | 15% | 5% |
| Malawi | 10.8% | 13% | 5% |
| Uganda | 7.5% | 15% | 6% |
| Tanzania | 5.1% | 11% | 5% |

*Data from* UNICEF. Measuring the determinants of childhood vulnerability. 2014. Available at: http://data.unicef.org/corecode/uploads/document6/uploaded_pdfs/corecode/Measuring-the-Determinants-of-Childhood-Vulnerability_Final-Report-5_8-LR-_172.pdf. Accessed June 9, 2015.

HIV, orphan prevalence, and orphans living in poverty). Extreme poverty creates multiple, overlapping deprivations that remain with children across their life course. These deprivations, as outlined by UNICEF, are aligned with the core needs that must be met for a child to achieve his or her full potential: nutrition, health, water, sanitation, housing, protection from violence, education, and information.[18] Multiple deprivation analysis using Demographic Health Survey and Multiple Indicator Cluster Survey data from 30 SSA countries shows that 67% of children under age 18 experience multiple deprivations during childhood and adolescence.

### Attending and Completing School

Most countries in SSA have adopted universal primary school education policies giving all children the right to free primary education and children affected by HIV cannot be openly excluded from enrolling in or attending school.[7] Most SSA countries have met and exceeded the Millennium Development Goal to increase primary school enrollment to 80%. The countries with primary school enrollment well above 95% are Rwanda, Tanzania, Malawi, Zambia, Togo, Cape Verde, and Cameroon.[19] These "spectacular leaps," as described by the 2014 Millennium Development Goal Report, are indeed a critical success for all children living in poverty. Yet the poorest and most vulnerable, including those affected by HIV, are still left behind in that they may be enrolled in school but not attending due to inability to pay school fees other than tuition, the need to work, or a requirement to take care of younger siblings or other family members. Overall, 22 million children do not complete primary school and, even though enrollment rates have risen, SSA continues to have the lowest primary school completion rates in the world with an overall average of 60%.[19]

Before large infusions of donor funding targeting care and support, OVC were 13% less likely to be enrolled in school than children not affected by HIV[7]; however, the degree to which being orphaned or affected by HIV is still a predictor of school nonattendance is unclear. UNICEF reported in 2014 that orphans in SSA are more likely to leave school than nonorphans,[10] but a study conducted in Uganda from 2011 to 2013 found that 79% of OVC were enrolled in school.[20] Likewise, a 2012 analysis of Demographic Health Survey data on access to primary school in East and Southern Africa by Family Health International 360 found orphan enrollment and attendance to be quite high and no worse than that of nonorphans.[21] Overall, this review notes that poverty rather than orphanhood is the strongest predictor of school nonattendance and that a broader definition of vulnerability (including children affected by HIV) will provide a more accurate picture of the impact of HIV on educational access and attainment.

Access to secondary school in SSA is extremely low, with 40% of children not attending school beyond primary in West Africa and 27% in East and Southern Africa.[22] Few countries offer universal access to secondary school and those that do still have relatively low enrollment due to distance and high costs other than tuition, with girls and youth living in rural areas having lower access than boys and urban youth.[22]

### Shelter and Care

OVC are often affected by homelessness and neglect. This is particularly true for double orphans but also for single orphans whose living parent may be too ill to provide for their needs. Children whose parents are involved in sex work, drug use, or behaviors that create an environment that puts a child at risk for abuse or other forms of harm may also be in need of alternative care provided by extended family, community members, or residential facilities. Government orphanages are often overcrowded and underfunded and may not be the best option for a child. However, the commonly found maxim among many child rights advocates, donors, and policy-makers, that residential care is the least desirable option needs to be reanalyzed in light of evidence emerging from SSA.[23–31]

The primary support for the position that residential care should always be avoided comes from the Bucharest Early Intervention Project, which measured health and well-being of children in Romanian orphanages who were institutionalized in warehouse-like government institutions during the Ceausescu era.[24,32] The same conditions do not necessarily apply in SSA. Quality of residential care can vary dramatically from institution to institution, based on the staff-to-child ratio; staff turnover; resources for food, health, and amenities; and the degree to which the programming is child-centered with a focus on building social and emotional attachments and supporting cognitive development. In child-centered institutions, children have been shown to thrive in residential care in a way they could not in the homes of extended family or community members that are economically overstretched.[23,29,30] The longitudinal Positive Outcomes for Orphans Study looked at children from 5 countries in SSA and concluded that children living in institutional care had statistically better health and nutrition outcomes than those raised by extended family. The same study also noted that caregivers in family settings were more likely to exhibit discrimination and propagate stigma than their counterparts in institutions.[26,33–35]

In SSA, OVC are often absorbed into the extended family. However, in those countries most affected by the pandemic, a generation of working-age adults has died of AIDS-related illnesses. This often leaves elderly grandparents responsible for the care of multiple children, overwhelming their meager resources and catapulting them into poverty, and forcing children into residential care. Extended families and neighbors often provide informal foster care for orphans and children who can no longer live in their parents' home. However, few SSA countries have a national system for recruiting foster families in which children can be placed and their health and wellbeing monitored. Similarly, legal adoption of children within many SSA countries is neither common nor easy. Ethiopia went through an extended period of facilitating international adoptions of orphans but has decreased the number dramatically in the last 10 years due to a combination of corrupt systems, evidence of parents being coerced into putting children up for adoption, and a desire by government to keep children in the county.[36]

Children in foster care can also experience trauma from physical and emotional abuse and labor exploitation because fostered children are sometimes expected to carry a heavier burden of housework than other children living in the household. As Lugalla[37] notes of children orphaned by HIV in Tanzania, "Cases of orphans being abused by foster parents, adults or guardians are not hard to find. ...Most orphans neither know what abuse is and what it is not. Even when they are severely abused they do not know where they can report for assistance."

Faith and community-based organizations have come to play a major role in residential or community care of OVC. These organizations usually provide temporary care for children in crisis and try to reunite them with extended family and place them back in the community. A small but growing number of organizations provide permanent care to children throughout adolescence and assist them with the transition into early adulthood and independent living.[23] Nonresidential community-based care approaches have proliferated in the last 10 years. Examples include daycare centers for very young children, drop-in centers for all family members, night shelters for the children of sex workers, safe houses for parents or children at risk of abuse, and a variety of special support services to child-headed households.

Several human rights documents guide decisions concerning how best to care for children orphaned and made vulnerable by HIV. The most prominent among them are the 1989 United National International Convention on the Rights of the Child[38] and the 2009 Guidelines for the Alternative Care of Children.[39] Both documents emphasize that all decisions "should be carried out on a case-by-case basis," and decisions "should involve full consultation at all stages with the child, according to his or her evolving capacities.

### Psychological Distress and Resilience

HIV can have several implications for the mental health of affected children as well as for their caretakers. These mental health risks are well-documented in the global literature, but with 2 important, related caveats. First, risk does not guarantee a negative outcome in that vulnerabilities can be mediated by several internal and external factors.[13] Internal factors include active coping mechanisms that enable resilience such as hope for the future, self-esteem, talking about feelings, and having a sense of humor. External sources of coping and resilience include parental attention and attachment; harmonious family relations; perceived peer, family, and community support; and access to education and financial resources.[40] Second, in the absence of factors supporting coping and resilience, all children are at risk for psychological and emotional distress. In other words, the multiple overlapping deprivations, discussed earlier,[18] of extreme poverty, food insecurity, lack of access to school and other economic and social resources, and experience of domestic violence or abuse have a significant impact on a child's capacity for resilience regardless of the presence of HIV. For example, a child affected by HIV who is well-fed and loved by family and friends may have greater capacity for resilience and positive adaptive behavior than a child unaffected by HIV who lives in an impoverished, food-insecure home or who has been exposed multiple adverse childhood experiences.

The focus on sources of resilience is a relatively new trend in the OVC literature, which builds on a strong foundation of research documenting the many vulnerabilities and forms of distress faced by children affected by HIV.[40–42] HIV + children also face cognitive delays which can have a strong impact on educational attainment, mental health, coping, and resilience.[13]

Longitudinal findings from Kwa-Zulu Natal add yet more complexity in that both orphans and nonorphans showed relatively low levels of anxiety, depression, oppositional behavior, and low self-esteem at baseline. Later rounds of data collection found slightly higher levels of distress but still no differences based on orphan status. Overall, girls were more likely to experience depression, anxiety, and low self-esteem. Other predictors of distress included number of children in the house, being very ill, alcohol use by a household member, and food insecurity. Food insecurity was by far the strongest predictor of distress. Having a higher level of household assets and high levels of perceived social support were associated with lower levels of distress.[43]

### Special Needs of Adolescents

Four million HIV + adolescents are living in SSA. Most of them were infected perinatally and have survived due to the availability of pediatric ART.[44] As vertically infected children age into adolescence, they need specialized support targeted to their developmental stage and maturity level. Such specialized training includes guidance on delaying sexual debut, disclosing serostatus to potential sex partners, and using safe sex practices to protect their partners and themselves. HIV-affected youth may also need educational counseling and support as they enter secondary schools or higher education, and assistance finding vocational training or formal professional opportunities. HIV-affected teens have also been found to be at 3-fold higher risk of emotional and physical abuse and 6-fold risk of engaging in transactional sex than those not affected by HIV.[45] Teens who had previous exposure to abuse, extreme poverty, and food insecurity were most vulnerable to ongoing abuse and the decision to engage in survival sex.

Many countries have not been able to adjust to this new reality and throughout the world adolescents are received and counseled at adult treatment centers[46] by staff members who are unfamiliar with their specialized needs. This in turn results in dissatisfaction among adolescent clientele and avoidance of treatment centers.[47,48] HIV-infected and affected youth also face challenges when they turn 18, which is when many OVC-specific programs stop providing care. These youth are eligible for adult ART and other support programs but often receive little help negotiating this transition, putting them at risk for missing their medicines and rendering them no-longer eligible for educational and other support.

## ADDRESSING CHILDREN'S NEEDS IN THE CONTEXT OF HIV

The global strategy to provide treatment, care, and support to children infected with or affected by HIV falls into 4 categories: (1) prevention of mother-to-child transmission during pregnancy, delivery, and breastfeeding; (2) treatment of HIV + children with ART; (3) mitigation of impact of HIV on infected and affected children to ensure that they achieve their maximum potential across their life course; and (4) advocacy for social change to reduce HIV-related poverty, stigma, and discrimination. The following sections will look at the global OVC response by looking in depth at accomplishments and challenges faced in each of these categories.

### Prevention of Mother-To-Child Transmission

PMTCT requires the following:

- Primary prevention of HIV in women of childbearing age
- Prevention of unintended pregnancies in women with HIV infection
- Prevention of HIV transmission from women to their infants via use of antiretroviral drugs
- Provision of lifelong treatment, care, and support to women with HIV and to their families.[49]

Most emphasis has been placed on the use of ART to prevent transmission from mothers with HIV to their infants because services centered on ART offered in prenatal, perinatal, and postnatal care together can reduce the risk of mother-to-child transmission to less than 5% in breastfeeding populations and less than 2% in non-breastfeeding populations. To achieve this, programs must be designed so that pregnant women who are HIV + attend prenatal care; are offered, accept, and receive the results of a HIV test; and accept and adhere to antiretroviral-drug prophylaxis for themselves and their exposed infant. This is often referred to as the PMTCT cascade.[50] Current guidelines for PMTCT by the World Health Organization (**Box 1**) emphasize the importance of providing lifelong ART to pregnant women, with the ideal situation being lifelong treatment of all HIV + pregnant women (Option B+).

Progress toward achieving 100% coverage with PMTCT has been encouraging, with 67% of HIV + pregnant women globally receiving 1 of the 3 options (although the majority still receive the less effective Option A). SSA lags behind the rest of the world, with only 52% of eligible mothers receiving treatment.[2] (**Box 2**).

---

**Box 1**
**World Health Organization guidelines for prevention of mother-to-child transmission of human immunodeficiency virus**

Option A: Triple-combination ART for mothers with a CD4 count below 350, starting as soon as diagnosed. For pregnant women with a CD4 count above 350, antepartum zidovudine (AZT), intrapartum single-dose of nevirapine (NVP) and first dose of AZT-lamivudine (AZT/3TC), and postpartum daily AZT/3TC for 7 days. Daily doses of NVP are provided to infants from birth until 1 week after breastfeeding ceases

Option B: Triple-combination ART for mothers with a CD4 count below 350 to start on detection of HIV and continued for life, and for pregnant women with a CD4 count above 350 on detection through cessation of breastfeeding. Daily doses of ART are provided for infants through 4 to 6 weeks regardless of feeding method.

Option B+: Lifelong ART for pregnant women, regardless of CD4 count, and daily dosing of infants through 4 to 6 months.

*Data from* World Health Organization. Programmatic update: use of antiretroviral drugs for treating pregnant women and preventing HIV Infection in infants. Geneva (Switzerland): WHO Press; 2012.

---

## Adult and Pediatric Access to Antiretroviral Therapy

Free access to ART became increasingly available to adults in much of SSA during the first decade of the twenty-first century with funding from the global community, and the goal of achieving universal access by the end of 2015. Pediatric treatment has been slower to be adopted because of the toxicity of many first-line ART agents, the difficulties in creating pediatric formulations, and the complexity of monitoring the clinical status of children. However, the international, multisectorial movement toward an AIDS-free generation, has emphasized the importance of simplified, less toxic drug regimens that require minimal clinical monitoring while maintaining clinical efficacy.[47]

---

**Box 2**
**World Health Organization guidelines for preferred and alternative first-line regimens for children**

*Children younger than 3 years old*

Preferred first-line regimens: abacavir (ABC) or AZT + 3TC + lopinavir-ritonavir (LPV/r)

Alternative first-line regimens: ABC or AZT + 3TC + NVP

*Children 3 to 9 years old and adolescents less than 35 kg*

Preferred first-line regimens: ABC + 3TC + efavirenz (EFV)

Alternative first-line regimens: ABC or AZT or tenofovir (TDF) + 3TC (or emtricitabine [FTC]) + NVP or EFV

*Adolescents (10–19 years) >35 kg*

Preferred first-line regimens: TDF + 3TC (or FTC) + EFV

Alternative first-line regimens: ABC or AZT or TDF + 3TC (or FTC) + NVP or EFV

*Data from* World Health Organization. March 2014 supplement to the 2013 consolidated guideline on use of antiretroviral drugs for treating and preventing HIV infection. 2014. Available at: http://www.who.int/hiv/pub/guidelines/arv2013/arvs2013upplement_march2014/en/. Accessed July 27, 2015.

Treatment-eligible children living with HIV in SSA are half as likely to receive ART as HIV + adults,[51] and yet the effectiveness of ART in extending children's lives into adolescence and adulthood is well-documented.[52] Scaling up universal access to pediatric ART will reduce deaths, extend longevity, and improve the quality of life for both children and their families; however, the higher cost of the most effective regimes may lead to many countries choosing cheaper but less effective ART.[53]

### Mitigation of the Impacts of Human Immunodeficiency Virus on Children and Families

The vigorous global policy and foreign-assistance response to address vulnerabilities faced by OVC has led to numerous innovative programs focused on providing care and support through household financial assistance, community-based and residential care for children without an able adult caretaker, and access to education.

#### International policy and donor response

In March 2004, the Joint United Nations Programme on HIV and AIDS (UNAIDS) Committee of Cosponsoring Organizations endorsed a Framework for the Protection, Care, and Support of Orphans and Vulnerable Children Living In a World with HIV and AIDS.[54] This consensus document identified the following key strategies to address the growing crisis around the world and particularly in Africa:

1. Strengthen the capacity of families to protect and care for OVC by prolonging the lives of parents and providing economic, psychosocial, and other support
2. Mobilize and support community-based responses to provide both immediate and long-term support to vulnerable households
3. Ensure access for OVC to essential services, including education, health care, birth registration, and others
4. Ensure that governments protect the most vulnerable children through improved policy and legislation and by channeling resources to communities
5. Raise awareness at all levels through advocacy and social mobilization to create a supportive environment for children affected by HIV.

International donors have largely funded the response to the OVC crisis in SSA. The Global Fund to Fight AIDS, Malaria, and Tuberculosis was created in 2002 as a mechanism through which wealthy countries could contribute to a general fund and governments of countries hit hard by these diseases could submit proposals for funding to treat and care for people living with HIV, and build in-country health-systems capacity.

In 2003, the United States implemented the President's Emergency Fund for AIDS Relief (PEPFAR) to provide support for OVC in 7 priority areas: education, psychosocial care and support, household economic strengthening, social protection, health and nutrition, child protection, and legal protection.[55] PEPFAR funding is largely distributed to civil society partners to improve care and support services implemented by community, faith-based, and other nongovernmental organizations that deliver the bulk of care and support for OVC. PEPFAR provides services to more than 5 million HIV-affected children per year[56] and has been described as the largest relief effort by a single nation that the world has ever seen.[57] Further funding for OVC programming comes from other bilateral country partners, private corporations and foundations, religious bodies, and individual citizens around the world.

Although the international response to mitigating the impact of HIV in SSA and other high-prevalence regions has been remarkable, the dependence of most OVC care and support programs on donor assistance is a critical vulnerability. In recent years, donor organizations have turned their focus to building local capacity with the goal that these organizations become self-sustaining. However, the extent to which support for children and families can be maintained at the level needed by individual governments and local organizations remains to be seen.

### Poverty alleviation and social protection

African countries, as well as donor organizations, have begun to invest in social welfare and protection programs with the broad goals of reducing poverty, improving school enrollment and attendance, improving nutrition, and overall improved health of children and families. In particular, cash transfer programs have become an increasingly popular form of social protection and have been shown to be an effective method of reducing poverty, improving school attendance, and improving healthy behaviors in number of contexts. There are 2 types of cash transfer programs: unconditional and conditional.

Unconditional cash transfers (UCTs) involve regular dispersals of cash (usually 10–25 USD per month) to extremely poor households with the goal of improving food security and access to education for children and to help families meet their other most basic requirements for survival. Families use the money in whatever way they see fit, including investing in income-generating endeavors or savings. Thirty-seven SSA countries have unconditional cash transfer programs,[58] though most of these are funded in large part by donors with a few exceptions. For example, South Africa has a long-standing, extensive social grants system and Zambia funds 80% of its cash transfer program.[59]

Conditional cash transfers (CCTs) offer individuals or households a regular sum of money for specified purposes or to create incentives for engaging in desired behaviors that promote health and well-being. Disbursals may depend on school attendance, remaining free of HIV or sexually transmitted infections, using condoms, maintaining child weight for height, immunization, and the like. Overall, both UCTs and CCTs have been shown to improve school enrollment and attendance, reduce poverty, and improve child nutritional status.[60] However, few studies have shown that CCTs reduce HIV infection though they have been associated with decreases in sexual risk-taking.[61]

Cash transfer programs have been tested only minimally in the context of high HIV-related orphaning and vulnerability. Kenya's cash transfer program, which started in 2004, specifically targets OVC and has been found to improve overall child and household wellbeing.[59] Shifts in spending patterns show more money spent on food, clothing, and health; and less on alcohol.[61] Households with OVC experienced a 13% decline in poverty,[59,62] and adolescent and young adults in households receiving cash were 31% less likely to report sexual debut between the 2007 baseline and the third round of data collection in 2011 than their peers from nonintervention households.[63]

Many evaluations have been done of various types of cash transfer programs around the world. However, drawing a broadly generalizable conclusion about effectiveness or potential utility in a new context or across multiple contexts is not possible. Effectiveness in changing the lot of the most vulnerable families depends on sophisticated targeting to find the poorest of the poor with outcomes that depend on amount, frequency of disbursals, and other determinants.[35] With CCTs, frequency and stringency of monitoring and enforcing conditions also influence evaluation outcomes.[64]

### Advocacy for Social Change to Reduce Social Marginalization, Stigma, and Discrimination

The evidence base developed during the last 30 years of the HIV pandemic suggests that the key responses must address actionable causes.[65] Specifically

- Ignorance about the harm of stigma
- Continuing irrational fears of infection
- Moral judgment.

The most commonly used approaches that have been shown to be successful in reducing stigma and discrimination include formalizing community interaction between people living with HIV and those vulnerable to HIV infection, using media to educate the broad population through TV and radio, and developing engaging programming that normalizes HIV. MTV's Staying Alive Foundation has sponsored a wide variety of programming, including the popular, multiseason television and radio drama *Shuga*, and the use of high visibility entertainers and musicians in 40 high-incidence countries.[66] Other successful programs engage religious and community leaders, national or international celebrities, and peer mobilization by people living

| Table 4 | |
|---|---|
| **Caring for orphans and vulnerable children** | |
| **Area of Vulnerability** | **Key Strategies for OVC Programming** |
| Attending and completing school | Payment of school fees (primary and secondary school), provision of school uniforms and classroom materials, and infrastructure development |
| Psychological Distress and Resilience | Psychosocial care and support such as succession planning and dealing with loss of a parent, disclosure of HIV status, counseling and treatment for depression, enhancing coping mechanisms, identifying and supporting sources of resilience, and providing targeted services to survivors of abuse |
| Poverty | House economic strengthening through CCTs or UCTs, income-generation for caregivers of households with OVC, and development of income-generating skills for OVC themselves |
| Shelter and Care | Social protection strategies ensuring safe shelter and care, services for homeless and street children, alternative methods of care, such as finding foster homes, community shelters, or orphanages, and community engagement to provide income for OVC |
| Poor nutrition | Support for breastfeeding or providing alternative milk if indicated, heightened growth monitoring, school nutrition services, and cash transfer programs |
| Social isolation, stigma, discrimination | Legal protections to prevent discrimination in school or work, community education to address the roots of discrimination, empowerment of OVC by birth registration, negotiating skills, and community peer groups |
| Trafficking, transactional and survival sex, child marriage | Child protection services to supplement the legal framework to identify children being trafficked, exploited at home or work, and ensure that child rights are maintained |
| Access to treatment, care, and support | Capacity building of service providers in government and nongovernmental sectors, health systems strengthening, and workforce development |

*Data from* PEPFAR. Guidance for Orphans and Vulnerable Children. 2012. p. 1–89. Available at: http://www.pepfar.gov/documents/organization/195702.pdf. Accessed July 27, 2015.

with HIV. Advocacy for nondiscrimination and incorporation of human rights principles in schools, health care, and workplaces are also vital.[65]

## FUTURE DIRECTIONS

The multidimensional nature of programming for OVC requires long timelines, focused on achieving multiple outcomes.[67] In the first decade of the twenty-first century, the global emergency response to HIV had an with insufficient focus on measuring effectiveness or impact of services offered.[67,68] Since 2011, OVC programming has been increasingly evidence-based, developed through rigorous evaluation of early work.[33,67–70] These new approaches strive to take into account the developmental stages of children especially as they enter adolescence, focus on child and family-centered care, and address underlying poverty. **Table 4** summarizes the key vulnerabilities of children in SSA, and the future directions of OVC programming.

## SUMMARY

Children infected with, orphaned, or made vulnerable by HIV in SSA require strong health systems, effective social support networks, and economic support. Yet these crucial supports are often lacking. Prevention of pediatric infection, and treatment with ART are 2 interventions that have been shown to be highly effective in reducing the incidence of HIV in children, and further rapid progress is expected. However, children infected with HIV represent a tiny minority of those orphaned or made vulnerable by HIV. These children are exposed to significant societal discrimination, and are often pushed into extreme poverty by the presence of HIV in the household. Broad, society-wide interventions are necessary to address the physical and mental health of these children, while building a strong educational foundation for their progress through adolescence and into a safe, secure, and productive adulthood.

It is equally important to bear in mind that children orphaned or made vulnerable by HIV only represent 16% of vulnerable children in SSA. Multidimensional poverty continues to be the most common, preventable predictor of negative outcomes for children. Caregivers, service providers, governments, and donors, must use the current focus on children orphaned and made vulnerable by HIV to strengthen the societal mechanisms that will address the needs of all vulnerable children in SSA.

## REFERENCES

1. UNAIDS. Report on the AIDS epidemic 2013. Available at: http://www.unaids.org/sites/default/files/en/media/unaids/contentassets/documents/epidemiology/2013/gr2013/UNAIDS_Global_Report_2013_en.pdf. Accessed May 18, 2015.
2. UNICEF. Towards an AIDS-free generation - Children and AIDS - Sixth Stocktaking Report, 2013. Available at: http://www.unicef.org/publications/index_70986.html. Accessed July 26, 2015.
3. UNAIDS. Children and HIV. In: UNAIDS Fact sheet 2014. Available at: http://www.unaids.org/en/resources/documents/2014/20140508_FactSheet_Children. Accessed June 23, 2015.
4. UNICEF. Progress for Children. Beyond Averages: Learning from the MDGs. 2015. Available at: http://www.unicef.org/publications/files/Progress_for_Children_No._11_22June15.pdf. Accessed July 28, 2015.
5. UNICEF/UNAIDS/USAID. Children on the brink 2004: A joint report of new orphan estimates and a framework for action. 2004 Available at: http://www.unicef.org/publications/index_22212.html. Accessed July 27, 2015.

6. World Health Organization. Treatment of children living with HIV. In WHO HIV update May 2015. Available at: http://www.who.int/hiv/topics/paediatric/en/. Accessed July 26, 2015.

7. Bryant M, Brooks B, Shann M, et al. Evaluating the effectiveness of educational block grants to orphans and vulnerable children. In OVC-CARE Project Reports. Available at: http://www.bu.edu/cghd/publication/evaluating-the-effectiveness-of-educational-block-grants-to-orphans-and-vulnerable-children-final-report/. Accessed July 26, 2015.

8. World Bank. OVC Toolkit. Available at: http://info.worldbank.org/etools/docs/library/138974/toolkit/howknow/definitions.htm. Accessed May 18, 2015.

9. UNAIDS. UNAIDS Terminology Guidelines, 2011. Available at: http://www.unaids.org/sites/default/files/media_asset/JC2118_terminology-guidelines_en_0.pdf. Accessed July 27, 2016.

10. UNICEF. Measuring the determinants of childhood vulnerability. 2014. Available at: http://data.unicef.org/corecode/uploads/document6/uploaded_pdfs/corecode/Measuring-the-Determinants-of-Childhood-Vulnerability_Final-Report-5_8-LR-_172.pdf. Accessed June 9, 2015.

11. UNAIDS. The gap report, 2014. Available at: http://www.unaids.org/en/media/unaids/contentassets/documents/unaidspublication/2014/UNAIDS_Gap_report_en.pdf. Accessed July 27, 2015.

12. World Bank. Poverty & Equity Data | Sub-Saharan Africa | The World Bank. Available at: http://povertydata.worldbank.org/poverty/region/SSA. Accessed June 10, 2015.

13. Sherr L, Cluver LD, Betancourt TS, et al. Evidence of impact: health, psychological and social effects of adult HIV on children. AIDS 2014;28(Suppl 3):S251–9.

14. Cluver L, Orkin M, Boyes ME, et al. Pathways from parental AIDS to child psychological, educational and sexual risk: developing an empirically-based interactive theoretical model. Soc Sci Med 2013;87:185–93.

15. Cluver L, Operario D, Gardner F. Parental illness, caregiving factors and psychological distress among children orphaned by acquired immune deficiency syndrome (AIDS) in South Africa. Vulnerable Child Youth Stud 2009;4(3):185–98.

16. Bachman-DeSilva M, Skalicky A, Beard J, et al. Early impacts of orphaning: health, nutrition, and food insecurity in a cohort of school-going adolescents in South Africa. Vulnerable Child Youth Stud 2012;7(1):75–87.

17. Onyango MA, Adu-Sarkodie Y, Agyarko-Poku T, et al. "It's all about making a life": poverty, HIV, violence, and other vulnerabilities faced by young female sex workers in Kumasi, Ghana. J Acquir Immune Defic Syndr 2015;68(Suppl 2):S131–7.

18. UNICEF. Multiple overlapping deprivation analysis for children. Available at: http://www.unicef-irc.org/MODA/. Accessed June 22, 2015.

19. United Nations. Millennium Development Goals Report 2014. Available at: http://www.un.org/millenniumgoals/2014.MDGreport/MDG.2014.Englishweb.pdf. Accessed June 22, 2015.

20. Olanrewaju AD, Jeffery C, Crossland N, et al. Access to education for orphans and vulnerable children in Uganda: a multi-district, cross-sectional study using lot quality assurance sampling from 2011 to 2013. PLoS One 2015;10(7):e0132905.

21. Smiley A, Omoeva C, Sylla B, et al. Orphans and vulnerable children: trends in school access and experience in Eastern and Southern Africa. Washington,

DC: Education Policy and Data Centre, FHI360; 2012. Available at: https://www.mendeley.com/research/orphans-vulnerable-childre-trends-school-access-experience-eastern-southern-africa/?utm_source=desktop&utm_medium=1.13.8&utm_campaign=open_catalog&userDocumentId=%7B491327bc-2725-4925-bcbe-5ddf95292dc5%7D. Accessed June 16, 2015.

22. UNICEF. UNICEF statistics on secondary education. Web site. Available at: http://data.unicef.org/education/secondary. Accessed July 28, 2015.

23. Irwin A, Adams A WA. Home truths: facing the facts on children, AIDS, and poverty. Final Report of the Joint Learning Initiative on Children and HIV/AIDS. Boston (MA): Association Francois-Xavier Bagnold, Harvard University; 2009.

24. Morrison L. Ceausescu's legacy: family struggles and institutionalization of children in Romania. J Fam Hist 2004;29(2):168–82.

25. Zeanah CH, Egger HL, Smyke AT, et al. Institutional rearing and psychiatric disorders in Romanian preschool children. Am J Psychiatry 2009;166(7):777–85.

26. Whetten K, Ostermann J, Whetten RA, et al. A comparison of the wellbeing of orphans and abandoned children ages 6–12 in institutional and community-based care settings in 5 less wealthy nations. PLoS One 2009;4(12):e8169.

27. Zimmerman B. Orphan living situations in Malawi: a comparison of orphanages and foster homes. Rev Policy Res 2005;22(6):881–917.

28. Wolff PH, Tesfai B, Egasso H, et al. The orphans of Eritrea: a comparison study. J Child Psychol Psychiatry 1995;36(4):633–44.

29. Wolff PH, Fesseha G. The orphans of Eritrea: are orphanages part of the problem or part of the solution? Am J Psychiatry 1998;155(10):1319–24.

30. Wolff PH, Fesseha G. The orphans of Eritrea: a five-year follow-up study. J Child Psychol Psychiatry 1999;40(8):1231–7.

31. Wolff PH, Fesseha G. The orphans of Eritrea: what are the choices? Am J Orthop 2005;75(4):475–84.

32. Zeanah CH, Fox NA, Nelson CA. The Bucharest Early Intervention Project: case study in the ethics of mental health research. J Nerv Ment Dis 2012;200(3):243–7.

33. Whetten K, Ostermann J, Pence BW, et al. Three-year change in the wellbeing of orphaned and separated children in institutional and family-based care settings in five low- and middle-income countries. PLoS One 2014;9(8):e104872.

34. Whetten K, Ostermann J, Whetten R, et al. More than the loss of a parent: potentially traumatic events among orphaned and abandoned children. J Trauma Stress 2011;24(2):174–82.

35. Whetten R, Messer L, Ostermann J, et al. Child work and labour among orphaned and abandoned children in five low and middle income countries. BMC Int Health Hum Rights 2011;11(1):1.

36. UNICEF. In Ethiopia, placing institutions and adoption practices under scrutiny - and reuniting children with their families, Web site. Available at: http://www.unicef.org/protection/ethiopia_66598.html. Accessed June 22, 2015.

37. Lugalla JLP. AIDS, orphans, and development in Sub-Saharan Africa: a review of the dilemma of public health and development. Dev Stud 2003;19(1):26–46.

38. United Nations. The Convention: on the rights of the child. 1989. Available at: http://www.ohchr.org/en/professionalinterest/pages/crc.aspx. Accessed June 22, 2015.

39. United Nations. Guidelines for the alternative care of children. 2010 Available at: http://www.unicef.org/protection/alternative_care_Guidelines-English.pdf. Accessed June 22, 2015.

40. Betancourt TS, Meyers-Ohki SE, Charrow A, et al. Annual research review: mental health and resilience in HIV/AIDS-affected children—a review of the literature and recommendations for future research. J Child Psychol Psychiatry Allied Discip 2013;54(4):423–44.

41. Beard J, Biemba G, Brooks MI, et al. Children of female sex workers and drug users: a review of vulnerability, resilience and family-centred models of care. J Int AIDS Soc 2010;13(Suppl 2):S6.

42. Heath MA, Donald DR, Theron LC, et al. AIDS in South Africa: therapeutic interventions to strengthen resilience among orphans and vulnerable children. Sch Psychol Int 2014;35(3):309–37.

43. Bachman Desilva M, Skalicky AM, Beard J, et al. Longitudinal evaluation of the psychosocial wellbeing of recent orphans compared with non-orphans in a school-attending cohort in KwaZulu-Natal, South Africa. Int J Ment Health Promot 2012;14(3):162–82.

44. Lee VC, Muriithi P, Gilbert-Nandra U, et al. Orphans and vulnerable children in Kenya: results from a nationally representative population-based survey. J Acquir Immune Defic Syndr 2014;66(Suppl 1):S89–97.

45. Cluver L, Orkin M, Boyes M, et al. Transactional sex amongst AIDS-orphaned and AIDS-affected adolescents predicted by abuse and extreme poverty. J Acquir Immune Defic Syndr 2011;58(3):336–43.

46. National AIDS Control Organization. Operational Guidelines for Care & Support Centres Operational Guidelines for Care & Support Centres. 2013. Available at: http://www.naco.gov.in/upload/NACP-IV/18022014.CST/CSC.Guidelines.pdf. Accessed July 27, 2015.

47. World Health Organization. Paediatric ARV drug optimization. Geneva (Switzerland): WHO Press; 2014.

48. World Health Organization. Treatment of children living with HIV. [cited June 23, 2015]; Available at: http://www.who.int/hiv/topics/paediatric/en/. Accessed July 28, 2015.

49. World Health Organization. Guidance on global scale-up of the prevention of mother to child transmission of HIV: towards universal access for women, infants and young children and eliminating HIV and AIDS among children/Inter-Agency Task Team on Prevention of HIV Infection in Pregnant Women, Mothers and their Children. Geneva (Switzerland): WHO Press; 2007. p. pp1–40.

50. Padian NS, McCoy SI, Karim SSA, et al. HIV prevention transformed: the new prevention research agenda. Lancet 2011;378(9787):269–78.

51. UNAIDS. United Nations General Assembly High Level Meeting Reports (2010-2015. Web site. Available at: http://www.unaids.org/en/dataanalysis/knowyour response/countryprogressreports/2015countries/Special SessionCommission. Accessed July 27, 2015.

52. Pegurri E, Konings E, Crandall B, et al. The missed HIV-positive children of Ethiopia. PLoS One 2015;10(4):e0124041.

53. Ciaranello AL, Doherty K, Penazzato M, et al. Cost-effectiveness of first-line antiretroviral therapy for HIV-infected African children less than 3 years of age. AIDS 2015;29(10):1247–59.

54. UNICEF. The framework for the protection, care, and support of orphans and vulnerable children living in a world with HIV and AIDS. 2004. Available at: http://www.unicef.org/aids/files/Framework_English.pdf. Accessed July 27, 2015.

55. PEPFAR. Guidance for orphans and vulnerable children. 2012;1–89. Available at: http://www.pepfar.gov/documents/organization/195702.pdf. Accessed July 27, 2015.

56. PEPFAR. Latest PEPFAR Program Results. In the United States President's Emergency Plan For AIDS Relief: 2014 results update. 2015. Available at: http://www.pepfar.gov/funding/results/. Accessed June 22, 2015.

57. US Government. Congressional budget justification: supplement. Fiscal year 2015 Pub 2014. Available at: http://www.pepfar.gov/documents/organization/236283.pdf. Accessed June 10 2015.

58. Pettifor A, MacPhail C, Nguyen N, et al. Can money prevent the spread of HIV? A review of cash payments for HIV prevention. AIDS Behav 2012;16(7):1729–38.

59. Bryant JH. Kenya's cash transfer program: protecting the health and human rights of orphans and vulnerable children. Health Hum Rights 2009;11(2):65–76.

60. Fiszbein A, Schady N. Conditional cash transfers: reducing present and future poverty. New York: World Bank; 2009. Available at: https://openknowledge.worldbank.org/bitstream/handle/10986/2597/476030PUB0Cond101Official0Use0Only1.pdf?sequence=1. Accessed July 28, 2015.

61. University of North Carolina. The impact of Kenya's cash transfer for orphans and vulnerable children on human capital. J Dev Eff 2012;4(1):38–49.

62. Branson N, Hitchin J. Cash transfers: Indebted to donors. In Africa Research Institute: Understanding Africa today. 2014. Available at: http://www.africaresearchinstitute.org/blog/cash-transfers-indebted-to-donors/. Accessed July 27, 2015.

63. Handa S, Halpern CT, Pettifor A, et al. The Government of Kenya's cash transfer program reduces the risk of sexual debut among young people age 15-25. PLoS One 2014;9(1):e85473.

64. Garcia M, Moore CM. The cash dividend: the rise of cash transfer programs in Sub-Saharan Africa. World Bank; 2012. Available at: https://openknowledge.worldbank.org/handle/10986/2246.License: CCBY3.0IGO. Accessed July 27, 2015.

65. UNAIDS. Key programmes to reduce stigma and discrimination and increase access to justice in national HIV responses. 2012. Available at: http://www.unaids.org/sites/default/files/media_asset/Key_Human_Rights_Programmes_en_May2012_0.pdf. Accessed July 27, 2015.

66. Staying Alive Foundation web site. Available at: http://stayingalivefoundation.org/. Accessed June 22, 2015.

67. Bryant M, Beard J, Sabin L, et al. PEPFAR's support for orphans and vulnerable children: some beneficial effects, but too little data, and programs spread thin. Health Aff 2012;31(7):1508–18.

68. Larson B, Wambua N, Masila J, et al. Exploring impacts of multi-year, community-based care programs for orphans and vulnerable children: a case study from Kenya. Aids Care 2013;25:S40–5.

69. Nyberg BJ, Yates DD, Lovich R, et al. Saving lives for a lifetime: supporting orphans and vulnerable children impacted by HIV/AIDS. J Acquir Immune Defic Syndr 2012;60(Suppl 3):S127–35.

70. Santa-Ana-Tellez Y, DeMaria LM, Galárraga O. Costs of interventions for AIDS orphans and vulnerable children. Trop Med Int Health 2011;16(11):1417–26.

# Children's Environmental Health

## Beyond National Boundaries

Mark D. Miller, MD, MPH[a,b,*], Melanie A. Marty, PhD[c],
Philip J. Landrigan, MD, MSc[d]

## KEYWORDS

- Children • Environment • Air pollution • E-waste • Pesticides • Lead
- Climate change • Developing nations

## KEY POINTS

- Children are especially vulnerable to environmental pollution, which is a major cause of childhood disease and disability in countries at every level of socioeconomic development.
- Environmental threats to children include air and water pollution, toxic industrial chemicals, pesticides, heavy metals, hazardous wastes and global climate change.
- Global climate change is expected to amplify environmental threats to child health.
- The World Health Organization estimates that environmental pollutants cause more deaths than human immunodeficiency virus, acquired immunodeficiency syndrome (HIV/AIDS), tuberculosis, and malaria combined.

*Continued*

Disclosure Statement: The authors have nothing to disclose. This publication was supported by the cooperative agreement award number 1 U61TS000237-01 from the Agency for Toxic Substances and Disease Registry. Its contents are the responsibility of the authors and do not necessarily represent the official views of the Agency for Toxic Substances and Disease Registry (ATSDR), State of California, or the California Environmental Protection Agency.
The US Environmental Protection Agency (EPA) supports the PEHSU by providing partial funding to ATSDR under Inter-Agency Agreement number DW-75-92301301. Neither EPA nor ATSDR endorse the purchase of any commercial products or services mentioned in PEHSU publications.

[a] Children's Environmental Health Program, Office of Environmental Health Hazard Assessment, California EPA, 1515 Clay Street, 16th Floor, Oakland, CA 94612, USA; [b] Western States Pediatric Environmental Health Specialty Unit at UCSF, SFGH, Occupational Environmental Medicine, Box 0843, San Francisco, CA 94143-0843, USA; [c] Office of Environmental Health Hazard Assessment, California Environmental Protection Agency, 1001 I Street, Sacramento, CA 95814, USA; [d] Arnhold Institute for Global Health, Icahn School of Medicine at Mount Sinai, 17 East 102nd Street, Room D3-145, New York, NY 10029-6574, USA
* Corresponding author. Children's Environmental Health Program, Office of Environmental Health Hazard Assessment, California EPA, 1515 Clay Street, 16th Floor, Oakland, CA 94612.
*E-mail address:* ucsfpehsumiller@gmail.com

Pediatr Clin N Am 63 (2016) 149–165
http://dx.doi.org/10.1016/j.pcl.2015.08.008      **pediatric.theclinics.com**
0031-3955/16/$ – see front matter © 2016 Elsevier Inc. All rights reserved.

*Continued*

- Pollution caused by toxic chemicals is a growing problem in low-income and middle-income countries, resulting in acute and chronic disease in children and undermining programs for national and international development.
- Pediatricians have an opportunity to reduce environmental health impacts with the aid of many organizations working on these issues worldwide.

## INTRODUCTION

Children today live in a world with increasing exposure to environmental hazards. Environmental stressors have increased as the world's population has increased from 2.5 billion in 1950 to 7 billion today.[1] A global trend toward urbanization is further accelerating children's exposures to environmental hazards, especially in the world's poorer countries. By 2050, it is projected that 66% of the world's population will reside in cities.[2]

Environmental pollution in both urban and rural settings has become a major cause of disease in children.[3] Along with traditional hazards of indoor air pollution and contaminated drinking water, children today are exposed to newer environmental threats such as urban air pollution, global climate change, toxic industrial chemicals, pesticides, heavy metals, and hazardous wastes.[4,5] All of these global environmental changes have major implications, positive as well as negative, for the health of children.

The World Health Organization (WHO) estimates that 17% of deaths of children in developed nations are attributable to environmental exposures compared with 24% in developing nations.[6] Environmental exposures result in more deaths (adults and children) than are caused by human immunodeficiency virus (HIV)/AIDS, tuberculosis, and malaria combined.[7] The diseases caused by traditional forms of environmental pollution (eg, coliforms in water or air pollution from solid fuels) are predominantly diarrhea, pneumonia, and other infectious diseases. Modern environmental threats, by contrast, are linked mainly to chronic diseases: asthma, neurodevelopmental disorders, birth defects, obesity, diabetes, cardiovascular disease, mental health problems, and pediatric cancer. Children in rapidly industrializing countries are simultaneously confronted by both ancient and modern environmental threats to health.

In an ever more interconnected world, pediatricians need to be aware of current environmental threats to children's health, locally as well as globally. Highly toxic pesticides no longer permitted in the United States are still used in countries around the world and can expose North American children who eat imported fruits and vegetables. Recent immigrants bring hazards from their home countries such as lead-contaminated cosmetics or medications containing mercury.[8] Children adopted from foreign countries may have been exposed prenatally or during early childhood to chemical hazards more common in their country of origin. Awareness of hazards such as these and openness to the discovery of new environmental threats to children's health will enhance pediatricians' ability to diagnose, treat, and prevent disease in children.

## AIR

Air pollution is a complex mixture of gases, particles, and aerosols, and results from mobile sources, industrial facilities, home heating and cooking, and natural sources such as wildfires. The intense smog episodes in London in 1952, and similar episodes elsewhere, resulted in a large spike in deaths from cardiovascular and respiratory disease.[9] Since then, air pollution epidemiologists have identified many adverse health outcomes in both children and adults. Particulate matter (PM), also known as particulate air pollution, especially finer ambient particles, can penetrate deeply into the respiratory tract and is associated with cardiovascular morbidity and mortality in adults.[10] Ozone, nitrogen oxide (NOx), and other pollutants are similarly associated with increased mortality and morbidity.

The fetus, infants, and children are particularly susceptible to adverse effects of air pollution due to rapid cell division, differentiation, and the high demand for oxygen and nutrients to support growth. Studies report associations between air pollution, especially PM2.5 ($\leq$ 2.5 microns in diameter), and adverse birth outcomes, including

- Lower birth weight, intrauterine growth retardation, and preterm birth[11]
- Birth defects (mixed results)[12]
- Infant mortality (postneonatal respiratory infection).[13]

Researchers studying a cohort of children in southern California have demonstrated associations between reduced lung function growth and regional and traffic-related air pollution, including PM2.5, NOx, and ozone.[14] Reduced lung function at age 18 years is irreversible because lung function growth has stopped by that age. Compromised lung function in early adulthood is associated with risk for premature mortality and other adverse health outcomes throughout adult life.[15] A meta-analysis conducted by the Centers for Disease Control and Prevention (CDC) found traffic exposure in childhood to be associated with a 50% increase in childhood acute lymphoblastic leukemia.[16] Other studies have implicated traffic in risk for germ cell tumors and retinoblastomas in children.[17] In 2013, the International Agency for Research on Cancer (IARC) identified air pollution and PM as known human carcinogens based on sufficient evidence of lung cancer in adults.[18] Finally, research has shown associations between air pollution and adverse neurodevelopmental effects in children.[19,20]

Many studies have reported associations between regional and traffic-related air pollution, including diesel exhaust, and exacerbation and induction of asthma.[14]

Many governmental organizations have set standards for components of air pollution that serve as goals and promote innovation in pollution controls (**Table 1**). In the United States, both the California Environmental Protection Agency (EPA) and the US EPA have used considerable resources implementing regulatory actions to

**Table 1**
**Air quality standards and guidelines for key primary pollutants**

| Pollutant | Averaging Time | WHO ($\mu g/m^3$) | US EPA ($\mu g/m^3$) | California EPA ($\mu g/m^3$) |
|-----------|----------------|-------------------|----------------------|------------------------------|
| PM2.5 | Annual | 10 | 12 | 12 |
|  | 24 h | 25 | 35 | — |
| PM10 | Annual | 20 | — | 20 |
|  | 24 h | 50 | 150 | 50 |
| Ozone | 1 h | — | — | 180 |
|  | 8 h | 100 | 137 | 147 |
| $NO_2$ | 1 h | 200 | 188 | 339 |
|  | Annual | 40 | 100 | 57 |

*Abbreviations:* EPA, Environmental Protection Agency; $NO_2$, Nitrogen dioxide.

reduce air pollution. These efforts have paid off in terms of improving children's health. Investigators report improved lung function growth in successive cohorts of children in southern California as air quality has improved. Improvements in 4-year lung function growth during childhood, measured by forced expiratory volume (FEV)-1 and forced vital capacity (FVC), have coincided with lower ambient exposures to both NOx and PM pollution.[21] The proportion of children with clinically significant decrements in lung function at age 15 years declined from 7.9% to 3.6% from the mid-1990s to 2011. Previously, these investigators had shown that children who moved from a high pollution area to a lower pollution area experienced improvement in lung function growth. Clearly, regulations that reduce air pollution can be effective and result in health improvements for children. Regional, national, and global improvements are needed.

Airborne pollutants are transported around the world and can affect the health of children far from their point of origin. Industrial and traffic emissions from Asia add to exposures in the western United States; airborne particulate pollution from coal-burning power plants in the Ohio Valley adversely affect children on the east coast of the United States.[22]

Low- and middle-income countries (LMICs) are experiencing large increases in exposures to urban air pollution due to increased combustion of coal and other fossil fuels for industrial activities, as well as increasing car ownership. Globally, 88% of urban residents live in cities that fail to meet WHO air quality guidelines. The WHO compiles information on particulate matter concentrations from more than 1000 cities around the globe (**Table 2**).[23,24] This information indicates that LMICs generally have more particulate air pollution and, by inference, other air pollutants than high-income countries (HICs). Thus, children in LMICs are at much higher risk of adverse respiratory health effects from air pollution. Further, indoor air pollution can be very high in homes using biomass for cooking with inadequate ventilation. WHO attributes 334,000 deaths of children to household air pollution and 127,000 to outdoor air pollution worldwide annually, mostly from lower respiratory infections.[25] Efforts to reduce both indoor and outdoor air pollution globally are warranted.

Worldwide, 3 billion people use indoor, inefficient, solid fuel cookstoves or fires that cause more than 1.9 million deaths annually and are the fourth largest health risk in the developing world.[26,27] The Global Alliance for Clean Cookstoves is a public–private partnership working to get 100 million households to adopt clean and efficient

**Table 2**
**Examples of particulate matter concentrations in big cities around the globe**

| | Annual Average Outdoor Measurements, PM10 ($\mu g/m^3$) | Annual Average Outdoor Measurements, PM2.5 ($\mu g/m^3$) |
|---|---|---|
| Los Angeles, CA, USA (2012) | 33 | 20 |
| Beijing, China (2010) | 121 | 56 |
| Delhi, India (2011, 2013) | 286 | 153 |
| Mexico City, Mexico (2011) | 93 | 25 |
| Santiago, Chile (2011) | 69 | 26 |
| Cairo, Egypt (2011) | 135 | 73 |
| Abu Dhabi, UAE (2011) | 170 | 64 |
| Berlin, Germany (2011) | 24 | 20 |
| Dhaka, Bangladesh (2013) | 180 | 86 |

cookstoves by 2020 (**Box 1**). Helping a community transition to clean and efficient stove technologies will help improve immediate and long-term health and reduce production of greenhouse gases.

## WATER

In North America, drinking water generally presents a low risk for microbial infection due to engineering for hygiene. Federal and state agencies set standards for chemical contaminants of concern, including chemicals that affect infants and children, such as nitrates (methemoglobinemia), perchlorate (inhibition of iodine uptake by the thyroid), and lead (neurodevelopmental delay). Information pertaining to drinking water standards can be obtained online (see **Box 1**). Large water systems are routinely monitored in the United States but private wells serve a many people and are not monitored for contaminants. Emerging concerns include pharmaceuticals in drinking water, climate change–associated water quality and scarcity issues, and region-specific contaminants, including arsenic and radionuclides.

In many LMICs, availability of clean drinking water is among the most acute environmental health needs. Different strategies have been effective in different circumstances. New York City has used extensive watershed protection to maintain quality while reducing expenses by limiting the need for additional expensive water treatment.[28] This model is being used to protect urban water systems in projects around the world (see **Box 1**). Where there are no sanitary water systems, other novel approaches have been successful. More than 5 million people in 50 countries use solar disinfection (SODIS) to improve water quality and decrease diarrheal diseases.[29] Plastic bottles (polyethylene terephthalate [PET]) are filled with low turbidity water and placed in the sun for 6 to 48 hours (depending on weather). Ultraviolet-induced DNA alteration, thermal inactivation, and photo-oxidative destruction inactivate disease-causing organisms. Studies have demonstrated 9% to 86% reductions in diarrheal diseases.[30] Training and technical support for implementing SODIS programs are available (see **Box 1**).

## PESTICIDES

More than 700 pesticide chemicals, including insecticides, herbicides, rodenticides, and fungicides, are currently registered with US EPA. These are chemicals deliberately engineered to kill or repel living things and thus have inherent toxic potential.

Synthetic pesticides introduced after World War II are now ubiquitous. A 2000 US EPA survey demonstrated that 74% of US households use 1 or more pesticides around the home. Over time, insecticide use has evolved from chlorinated compounds such as dichlorodiphenyltrichloroethane (DDT) to organophosphates (OPs) and, more recently, pyrethroids. Though having low acute toxicity, organochlorine pesticides are persistent and associated with chronic health concerns. In making the switch to the OPs, we have substituted for the acute and neurodevelopmental toxicity of OPs. Due to regulatory actions based on demonstrated neurocognitive impacts, since the early 2000s, residential use of OPs has largely been replaced by pyrethroids. Initial concerns about pyrethroids being associated with allergic reactions have been accentuated with recent studies suggesting possible impacts on neurodevelopmental delay, autism, and male reproductive health.[31,32]

Newer, designer, pesticides have been introduced in recent years that target physiologic systems of insects and plants with the assumption that they would likely not have effects on human health. A prominent example is the neonicotinoid pesticides that target nicotinic acetylcholine receptors, which are different in insects than

**Box 1**
**Online children's environmental health resources**

*General children's environmental health*

- A *Story of Health*. Multimedia e-book explores how environments interact with genes to influence health across the lifespan. Free Continuing Medical Education credits available from the CDC (http://coeh.berkeley.edu/ucpehsu/soh.html)
- *Little Things Matter*. Video illustrates key concepts in children's environmental health in multiple languages (https://www.youtube.com/channel/UCblp9EePwfR8doGm9JbJOjA/videos).

*Air*

- California (http://www.arb.ca.gov/homepage.htm) and US EPA (http://www2.epa.gov/learn-issues/learn-about-air and http://www.epa.gov/air/peg/reduce.html) provide Web-based information on how regulatory efforts have reduced exposures and ways individuals can reduce pollution, primarily applicable to the developed world (http://www.arb.ca.gov/html/cando.htm); The WHO also has information on reducing air pollution (http://www.who.int/mediacentre/factsheets/fs313/en/)
- The Global Alliance for Clean Cookstoves is working to overcome the market barriers that currently impede the production, deployment, and use of clean cookstoves in developing countries (http://cleancookstoves.org).

*Pesticides*

- Guide to management of acute pesticide poisoning from the US EPA (http://www2.epa.gov/pesticide-worker-safety/recognition-and-management-pesticide-poisonings)
- *International Tools for Preventing Local Pesticide Problems: A Consolidated Guide to Chemical Codes and Conventions*. Editors, Goldenman G and Vera EP.
- European Center on Sustainable Policies for Human and Environmental Rights (http://www.pan-uk.org/publications/guide-to-the-chemical-codes-conventions)
- Information on obsolete pesticide management
  - The Food and Agriculture Organization of the United Nations (http://www.fao.org/agriculture/crops/obsolete-pesticides/prevention-and-disposal-of-obsolete-pesticides/en/)
  - Obsolete Pesticides works in Eastern Europe to Central Asia. The Web-site has information about other groups working in different parts of the world (https://obsoletepesticides.net/site/).

*Lead*

- Brief fact sheet, *Recommendations on Medical Management of Childhood Lead Exposure and Poisoning*, including low level exposure (http://www.pehsu.net/documents/medical-mgmnt-childhood-lead-exposure-June-2013.pdf)
- *Guidelines for the Identification and Management of Lead Exposure in Pregnant and Lactating Women* from the CDC (http://www.cdc.gov/nceh/lead/publications/leadandpregnancy2010.pdf).

*Climate change*

- WHO has many programs and an extensive set of resources (http://www.who.int/globalchange/environment/en/)
- *California's Climate Action Plan: Integrating Public Health into Climate Action Planning* provides background on public health and climate change, as well as model state and local activities addressing climate mitigation and adaptation (http://www.cdph.ca.gov/programs/CCDPHP/Documents/CAPS_and_Health_Published3-22-12.pdf)
- *The Challenges of Climate Change: Children on the Front Line*. Summary of climate impacts on children with a global perspective (http://www.unicef-irc.org/publications/pdf/ccc_final_2014.pdf).

*Water*

- Swiss Federal Institute of Aquatic Sciences and Technology and a nongovernmental organization (NGO) Helvetas Swiss Intercooperation provide technical and project management support for SODIS projects in 25 countries (http://www.sodis.ch/methode/index_EN)

- The US EPA provides information about contaminants in drinking water and drinking water regulations (http://water.epa.gov/drink/)

- The Natural Capital Project develops scientifically rigorous approaches worldwide to incorporate the value of nature into policy decisions; the Resource Investment Optimization System (RIOS) tool is used for watershed management (http://www.naturalcapitalproject.org/RIOS.html).

*E-waste*

- The NGO, Pure Earth, devises clean-up strategies, empowers local champions and secures support from national and international partnerships; 80 projects in 20 LMICs around the world are completed (http://www.pureearth.org).

mammals.[33] There are few epidemiologic studies of the health impacts of these chemicals (used in agriculture and as flea and tick pesticides for pets) on humans though limited evidence has suggested a possible impact on neurodevelopment.[34]

Pesticides may have developmental impacts via mechanisms distinct from their pesticidal action, as has been demonstrated for the organophosphate chlorpyrifos.[35]

Glyphosate, the herbicide with greatest use worldwide, was long considered a relatively innocuous pesticide. But in 2015, based on new evidence of carcinogenicity from both animal studies and epidemiologic investigations, the IARC identified glyphosate as "probably carcinogenic to humans."[36] Understanding of the health hazards associated with chemical exposures changes with evolving science.

In 2011, acute poisoning incidents from pesticides were responsible for more than 39,000 calls to poison centers in the United States.[37] An excellent manual, *Recognition and Management of Pesticide Poisonings*, is available from the US EPA online, in English and Spanish.[38] Low-dose exposures to certain pesticides during pregnancy and childhood are associated with increased risk for attention problems, lower intelligence quotient (IQ), behavioral changes, and pervasive developmental delay, altered brain architecture, asthma and respiratory symptoms, and childhood leukemia.

Though OP pesticides have largely been banned for residential use in the United States, they continue to be used in agriculture and their residues are found on food. Pesticide residues (eg, OPs and herbicides) on food contribute significantly to exposure in children, even those living in agricultural communities.[39] Consumption of fresh fruits and vegetables is a priority for children, thus selection of organic products should be weighed against their cost and availability. Nonetheless, the evidence of health effects from low-dose exposures to some pesticides indicates a need to reduce developmental exposure to pesticides as much as is practical. In 2012, 4.7% of imported and 0.9% of domestic foods sampled contained residues greater than allowable in the United States.[40] Some of the pesticides found on imported foods are not registered for use in the United States. Some products had high rates of unallowable residues. For example, more than 40% of imported Basmati rice was in violation. The Environmental Working Group uses federal agency data to determine fresh produce that has high (dirty dozen) and low (clean 15) pesticide loads.[41] Those concerned about exposure can use these aids in determining which produce might be preferable.

Residential use of pesticides is a major contributor to exposure. Integrated pest management (IPM) is an approach to minimizing pesticide use in residential, school, and agricultural settings. It integrates chemical and nonchemical methods to provide the least toxic control of pests. IPM has proven to be cost-effective and, at times, more effective at long-term control of pests while reducing pesticide exposure.[42,43] Unfortunately, adoption of IPM methods in LMICs has lagged behind that of HICs.[44]

Several billion pounds of pesticides are used annually worldwide, less than one-quarter of that in the United States.[45] The production and export of obsolete and persistent pesticides from developed to developing nations, though still a problem, has improved with international agreements and guidance.[46] These documents provide information and tools useful for health care workers in addressing public health and are well summarized in *International Tools for Preventing Local Pesticide Problems* (see **Box 1**).[47]

Whether in the United States or abroad, appropriate and safe use of pesticides depends on education and training of the workers or community members using them.[48] Children have been exposed when parents bring contaminated clothing home, use agricultural pesticides from work at home, use empty containers to hold water or food, and when children work in fields or apply pesticides. In many nations, pesticides are used in a setting of illiteracy and limited safety training.[49] Health care providers working in developing nations should be able to recognize and treat pesticide poisoning. They can provide education on the health effects of pesticides and how to prevent exposure. Sources such as *A Community Guide to Environmental Health* can help with simple low-literacy approaches to improving community health and can include pesticide education.[50] Both acute and chronic low-level exposures have resulted from misuse as well as careless use and accidents.[51] Contamination of water, soil, housing, and food with current and obsolete pesticides is not rare. Often, old obsolete pesticides have been stockpiled and inadequately stored (at times degrading to more hazardous material) in developing nations. Information on obsolete pesticide management is available from the United Nations and nongovernmental organizations (NGOs) such as ObsoletePesticides.net (see **Box 1**).

## METALS

Children are highly vulnerable to metals. Their unique patterns of exposure and developmentally determined susceptibilities make infants and children much more susceptible than adults to injury by toxic metals.

### Lead

Despite recent advances in prevention, acute and chronic lead poisoning remain problems of enormous importance for child health and development worldwide. Global consumption of lead is increasing today because of increasing demand for batteries and energy-efficient vehicles. An estimated 40% of the world's children have blood lead levels exceeding 5 µg/dL, 90% of whom live in developing nations.[52] In the United States, the CDC has reduced levels at which actions should be taken to 5 µg/dL and developed guidance for screening and treatment of pregnant and lactating women (see **Box 1**).

Patterns and sources of exposure to lead, prevalence rates of lead poisoning, and the severity of outcomes vary greatly (**Box 2**). Countries with strong prevention programs have imposed bans on certain uses of lead, have set environmental standards, and have deployed screening programs. Some countries have lead hot spots, such as battery recycling plants, smelters, refineries, mines, hazardous waste sites, and sites where waste is burned in the open.[53]

---

**Box 2**
**Sources of children's exposure to lead**

*The major current sources of children's exposure to lead are*

- Active industry, such as mining, smelting, and informal battery recycling
- Lead-based paints and pigments
- Lead solder in food cans
- Ceramic glazes
- Drinking-water systems with lead solder and lead pipes
- Products, such as herbal and traditional medicines, folk remedies, cosmetics, and toys
- Incineration of lead-containing waste
- Electronic waste (e-waste)
- Food chain and contaminated soil
- Contamination as a legacy of historical contamination from former industrial sites.[41]

---

Acute, symptomatic lead poisoning still occurs today in the United States but is most commonly detected in children in low-income countries and marginalized populations, or in children living in lead-polluted sites.

### Mercury

Mercury is a highly toxic metal. It occurs in the environment in several forms, of which methylmercury is the most hazardous. Methylmercury is a potent developmental neurotoxicant. Human exposure to methylmercury is of grave concern, especially exposures occurring during pregnancy. Methylmercury crosses the placenta, passes easily into the brains of fetuses and young children, and causes permanent injury to the developing human brain.[54]

Polluting industries are the main source of mercury emission to the environment and account for about 70% of the 5500 tons of mercury released around the world each year.[55] Four industries are especially problematic:

- Coal-burning electrical power plants, the major global source of mercury emission
- Waste incinerators, including hospital incinerators
- Chloralkali facilities that use metallic mercury as a catalyst to produce chlorine gas
- Artisanal gold mining that uses metallic mercury to form an amalgam to separate gold from ore.

Consumption of fish contaminated by methylmercury is the major route of human exposure. Mercury concentrates as it moves up the food chain to reach very high levels in the predatory fish at the top of the chain, such as yellowfin tuna, mackerel, and striped bass.[55] Fish are an important source of fatty acids and protein for many people. Despite mercury content, fish consumption has been shown to provide neurodevelopmental benefits. However, for each incremental benefit from consumption there is a decrease associated with any mercury content. With this in mind, reasonable advice is to encourage the consumption of fish but to choose those lower in mercury.[56] The US EPA and states provide guidelines as well as information about fishing advisories.

## Arsenic

Arsenic is a metalloid element that occurs naturally in the earth's crust. High concentrations are released into the environment by polluting industries. Worldwide, drinking water is the principal source of arsenic exposure, including in some areas of the United States, but inhalation can be an important exposure route for people living near smelters.

Inorganic arsenic is associated with several human cancers, including lung, bladder, and skin cancer.[52] Perinatal exposures to arsenic in drinking water have been linked to increases in late fetal, neonatal, and postneonatal mortality, as well as to neurodevelopmental abnormalities, adult cancers, and bronchiectasis.[57–60] The risks for lung and bladder cancer are 2 to 4 times greater for early life exposure than during later childhood or adulthood.[61]

## SPREAD OF TOXIC CHEMICALS TO DEVELOPING COUNTRIES

With globalization of trade and spread of the western life style, toxic chemicals that previously were found only in HICs have been entering LMICs with ever increasing rapidity.[62] The manufacture and use of chemicals are shifting to so-called pollution havens where labor costs are low and environmental and public health protections are often few.[63,64] Tragic episodes of environmental exposure to toxic chemicals include the Bhopal disaster in India in 1985 and the current exposure of more than 1 million persons in Asia and Sub-Saharan Africa to chrysotile asbestos.[65,66]

## E-Waste

The global movement of electronic waste (e-waste) from LMICs to HICs provides another example of poorly controlled and rapidly growing exposure to chemical contamination. More than 45 million tons of e-waste was generated globally in 2012.[67] In LMICs, recycling of valuable compounds from e-waste, such as copper and gold, has evolved into an important industry.

E-waste contains many hazardous chemicals, including lead, cadmium, mercury, nickel, barium, and lithium, as well as persistent organic pollutants, such as polychlorinated biphenyls (PCBs) and brominated flame retardants.[67] Unsafe recycling activities, such as open burning of e-waste, produce toxic combustion products including dioxin-like PCBs and polychlorinated dibenzo-dioxins and -furans (PCDD/Fs).[68]

E-waste may pose significant health risks to children, especially child workers in the recycling industry. Children at e-waste sites have been reported to display elevated levels of multiple toxic chemicals, including lead, nickel, manganese, and chromium.[69] The Basel Convention, an international treaty, restricts transfer of hazardous waste between countries but the United States has not ratified this 1989 treaty. Various governmental entities and NGOs work with poor communities around the world by evaluating and remediating toxic contamination. These organizations are resources for clinicians working with contaminated communities (see **Box 1**).

## CLIMATE CHANGE

The concept of "our shrinking globe" may be best illustrated by climate change. The impacts will be most fully experienced by children and people in poverty. The Save the Children Fund has estimated that as many as 175 million children will experience climate-related disasters each year during this decade.[70] Those who have underlying health conditions and limited access to essentials necessary for life will be least resilient. Already one-third of the global disease burden of children younger than 5 years of age is attributable to maternal and child malnutrition.[71] The health care community has a critical role to play in addressing climate change, adding credibility, and explaining the connections between emerging threats and health.

The impacts on health can be divided into direct and indirect effects (**Table 3**). Sustained high temperatures, air pollution, infectious diseases, and extreme weather and natural disasters will directly affect health. Climate change will also affect agriculture, access to clean water, social unrest, and migration, all of which, in turn, may endanger child health and welfare. For example, increasing carbon dioxide concentrations result in declines in the protein, iron, and zinc content of staple $C_3$ (carbon fixation) grains and legumes such as wheat, rice, soybeans, and peas (but not $C_4$ crops such as corn).[72] An estimated 2 billion people (including children) already suffer from deficiencies of zinc and iron with a resulting estimated 63 million life-years lost annually. This can be expected to increase significantly as food quality and yields decline. Indirect effects may be cascading. The incidence of preeclampsia in Bangladesh has been associated with rising salinity of drinking water as a result of seawater intrusion into groundwater.[73] Seawater intrusion is expected to be a problem of coastal areas around the world as a result of climate change.

Climate change mitigation includes altering factors (eg, greenhouse gas emissions, black carbon) associated with climate change and ecosystem degradation. Adaptation strategies aim to make changes that will moderate harm and exploit beneficial opportunities under changing conditions. An example of the range of local responses possible is found in *Climate Action for Health: Integrating Public Health into Climate Action Planning*, from the California Department of Public Health (see **Box 1**). Many programs reduce emissions and also have co-benefits that improve health immediately. Encouraging and designing for active transport (eg, walking, biking, public transport) reduces emissions and increases exercise. Thus, active transport programs will both reduce greenhouse gas production and benefit health by reducing air pollutants, obesity, and cardiovascular disease.

The WHO has many programs addressing climate change and human health, including programs on climate adaptation in LMICs. An example is the project in

**Table 3**
**Direct and indirect effects of climate change**

| Direct Impacts | Indirect Impacts |
|---|---|
| Heat Stress <br> • Premature delivery <br> • Dehydration, hyperthermia | Water Security <br> • Need for increasing agriculture production despite current overuse |
| Air Pollution and Increase in Allergens <br> • Asthma <br> • Exacerbation other lung disease <br> • Impaired lung development | Malnutrition <br> • Shortage in supply, decreases in food quality or protein content of staple grains and legumes |
| Infectious Disease <br> • Vector borne disease (eg, malaria, West Nile, viral encephalitides, dengue) <br> • Diarrheal illnesses | Population Displacement <br> • Malnutrition <br> • Psychosocial stress <br> • Armed conflict, societal breakdown <br> • Increases in child abuse/neglect |
| Extreme Weather Events <br> • Heavy precipitation and flood, drought, hurricanes, monsoons, heat waves | Unexpected impacts for which the understanding is now evolving (eg, preeclampsia from increased water salinity) |

Barbados, already designated a water-scarce nation.[74] Sea level rise is expected to exacerbate this condition with saltwater intrusion into the water supply. In addition, they have the highest rate of dengue fever in the Americas. The program has 2 goals: use treated wastewater to recharge the aquifer and to improve rainwater storage to decrease dengue transmission while still capturing this vital resource. Physicians working in or collaborating with an LMIC should look for opportunities to improve immediate and long-term health through encouraging climate adaptation programs and associated co-benefits.

## THE HIGH COSTS OF CHEMICAL POLLUTION

Cost is an inevitable, but often overlooked and undercounted, consequence of environmental pollution.[75] A recent estimate of the costs of environmental pollution in American children found that lead poisoning, prenatal methylmercury exposure, childhood cancer, asthma, intellectual disability, autism, and attention deficit hyperactivity disorder of environmental origin costs the United States $76.6 billion each year.[76] The costs of pollution are both direct and indirect and can blunt the trajectory of economic productivity and national development (**Box 3**).

## FUTURE RESEARCH NEEDS

Research to better define the impacts of the environment on children's health is urgently needed in several areas. Etiologic research is one great need. Research is limited on the complex mechanisms involved in environmentally induced diseases.[77] The mechanisms of toxic chemicals vary widely and include binding to cellular macromolecules resulting in dysfunctional proteins and DNA damage, induction of reactive oxygen and nitrogen species, and epigenetic alterations. Interactions among chemicals and other environmental stressors and age-specific physiologic sensitivities influence toxic response. Cellular response to toxic insult may result in an inflammatory cascade, alterations in energy production, DNA damage repair, and changes in gene expression from epigenetic changes.[78,79] Because mitochondria play a vital

---

**Box 3**
**The costs of pollution**

- Direct medical costs.

- Indirect health-related costs: These costs include time lost from school and work, costs of rehabilitation, and costs of special education.

- Costs to health systems: Diseases caused by environmental pollution impose a heavy and unnecessary load on health care delivery systems particularly in poor countries that already are facing a human resources crisis in health sector. These diseases increase needs for health care staff, divert resources from other essential programs, and thus undercut efforts to advance development and improve health.

- Opportunity costs resulting from diminished economic productivity: In the United States, widespread low-grade lead poisoning is estimated to have resulted in a downward shift in societal mean IQ of about 5 points in the 1970s. This would reduce the number of people with gifted IQ levels (potential leaders) by about 50% and increase scores less than 70 by more than 50%. This increase in low IQ levels will impose a lifelong human and economic burden on societies.[39] Such widespread cognitive impairment can reduce the lifelong economic productivity of entire generations and blunt the trajectory of national development (see *Little Things Matter*, video listed in resources box).

role in cellular energy homeostasis, epigenetic regulation, and DNA damage repair, experts in the field have recommended future research in environmental mitochondriomics in children's environmental health.[78,79] Studies are needed to elucidate mechanisms of toxicity, interactions among environmental stressors, and also to link children's environmental exposures and health outcomes.[80] Public health research is another need. In many countries, basic systems for measuring environmental exposures, such as levels of air pollutants, and for counting the number of cases of disease caused by environmental contamination, are lacking and need to be put in place. Systematic information is needed also on the types and quantities of hazardous materials, such as asbestos and highly hazardous pesticides that are imported into countries around the world. This information is critical for defining environmental threats to children's health and for setting public health and pediatric priorities.

## SUMMARY

Environmental pollution is a major problem in countries around the world today. In this interconnected world, pollution in other countries can directly (by virtue of adoption, travel, and migration) or indirectly (by movement of products and pollution around the world) affect the health of children in distant parts of the globe. Alert pediatricians who obtain a brief history of environmental exposure have the opportunity to discover new links between environmental pollution and disease in children. Clinicians and educators involved in global health have the opportunity to address environmental health issues and can do so with the aid of many organizations working on these issues worldwide.

## REFERENCES

1. U.S. Census Bureau, International Database. Available at: https://www.census.gov/population/international/data/idb/worldpopgraph.php. Accessed June 15, 2015.
2. United Nations. World Urbanization Prospects, 2014 Revision. Available at: http://esa.un.org/unpd/wup/Highlights/WUP2014-Highlights.pdf. Accessed June 15, 2015.
3. Landrigan PJ, Fuller R. Environmental pollution: an enormous and invisible burden on health systems in low- and middle-income countries. World Hosp Health Serv 2014;50(4):35–40.
4. Barreto SM, Miranda JJ, Figueroa JP, et al. Epidemiology in Latin America and the Caribbean: current situation and challenges. Int J Epidemiol 2012;41:557–71.
5. Pan American Health Organization. The environment and human security. In: Health in the Americas. Available at: http://www.paho.org/saludenlasamericas/index.php?option=com_content&view=article&id=56&Itemid=52&lang=en. Accessed June 15, 2015.
6. World Health Organization (WHO). Preventing disease through healthy environments: Toward an estimate of the environmental burden of disease. Pruss-Ustun A, Corvalan C. 2006. Available at: http://www.who.int/quantifying_ehimpacts/publications/preventingdisease.pdf. Accessed June 16, 2015.
7. World Health Organization global health observatory data repository. Geneva (Switerland): WHO; 2015. Available at: http://www.who.int/gho/en/. Accessed June 8, 2015.
8. Saper RB, Phillips RS, Sehgal A, et al. Lead, mercury, and arsenic in US- and Indian-manufactured Ayurvedic medicines sold via the internet. JAMA 2008;300(8):915–23.

9. Davis D, Bell M, Fletcher T. A look back at the London Smog of 1952 and the half century since. Environ Health Perspect 2002;110(12):A734–5.

10. USEPA. Integrated science assessment for particulate matter. Washington, DC: U.S. Environmental Protection Agency; 2009. Available at: http://cfpub.epa.gov/ncea/cfm/recordisplay.cfm?deid=216546#Download. Accessed May 16, 2015.

11. Backes CH, Nelin T, Gore MW, et al. Early life exposure to air pollution: how bad is it? Toxicol Lett 2013;216(1):47–53.

12. Padula AM, Tagor IB, Carmichael SL, et al. Ambient air pollution and traffic exposures and congenital heart defects in the San Joaquin Valley of California. Paediatr Perinat Epidemiol 2013;27(4):329–39.

13. Scheers H, Mwalili SM, Faes C, et al. Does air pollution trigger infant mortality in Western Europe? A case-crossover study. Environ Health Perspect 2011;119: 1017–22.

14. Chen Z, Salam MT, Eckel SP, et al. Chronic effects of air pollution on respiratory health in Southern California children: findings from the Southern California Children's Health Study. J Thorac Dis 2015;7:46–58.

15. Schunemann HJ, Dorn J, Grant BJ, et al. Pulmonary function is a long-term predictor of mortality in the general population: 29-year follow-up of the Buffalo Health Study. Chest 2000;118:656–64.

16. Boothe VL, Boehmer TK, Wendel AM, et al. Residential traffic exposure and childhood leukemia a systematic review and meta-analysis. Am J Prev Med 2014; 46(4):413–22.

17. Heck JE, Wu J, Lombardi C, et al. Childhood cancer and traffic-related air pollution exposure in pregnancy and early life. Environ Health Perspect 2013;121: 1385–91.

18. International Agency for Research on Cancer. Scientific Publication No.61 Air Pollution and Cancer. 2014. Available at: http://www.iarc.fr/en/publications/books/sp161/index.php. Accessed June 16, 2015.

19. Jedrychowski WA, Perera FP, Camann D, et al. Prenatal exposure to polycyclic aromatic hydrocarbons and cognitive dysfunction in children. Environ Sci Pollut Res 2015;22:3631–9.

20. Lin CC, Yang SK, Lin KC, et al. Multilevel analysis of air pollution and early childhood neurobehavioral development. Int J Environ Res Public Health 2014;11: 6827–41.

21. Gauderman WJ, Urman R, Avol E, et al. Association of improved air quality with lung development in children. N Engl J Med 2015;372:905–13.

22. National Academy of Sciences. Global sources of local pollution: an assessment of long-range transport of key air pollutants to and from the United States. Washington, DC: National Academies Press; 2009.

23. WHO. World Health Organization Health Topics. Ambient (outdoor) Air Pollution. 2014. Available at: http://www.who.int/topics/air_pollution/en/. Accessed June 16, 2015.

24. WHO. World Health Organization. Ambient (outdoor) Air Pollution in Cities Database, 2014. 2014. Available at: http://www.who.int/phe/health_topics/outdoorair/databases/cities/en/. Accessed June 16, 2015.

25. World Health Organization. Burden of Disease for Household Air Pollution from 2012. Available at: http://www.who.int/phe/health_topics/outdoorair/databases/FINAL_HAP_AAP_BoD_24March2014.pdf?ua=1. Accessed June 16, 2015.

26. National Institute of Environmental Health Sciences. Cookstoves and Indoor Air. Available at: http://www.niehs.nih.gov/research/programs/geh/cookstoves/. Accessed June 9, 2015.

27. Global Alliance for Clean Cookstoves Factsheet. Available at: http://www.niehs.nih. gov/research/programs/geh/cookstoves/global_alliance_for_clean_cookstoves_fact_sheet_508.pdf. Accessed June 9, 2015.
28. Pires M. Watershed protection for a world city: the case of New York. Land Use Policy 2004;21:161–75.
29. McGuigan KG, Conroy RM, Mosler HJ, et al. Solar water disinfection (SODIS): a review from bench-top to roof-top. J Hazard Mater 2012;235-236:29–46.
30. CDC Solar Disinfection. Available at: http://www.cdc.gov/safewater/ solardisinfection.html. Accessed June 13, 2015.
31. Saillenfait A, Ndiaye D, Sabate J. Pyrethroids: exposure and health effects—an update. Int J Hyg Environ Health 2015;218(3):281–92.
32. Shelton JF, Geraghty EM, Tancredi DJ, et al. Neurodevelopmental disorders and prenatal residential proximity to agricultural pesticides: the CHARGE study. Environ Health Perspect 2015;122:1103–9.
33. Casida JE, Durkin KA. Neuroactive insecticides: targets, selectivity, resistance and secondary effects. Annu Rev Entomol 2013;58:99–117.
34. Keil AP, Daniels JL, Hertz-Picciotto I. Autism spectrum disorder, flea and tick medication, and adjustments for exposure misclassification: the CHARGE (Childhood Autism Risks from Genetics and Environment) case –control study. Environ Health 2014;13:3.
35. Adigun AA. Organophosphate exposure during a critical developmental stage reprograms adenylyl cyclase signaling in PC12 cells. Brain Res 2010;1329: 36–44.
36. Guyton KZ, Loomis D, Grosse Y, et al. Carcinogenicity of tetrachlorvinphos, parathion, malathion, diazinon, and glyphosate. Lancet Oncol 2015;16(5): 490–1.
37. Bronstein AC, Spyker DA, Cantilena LR, et al. 2011 annual report of the American Association of Poison Control Centers' National Poison Data System (NPDS): 29th annual report. Clin Toxicol (Phila) 2012;50:911–1164.
38. Reigart JR, Roberts JR, United States Environmental Protection Agency. Recognition and management of pesticide poisonings. 6th edition. Washington, DC: U.S. Environmental Protection Agency; 2013. Available at: http://www2.epa. gov/pesticide-worker-safety/recognition-and-management-pesticide-poisonings. Accessed June 15, 2015.
39. Bradman A, Quiros-Alcala L, Castorina R, et al. Effect of organic diet intervention on pesticide exposures in young children living in low-income urban and agricultural communities. Environ Health Perspect 2015. http://dx.doi.org/10.1289/ehp. 1408660.
40. US Food and Drug Administration. FDA Pesticide Monitoring Program – Fiscal Year 2012 Pesticide Report. Available at: http://www.fda.gov/downloads/Food/ FoodborneIllnessContaminants/Pesticides/UCM432758.pdf Accessed May 11, 2015.
41. Environmental Working Group. 2015 Shopper's Guide to Pesticides in Produce. Available at: http://www.ewg.org/foodnews/summary.php. Accessed June 9, 2015.
42. Williams MK, Barr DB, Camann DE, et al. An intervention to reduce residential insecticide exposure during pregnancy among an inner-city cohort. Environ Health Perspect 2006;114:1684–9.
43. Brenner B, Markowitz S, Rivera M, et al. Integrated pest management in an urban community: a successful partnership for prevention. Environ Health Perspect 2003;111:1649–53.

44. Parsa S, Morse S, Bonifacio A, et al. Obstacles to integrated pest management adoption in developing countries. Proc Natl Acad Sci U S A 2014;111(10): 3889–94.

45. US EPA. Pesticides Industry Sales and Usage: 2006 and 2007 Market Estimates. 2011. Washington, DC. Available at: http://www.epa.gov/opp00001/pestsales/07pestsales/table_of_contents2007.htm. Accessed June 15, 2015.

46. Food and Agriculture Organization of the United Nations. International Code of Conduct on the Distribution and Use of Pesticides. Rome, 2003. Available at: http://www.fao.org/docrep/005/Y4544E/Y4544E00.HTM. Accessed June 15, 2015.

47. International Tools for preventing local pesticide problems: a consolidated guide to chemical codes and conventions. In: Goldenman G, Vera EP (editor). European Centre on Sustainable Policies for Human and Environmental Rights. Available at: http://www.pan-uk.org/publications/guide-to-the-chemical-codes-conventions. Accessed June 15, 2015.

48. WHO. Childhood Pesticide Poisoning Information for Advocacy and Action United Nations Environment Programme. May 2004. Available at: http://www.who.int/ceh/publications/pestipoison/en/. Accessed June 11, 2015.

49. Naidoo S, London L, Burdorf A, et al. Pesticide safety training and practices in women working in small-scale agriculture in South Africa. Occup Environ Med 2010;67:823e828.

50. Conant J, Fadem PA. A community guide to environmental health. Berkeley (CA): Hesperian Foundation; 2004.

51. United Nations. Childhood Pesticide Poisoning Information for Advocacy and Action United Nations Environment Programme May 2004. Available at: http://www.who.int/ceh/publications/pestipoison/en/. Accessed June 9, 2015.

52. Fewtrell LJ, Prüss-Ustün A, Landrigan P, et al. Estimating the global burden of disease of mild mental retardation and cardiovascular diseases from environmental lead exposure. Environ Res 2004;94:120–33.

53. WHO (World health Organization). Childhood lead poisoning. Geneva (Switerland): WHO; 2010.

54. Kjellstrom T, Kennedy P, Wallis S, et al. Physical and mental development of children with prenatal exposure to mercury from fish. Stage II: interviews and psychological tests at age 6. Solna (Sweden): National Swedish Environmental Protection Board; 1989. Report 3642.

55. National Research Council. Toxicological effects of methylmercury. Washington, DC: National Academy Press; 2000.

56. Oken E, Choi AL, Karagas MR, et al. Which fish should I eat? Perspectives influencing fish consumption choices. Environ Health Perspect 2012;120: 790–8.

57. Hopenhayn-Rich C, Browning SR, Hertz-Picciotto I, et al. Chronic arsenic exposure and risk of infant mortality in two areas of Chile. Environ Health Perspect 2000;108:667–73.

58. von Ehrenstein OS, Poddar S, Yuan Y, et al. Children's intellectual function in relation to arsenic exposure. Epidemiology 2007;18:44–51.

59. Wasserman GA, Liu X, Parvez F, et al. Water arsenic exposure and children's intellectual function in Araihazar, Bangladesh. Environ Health Perspect 2004;12: 1329–33.

60. Smith AH, Marshall G, Liaw J, et al. Mortality in young adults following in utero and childhood exposure to arsenic in drinking water. Environ Health Perspect 2012;120:1527–31.

61. Steinmaus C, Ferreeccio C, Acevedo J, et al. Increased lung and bladder cancer incidence in adults after in utero and early-life arsenic exposure. Cancer Epidemiol Biomarkers Prev 2014;23(8):1529–38.

62. Spitz P. Chemical industry at the millennium: maturity, restructuring and globalization. Philadelphia: Chemical Heritage Foundation; 2003.

63. Cole MA, Elliott RJR, Okubo T. Trade, environmental regulations, and industrial mobility: an industry-level study of Japan. Ecological Economics 2010;69:1995–2002.

64. Kearsley A, Riddel M. A further inquiry into the *pollution haven hypothesis and the environmental Kuznets curve.* Ecological Economics 2010;69:905–19.

65. Dhara VR, Dhara R, Acquilla SD, et al. Personal exposure and long-term health effects in survivors of the union carbide disaster at Bhopal. Environ Health Perspect 2002;110:487–500.

66. Frank A, Joshi TK. The global spread of asbestos. Ann Glob Health 2014;80(4):257–62.

67. Lundgren K. The global impact of e-waste: addressing the challenge. Geneva (Switerland): Programme on Safety and Health at Work and the Environment (SafeWork), Sectoral Activities Department (SECTOR) International Labour Office; 2012. Available at: http://www.ilo.org/sector/Resources/publications/WCMS_196105/lang-en/index.htm. Accessed June 10, 2015.

68. Frazzoli CO, Orisakewe OE, Dragone R, et al. Diagnostic health risk assessment of electronic waste on the general population in developing countries scenarios. Environ Impact Assess Rev 2010;30:388–99.

69. Zheng G, Xu X, Li B, et al. Association between lung function in school children and exposure to three transition metals from an e-waste recycling area. J Expo Sci Environ Epidemiol 2013;23:67–72.

70. UNICEF Office of Research. 'The challenges of climate change: children on the front line', innocenti insight. Florence (Italy): UNICEF Office of Research; 2014.

71. Black RE, Allen LH, Bhutta ZA, et al. Maternal and child undernutrition: global and regional exposures and health consequences. Lancet 2008;371:243–60.

72. Myers SS, Zanobetti A, Kloog I, et al. Increasing CO2 threatens human nutrition. Nature 2014;510(7503):139–42.

73. Khan AE, Scheelbeek PFD, Shilpi AB, et al. Salinity in drinking water and the risk of (pre)eclampsia and gestational hypertension in coastal Bangladesh: a case-control study. PLoS One 2014;9(9):e108715.

74. WHO. Climate Change Adaptation to Protect Human Health, Barbados Project Profile. Available at: http://www.who.int/globalchange/projects/adaptation/en/index1.html. Accessed May 20, 2015.

75. Grosse SD, Matte T, Schwartz J, et al. Economic gains resulting from the reduction in children's blood lead in the United States. Environ Health Perspect 2002;110:721–8.

76. Trasande L, Liu Y. Reducing the staggering costs of environmental disease in children, estimated at $76.6 billion in 2008. Health Aff (Millwood) 2011;30:863–70.

77. Brunst KJ, Baccarelli AA, Wright RJ. Integrating mitochondriomics in children's environmental health. J Appl Toxicol 2015;35(9):976–91.

78. Byun HM, Baccarelli AA. Environmental exposure and mitochondrial epigenetics: study design and analytical challenges. Hum Genet 2014;133(3):247–57.

79. Shaughnessy DT, McAllister K, Worth L. Mitochondria, energetics, epigenetics, and cellular response to stress. Environ Health Perspect 2014;122:1271–8.

80. Vanos JK. Children's health and vulnerability in outdoor microclimates: a comprehensive review. Environ Int 2015;76:1–15.

# Our Shrinking Globe
## Implications for Child Unintentional Injuries

Olakunle Alonge, MBBS, MPH, PhD[a],*, Uzma R. Khan, MBBS, MSc[b],
Adnan A. Hyder, MD, MPH, PhD[a]

KEYWORDS

- Unintentional injuries • Children • Low- and middle-income countries
- Road transport injuries • Globalization

KEY POINTS

- Unintentional injuries are a major global health problem resulting in high morbidity and mortality among children of all ages.
- The burden of preventable childhood unintentional injuries is disproportionately borne by low- and middle-income countries (LMIC).
- Drowning and road transport injuries account for most unintentional injuries deaths for children.
- Globalization creates inequalities in the distribution of economic gains, risks, and opportunities for preventing child unintentional injuries between high-income countries and LMIC.
- Key strategies for injury prevention in LMIC in a globalized economy include advocacy, extending complex international laws that protect free market to ensure and enforce safety standards, improved surveillance, human resource capacity building, and further research on evidence-based interventions.
- Pediatricians should include unintentional injury prevention counseling as part of routine anticipatory guidance for infants, children, and adolescents.

## INTRODUCTION

Unintentional injuries are a leading cause of death for children of all ages. Globally, they accounted for 15.4% of about 2.6 million deaths recorded among children aged 1 to 14 years in 2013.[1] Although proportionate child mortality due to unintentional

[a] International Injury Research Unit, Department of International Health, Johns Hopkins University Bloomberg School of Public Health, 615 N Wolfe Street E8622, Baltimore, MD 21205, USA; [b] Department of Emergency Medicine, Aga Khan University, Stadium Road, Karachi 74800, Pakistan
* Corresponding author.
*E-mail address:* oalonge1@jhu.edu

Pediatr Clin N Am 63 (2016) 167–181
http://dx.doi.org/10.1016/j.pcl.2015.08.009 **pediatric.theclinics.com**

injuries is higher among high-income countries (HIC), the absolute count of death and mortalities due to unintentional injuries are higher in low- and middle-income countries (LMIC).[2] Hence, unintentional injuries kill more children and at a faster rate in LMIC relative to HIC. The term unintentional injuries in this context is defined as injury or poisoning that is not inflicted by deliberate means,[2] whereas injury itself is defined as "the physical damage that results when a human body is suddenly subjected to energy in amounts that exceed the threshold of physiologic tolerance—or else the result of a lack of one or more vital elements, such as oxygen."[3]

The risks of unintentional injuries among children are mainly defined by individual factors (behaviors and attributes), presence or absence of supervision and safety equipment, vehicle safety, as well as other factors within a child's social and physical environment.[4] These additional factors are not static and change over time because of multiple reasons. Globalization, defined as "a process of greater integration within the world economy through movements of goods and services, capital, technology and (to a lesser extent) labor, which lead increasingly to economic decisions being influenced by global conditions,"[5] cause significant environmental and behavioral changes among populations.[6] These changes have implications for the distribution of risk factors and preventative strategies for child unintentional injuries especially in LMIC.[4]

The goal of this article is to highlight the implications of globalization for child unintentional injury causation and prevention in LMIC. First, the article describes the burden of child unintentional injuries using the most recent global burden of disease data, highlighting the countries with the highest death count and mortalities due to child unintentional injuries in 2013. Second, the article describes the risk factors and preventative strategies for the leading injury mechanisms of child unintentional injury deaths. Third, the article presents a framework showing key manifestations of globalization and describes the positive and negative consequences of these features on the risk factors and prevention of child unintentional injuries in LMIC. Finally, the article suggests pathways for harnessing the positive consequences of globalization in reducing the burden of child unintentional injuries in LMIC.

## GLOBAL BURDEN OF CHILD UNINTENTIONAL INJURIES

Using the 2013 global burden of disease data,[1] the absolute death count and mortality for unintentional injuries[a] among children aged 1 to 14 years[b] were estimated and ranked for all countries (**Table 1**).[2,7] The 12 countries in **Table 1** account for 58% of the estimated 406,442 deaths due to unintentional injuries recorded among children aged 1 to 14 years globally in 2013. It is important to note that of these 12 countries, 8 are middle-income economies,[8] 2 (Equatorial Guinea and Russian Federation) are HIC, and 2 (Bangladesh and Afghanistan) are low-income economies. India has the highest absolute death count of 74,612, whereas Equatorial Guinea with 86.9 deaths

---

[a] Unintentional injuries include injury from the following mechanisms: road transport injury (pedestrian road injury, bicycle road injury, 2-wheel road injury, 4-wheel road injury, other road injury); other transport injury; falls; drowning; fire/burns; poisonings; exposure to firearm (accidental discharge); exposure to other mechanical forces (sharp objects, machine); adverse medical treatment (injuries from error in medical and surgical procedures).[2]

[b] Children are typically defined as individuals less than 18 years of age. However, because most global burden of disease data lumps individuals within ages 15 and 18 years into older age groups, the authors decided to restrict the analysis to those less than 15 years. Also, the proportionate mortality due to injuries among children 0 to 11 months is less than 2.5%.[2] Hence, this age group was also excluded from the analysis.

**Table 1**
Countries with the highest burden of unintentional injuries for children aged 1 to 14 years in 2013

| World Health Organization Region | Countries | Population | Absolute Count of Deaths Due Unintentional Injuries | Unintentional Injuries Mortality Rates/100,000 Population |
|---|---|---|---|---|
| Highest burden for unintentional injuries by absolute death count | | | | |
| Africa | Nigeria | 70,000,000 | 52,359 | 74.8 |
| South-East Asia | India | 339,500,000 | 74,612 | 22.0 |
| Europe | Russia | 20,303,452 | 3464 | 17.1 |
| Eastern Mediterranean | Pakistan | 57,200,000 | 17,512 | 30.6 |
| Western Pacific | China | 231,200,000 | 52,811 | 22.8 |
| Americas | Brazil | 45,400,000 | 4846 | 10.7 |
| Highest burden for unintentional injuries by mortalities | | | | |
| Africa | Equatorial Guinea | 271,641 | 236 | 86.9 |
| South-East Asia | Bangladesh | 43,900,000 | 15,838 | 36.1 |
| Europe | Turkmenistan | 1,404,346 | 485 | 34.5 |
| Eastern Mediterranean | Afghanistan | 13,287,813 | 9797 | 73.7 |
| Western Pacific | Mongolia | 706,954 | 298 | 42.2 |
| Americas | Bolivia | 3,467,534 | 1742 | 50.2 |

per 100,000 populations has the highest mortality. In general, these unintentional injury mortalities in each of the 12 countries are higher compared with the global average of 16.1 deaths per 100,000 (except in Brazil) (see **Table 1**).

Unintentional injuries account for more than 10% of all deaths among children aged 1 to 14 years for each of the 12 countries in 2013 (**Table 2**). The proportionate mortality ranges from 11% in Nigeria to as high as 49% in China and 48% in Russia. Globally, in 2013, most unintentional injuries deaths for children 1 to 14 years result from drowning (31%) and road transport injuries (RTI) (29%). These results are also the leading mechanisms for unintentional injuries deaths in each of the 12 countries. It is important to highlight the significance of drowning as a leading mechanism of death from unintentional injuries among children aged 1 to 14 years; when older children aged 15 to 19 years are included in the age category, RTI is often the leading mechanism.[2]

Globally, children aged 1 to 4 years have the highest all-cause and cause-specific mortalities for each of the leading injury mechanisms (**Table 3**). Both all-cause and cause-specific mortalities decline with age group for each of the leading injury mechanisms.

## RISK FACTORS AND PREVENTIVE STRATEGIES FOR CHILD UNINTENTIONAL INJURIES

Using a framework informed by the Haddon matrix for injury prevention,[9] the major risk factors for child unintentional injuries are summarized by injury mechanisms under 4 main categories: individual factors, vehicle/safety equipment, and the social and physical environment (**Table 4**).

Irrespective of the injury mechanism, being a male child, the young age of children related to cognitive and motor development, and lack of adequate supervision all play

**Table 2**
Proportionate mortality of deaths due to unintentional injuries by injury mechanisms for children aged 1 to 14 years for countries with the highest burden in 2013

| Country | All-Cause Death (n) | Proportionate Mortality Due to Unintentional Injuries (%) | % of RTI in Unintentional Injuries | % of Drowning in Unintentional Injuries | % of Burns in Unintentional Injuries | % of Falls in Unintentional Injuries | % of Poisoning in Unintentional Injuries |
|---|---|---|---|---|---|---|---|
| All | 2,639,232 | 15.4 | 29.2 | 31.5 | 8.3 | 6.8 | 2.8 |
| Nigeria | 468,818 | 11.2 | 50 | 12.1 | 8 | 6.5 | 3.7 |
| Equatorial Guinea | 1258 | 18.8 | 35.3 | 20.4 | 10.7 | 4.9 | 2.5 |
| India | 444,608 | 16.8 | 13.6 | 32.7 | 12.1 | 9.4 | 1.1 |
| Bangladesh | 42,457 | 37.3 | 5.3 | 82.3 | 0.8 | 4.4 | 0.2 |
| Russia | 7154 | 48.4 | 24.8 | 32.1 | 11.3 | 6.8 | 7.8 |
| Turkmenistan | 1913 | 25.3 | 15.8 | 51.7 | 12.7 | 4.9 | 2.4 |
| Pakistan | 106,768 | 16.4 | 18.8 | 28.3 | 9.0 | 7.6 | 10.3 |
| Afghanistan | 39,306 | 24.9 | 22.5 | 27 | 4.8 | 18.7 | 2.2 |
| China | 105,940 | 49.9 | 29 | 44.1 | 1.9 | 7.8 | 3.8 |
| Mongolia | 933 | 31.9 | 26.6 | 26.2 | 19.2 | 5.1 | 7.6 |
| Brazil | 15,517 | 31.2 | 45.3 | 29.7 | 3.6 | 4.6 | 0.5 |
| Bolivia | 4005 | 43.5 | 29.3 | 20.8 | 2.8 | 1.6 | 1.6 |
| USA | 10,026 | 38.9 | 44.6 | 20.8 | 11.8 | 2.5 | 1.2 |

**Table 3**
**Age-specific and cause-specific injury mortality per 100,000 populations in 2013**

| Global, y | All Unintentional Injuries Rate/ 100,000 | RTI Rate/ 100,000 | Drowning Rate/ 100,000 | Burns Rate/ 100,000 | Falls Rate/ 100,000 | Poisoning Rate/ 100,000 |
|---|---|---|---|---|---|---|
| 1–4 | 41.3 | 10.0 | 13.8 | 4.4 | 2.9 | 1.5 |
| 5–9 | 17.0 | 5.9 | 5.1 | 1.1 | 1.1 | 0.3 |
| 10–14 | 14.3 | 5.0 | 4.1 | 0.7 | 1.0 | 0.3 |

a determining role for unintentional injury events among young children.[4] It is important to recognize that most injury events among young children occur within the home settings[4]; hence, socioeconomic factors, including income and maternal education affecting choices in the home physical environment and the social living conditions of children, have important significance for child injury prevention.[4] Specific issues, such as child labor (eg, children working in agriculture and farming settings), work camps for the manufacture of goods and services intended for foreign markets, and externally influenced lack of regulations and standards to minimize production cost in some LMIC, are special cross-cutting risk factors for unintentional injuries[10]; they have cognizance for child injury prevention within a globalized economy.

Prevention and treatment options for each leading mechanism of child unintentional injuries are summarized according to the classical model for injury prevention in **Table 5.**[4] The 3 categories under the classical model are primary strategies: measures for preventing incidence of injuries; secondary strategies: measures for reducing the severity of injuries; and tertiary strategies: measures for decreasing the frequency and severity of disability after an injury.

It is important to note that these prevention options are mostly passive strategies and are not intended for instituting changes in behavior or socioeconomic conditions of population.[4] Also, the evidence supporting most these strategies is mainly from HIC, and few have been implemented and rigorously tested in LMIC, where most unintentional injuries occur.[4] A prevention strategy sometimes overlooked in both HIC and LMIC is for health workers, including pediatricians, to include unintentional injury prevention counseling as part of routine anticipatory guidance for infants, children, and adolescents.

### Implication of Globalization for Distribution of Child Unintentional Injury Risks and Prevention in Low- and Middle-Income countries

Globalization, as earlier defined, is not a natural process; the development of free market and interchange of ideas, as espoused in globalization, are maintained (sometimes enforced) by complex international laws and institutions.[11,12] Subsequently, there are potential winners and losers based on the operations of such international laws and institutions,[12] even though the actual process of globalization itself is neither inherently harmful nor beneficial.[13] Economic interest and dynamic interplay of political relations are the key drivers of globalization.[11] Hence, the benefits or harm of the process is often perceived in terms of economic loss or gain of countries and local economies without capturing the human cost.[14]

In order to outline the implications of globalization on the distribution of risks and prevention strategies for child unintentional injuries, 8 key manifestations of globalization are identified, which cut across economic, political, and social indicators.[5,12,13,15,16] Because the burden of child unintentional injuries is disproportionately borne by

**Table 4**
Risk factors for child unintentional injuries in low- and middle-income countries: examples

| Injury Mechanism | Individual Factors | Vehicle/Safety Equipment | Social Environment | Physical Environment |
|---|---|---|---|---|
| RTI | Speeding, drunk driving, cognitive development (younger children), increased risk-taking behaviors (older children) | Poor brakes, overloading, poor lighting, child restraint/seatbelts not provided or incorrectly fitted | Lack of road safety law and/or enforcement | Poor road design/condition, lack of separation for pedestrians and vehicles, mix of traffic |
| Drownings | Cognitive development, underlying medical conditions, lack of knowledge about water risk/survival skills, including swimming, alcohol consumption | Nonusage/lack of personal floatation devices, overloaded boats, unsafe watercrafts | Lack of pool-fencing legislation and/or enforcement | Unprotected water hazard in/around home environment, inadequate water infrastructure (eg, bridges), lack of barrier to unsafe water bodies |
| Burns | Pre-existing disability, lack of knowledge about fire, smoking in home/on the bed, inflammable clothes | Unsafe cooking stove, unsafe heat and light sources, fireworks, inadequate access to water supply | Absence of laws and regulations relating to building codes, smoke detectors, and flammable clothing, child labor | Nonseparation of cooking and living areas, overcrowded living conditions, unsafe storage of flammable substances |
| Falls | Pre-existing disability, evolving motor and cognitive skills | Unprotected staircase/balcony, windows, rooftops, trees; lack of protective equipment; stroller/walkers, highchairs/baby bouncers; bunk beds; products of leisure activities such as bicycles, scooters, swing ropes | Child labor, unsafe playgrounds | Lack of access to safe play areas/lack of impact-absorbing surfaces |
| Poisonings | Cognitive development | Toxicity of substance, liquid preparations, ease of opening a package, attractiveness, and inadequate labeling | Lack of regulation and standards for toxic products and packaging, lack of information or awareness on toxic substance | Ease of access and poor storage in home environment, indoor cooking fires, and indoor use of fuel-powered electricity-generating sets |
| Cross-cutting factors | Gender, age, lack of supervision | — | Poverty, single-parent family, large family size, poor maternal education | — |

**Table 5**
Preventive treatment strategies for child unintentional injuries in low- and middle-income countries: examples

| Injury Mechanism | Primary Prevention | Secondary Prevention | Tertiary Prevention |
|---|---|---|---|
| RTI | Graduated driver licensing system, reduction of speed around schools, residential and play areas, drinking age laws, blood alcohol concentration limits, separating different types of road users | Child restraints and seatbelts, wearing motorcycle and bicycle helmets, improved emergency response | Dedicated trauma centers and rehabilitation services |
| Drownings | Covering/removing water hazards, fencing around swimming pools, lifeguards at swimming areas, targeted awareness | Wearing flotation devices, training in resuscitation | Hospital care and rehabilitation services |
| Burns | Hot tap water legislation, smoke alarm laws, child-resistant lighters | First aid (apply cold water, remove clothing), fire-retardant household material | Burns centers, rehabilitation centers |
| Falls | Home visitation to identify hazards, redesigning nursery furniture and other products, playground standards such as surface material, height of equipment and maintenance, window guards | Improved emergency response | Pediatric acute care and rehabilitation services |
| Poisonings | Removing the toxic agent, child-resistant packaging of medicines and poisons | Immediate first aid | Early and accurate diagnosis, poison centers |

LMIC,[2] the authors projected on how these key manifestations of globalization impact on the distribution of risk factors and prevention strategies for child unintentional injuries in LMIC (**Table 6**).

Outsourcing production of goods and services to LMIC due to increased access to cheaper labor is perhaps one of the commonest features of globalization.[15] One of the negative consequences of outsourcing production when coupled with lax regulations on production and safety standards is that it creates an environment for increased child labor, reduction in parental supervision as labor participation increases, and poor and hazardous working conditions, which all may predispose to child unintentional injuries (**Box 1**).[10,17] The distribution of risk factors for child unintentional injuries further shifts to LMIC when international laws and institutions that maintain the process of globalization are not responsive to the rights of individuals in these countries[4] (**Fig. 1**).

Outsourcing production process to LMIC is associated with rapid movement of people, goods, and services,[12] which, coupled with weak transport infrastructure and road safety regulations, increases exposure to risk factors for RTI, such as exposure to high-capacity vehicles, overloading, and poor road conditions in these countries (**Box 2**).

The consequences of globalization on child unintentional injuries are not entirely negative. Some have argued that the increased labor access and transfer of wages to populations in LMIC help to improve living conditions and socioeconomic status in the countries.[18] These increased labor access and transfer of wages may be of significance for improving the home environment where most of the child unintentional injuries occur.

Globalization has also led to the emergence of global news media and global civil society organizations advocating for child unintentional injury prevention, which has led to increased awareness of the burden and risk factors, and availability of preventive services for child unintentional injuries in LMIC (**Box 3**, **Fig. 2**). For example, global network of nongovernmental organizations (NGO), such as the Global Alliance of NGOs for Road Safety, works collaboratively with government, academic institutions, and communities in LMIC to reduce child unintentional injuries from road transport.[19]

## DISCUSSION

The burden of child unintentional injuries is disproportionately borne by LMIC, and it seems that the highest burden concentrates in countries with middle income economies. Indeed, there is a correlation between economic development and increase in proportionate mortality from child unintentional injuries.[20] This correlation is driven in part by the forces of globalization maintained by complex international laws that increase labor and free market access, which disproportionately shifts economic gains and risk factors of child unintentional injuries between the HIC and LMIC. Recognizing the growing inequalities in the benefits of globalization between HIC and LMIC is at the crux of understanding pathways for leveraging globalization to reduce deaths and morbidity from child unintentional injuries. There is a need for major beneficiaries of globalization to recognize that economic gains from increased global trade come at a human cost.[14] This cost includes a net increase in the risk of child unintentional injuries in LMIC. Hence, the complex international laws and institutions that protect free market should also be extended to ensure and enforce safety standards in the production countries.[21]

Another pathway for leveraging globalization to reduce the burden of child unintentional injuries in LMIC is through improvement of socioeconomic conditions of families

**Table 6**
**Projected consequences of globalization on child unintentional injuries in low- and middle-income countries: examples**

| Key Manifestation of Globalization | Positive Consequences on Risk Factors of Child Injuries | Negative Consequences on Risk Factors of Child Injuries |
|---|---|---|
| 1 Rapid movement of goods and services[5] | Increased access to protective and safety devices | Increased risk from exposure to high-capacity vehicles, congested roads, and overloading of vehicles and watercraft; strain on transport infrastructure including roads and waterways, which increases risk; increased access to hazardous substances |
| 2 Rapid diffusion of computing, telecommunication, and information technology[12] | Improved access to information and awareness of risk factors; improved access to treatment options | Increased risk of injuries to children from distracted drivers while operating vehicle (mobile phones), reduction in direct supervision |
| 3 Labor access and changes in wages structure[15] | Increased wages in LMIC reduces extreme poverty and risks of child injuries related to socioeconomic status | Increased exposure to risk factors due to shift of production process to LMIC with poor/hazardous working conditions, increased child labor weaker controls, and enforcement on safety standards; increased risk due to reduction in direct parental supervision as labor participation increases among adults |
| 4 Growing income and health (access) inequalities[13] | Reduced risk of severe injuries related to poverty from improved living conditions and health access (for those with higher income) | Increased risk of severe injuries related to poverty (for those with worsening income opportunities); reduction in parental supervision; increase in affluence leads to exposure to risk from unsafe operations of newly acquired product/devices |
| 5 Emergence of global news media[16] | Increased visibility/awareness of burden and risk factors; directed funds and resources to addressing risk factors | None |
| 6 Spread of cultures (eg, music, art, sports)[16] | Spread of safe practices and standards in sporting and working conditions | Increased risk-taking behavior learned from entertainment media |
| 7 Global tourism[12] | Improvement in transport and other social infrastructure and standards in some LMIC, which reduces risk | Increased exposure to injury risk from child labor in hospitality industry; increased risk of injuries from child trafficking; lack of awareness of injury regulations/ standards among tourists in foreign countries |
| 8 Emergence of global civil society organization—with role in health delivery and human rights[12] | Increased policy engagement, education, and awareness on risk factors; facilitating transfer of financial resources and technical knowledge for tackling the risk factors; policy advocacy on child human rights | None |

> **Box 1**
> **Fire in export-based garment factory in Bangladesh**
>
> Factory fires in garment industries based in Bangladesh and Pakistan have gained a lot of media attention in recent times. These industries, although based in low- and middle-income countries, make clothes almost exclusively for markets and big stores in high-income countries, such as the United States, the Netherlands, United Kingdom, Germany, and France.
>
> In November 2012, fire razed a multistory garment factory just outside of Dhaka in Bangladesh killing more than 100 individuals working in the section where piles of yarn and fabric are kept. Two months before that incidence, another factory killed more than 280 individuals in a garment factory in Karachi, Pakistan.
>
> In the Dhaka fire incident, there were reports that fire exits had locks on that prevented trapped workers from exiting the burning building.[29] Also, another report claimed that this violation and other safety issues at the factory were identified before the fire incidence, but no reform or corrective actions were taken[30]; there are almost 4000 of similar factories throughout Bangladesh.
>
> Although Bangladesh earns more than $12.5 billion dollars from exports of garment products annually, the working conditions in some of these factories fall short of international standards.[29] Some months before the Dhaka fire, workers from more than 300 factories went on a strike to demand higher wages and better working conditions.[29]
>
> A report revealed that girls as young as 13 years of age work long hours at some of these garment factories in Bangladesh. In addition to being exposed to the kind of fire hazards witnessed at the Dhaka factory, these girls are also victims of physical and verbal abuse.[31]

and children in these countries.[4] Several studies have shown that low socioeconomic status is strongly associated with child unintentional injuries,[4,20,22] and that most child unintentional injuries occur within in home settings.[4] Hence, improving living wages for families who participate in the manufacture of goods and services intended for globalized markets would impact living conditions and potentially reduce the risk of child unintentional injuries.[23] Moreover, the cost of such improvement in living wages is likely to be minimal relative to the profit margins of the large conglomerates, and from a social justice perspective, this is a moral imperative.[23,24] Some policy advocates have called for the establishment of global living wages by the International

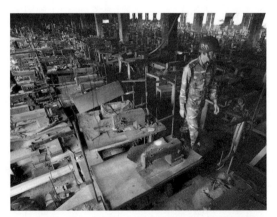

**Fig. 1.** A Bangladeshi police officer walks between rows of burned sewing machines in a garment factory outside Dhaka, Bangladesh, in November 2012. (AP Photo/Khurshed Rinku.)

> **Box 2**
> **Road traffic fatalities on Indian roads**
>
> India leads the rest of the world in the number of fatalities on its roads. The increase in these deaths correlates with the emergence of the country as a rapidly growing market in the global economy. The surge of cars and trucks on Indian roads, needed for rapid transport of goods and services, coupled with speed and poor law enforcement has been identified as some of the key contributory factors. Children are particularly vulnerable to road traffic fatalities in India because of the nonseparation of pedestrian and vehicles on busy roads. The following real-life stories are adapted from a *New York Times* article.[32]
>
> Akshay Singh, a 16-year-old boy from Uttar Pradesh was on his way to a wedding. He was struck by a truck that lost control while he was walking on a highway in Bijnor. Akshay died immediately, and he was crushed beyond recognition. The driver of the out-of-control truck took off and was never arrested until Rakesh Singh, Akshay's father, while still grieving his son, went searching for the truck driver. Rakesh had to take the investigating police in his own car to effect the arrest.
>
> Shivani, a 15-year-old girl, lived in Old Delhi and had to walk 1 km to school every day. She had to cross a busy highway every day on her to school. She was involved in a near fatal crash during one such attempt. She fractured her right leg and was in a coma for 4 days. According to Dr Mathew Varghese, the head of the Orthopedics Department of the hospital where Shivani received treatment, he saw many patients like Shivani every year, and in his own words, he believes that economic growth in India is being built on "the dead bodies of the poor on these highways."[32]

Labor Organization and the provision of employment benefits such as provision of crèche services (for child supervision while a parent participates in the labor market) and severance pay to workers in these countries.[24] Although such an intervention is a reasonable approach in the short term, it could lead to labor market distortions in LMIC and other unintended consequences.[25]

> **Box 3**
> **Impact of global media on childhood drowning-prevention policy in Bangladesh**
>
> In Bangladesh, childhood drownings, not the childhood cluster of infectious diseases, are the leading cause of deaths of children aged 1 to 4 years and a leading cause of death for children of all ages. Although the significant burden of childhood drowning has since been recognized by the government and other stakeholders, very little has been achieved in terms of a national policy for addressing this burden. All that changed after the British Broadcasting Corporation (BBC) News, a global news and media organization with reach in well over 75 countries, aired a special presentation in February 2015 on the magnitude of the burden of childhood drowning and prevention in Bangladesh.[33]
>
> The focus of the special presentation was the large-scale implementation of a research study on childhood drowning prevention being conducted by the Johns Hopkins Bloomberg School of Public Health's International Injury Research Unit in Baltimore, Maryland, USA along with the Center for Injury Prevention Research, Bangladesh and the International Center for Diarrheal Disease Research, Bangladesh. The project, sponsored by the Bloomberg Philanthropies, is providing 2 drowning-prevention interventions—the use of playpens and daycare services—to 80,000 toddlers in 7 subdistricts of Bangladesh.[34]
>
> Within 2 months of BBC News airing the presentation, the Education Ministry in Bangladesh announced a national policy making it mandatory for swimming lessons to be taught in schools throughout the country.[35] Although there are obvious challenges that the implementation of such a policy will face in the future, BBC News coming into the picture and drawing attention to the issue elicited an immediate response from the national government. This may be a step in the right direction.

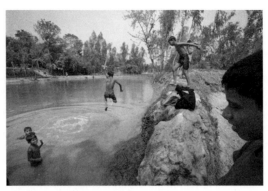

**Fig. 2.** Drowning risk in Bangladesh: children at play. (*Courtesy of* Bloomberg Philanthropies, New York, NY, with permission.)

Increasing corporate social responsibility[c] among major conglomerates is another pathway for leveraging globalization for reducing child unintentional injuries. Identifying actions by major firms that are both socially responsible (for child unintentional injury prevention) and privately responsible (to serve the firm's bottom line) is key to unlocking this pathway.[26] Although it may prove challenging to identify and motivate actions that serve such a dual role, a firm's reputation is often sufficient and a compelling enough reason to engage in purely socially responsible acts, such as investment in child unintentional injury prevention in LMIC.[26]

Activities of global civil society organizations and academic institutions could facilitate and direct global investments to areas of critical need in child unintentional injury prevention in LMIC. Indeed, the inequalities in risks and benefits of globalization extend into research and availability of treatment options for secondary and tertiary prevention of child unintentional injuries.[4] Government and private industry support child unintentional injuries prevention programs and research in LMIC through activities of global civil society organizations, and academic institutions could help in addressing these inequalities. In addition, global data collection for health could be targeted to capture these disparities and suggest priorities for intervention.[2]

There are a number of private global coalitions focused on reducing the burden of unintentional injuries in LMIC, including the Global Road Safety Partnership.[27] Some of the global companies that came together to establish these initiatives are closely associated with the transportation industry and recognized the centrality of the mobility to economic growth and the vulnerability of road users to fatal road crashes.[28] Hence, they are investing to promote safer roads and best practices for road injury prevention in some of the countries where they operate; this is a step in the right direction and could be further extended to addressing the issues around child unintentional injuries as well.

Cycles of globalization have been described to involve contemporary globalization (from the 1970s to preglobal financial crisis in 2007) and reverse globalization (postglobal financial crisis in 2007 to date). Contemporary globalization, characterized by increases in global trade through promotion of free market and private ownership

---

[c] Corporate social responsibility is defined as situations "where a firm goes beyond compliance and engages in actions that appear to further some social goods, beyond the interests of the firm and that which is required by the law."[26]

facilitated by trade liberalization, financial deregulation, and high-risk loan and grant precondition to LMIC,[12] informs the consequences of child unintentional injuries described in this article (see **Table 6**). It remains to be seen what the implication of reverse globalization, characterized by reduction in global trade (due to reduction in spending), market distortion leading to increasing financial regulation, increased protectionist measures by national governments, new trade barriers, and market fragmentation, would have on the distribution of child unintentional injuries risk factors and prevention efforts in LMIC.

Managing globalization and its impact in a way that is fair to all concerned presents complex challenges given the dynamic nature of the tradeoffs that drive it. Confronting these challenges may require efforts that go beyond global regulation and coordination of international standards and procedure. It may require multiple flexible solutions at various socioecologic levels that change with time and trend of globalization. Therefore, the key to managing globalization for fairness may lie in the ability to predict its impact through deliberate, intermittent, and independent assessments of key human and economic indicators and creating a platform for flexible decision-making at various policy levels.

In conclusion, globalization creates inequalities in the distribution of economic gains, risks, and opportunities for preventing child unintentional injuries between HIC and LMIC. Such inequalities contribute to the global burden of child unintentional injuries being disproportionately borne by LMIC. Globalization, however, also presents opportunities for addressing these inequalities—taking advantage of such opportunities would require an acknowledgment of the disparity and deliberate efforts among all stakeholders, including global companies, civil societies, and academic institutions.

## REFERENCES

1. Institute for Health Metrics and Evaluation (IHME). Global burden of disease study 2013 data. Seattle (WA): IHME; 2015.
2. Alonge O, Hyder AA. Reducing the global burden of childhood unintentional injuries. Arch Dis Child 2014;99(1):62–9.
3. Baker S. The injury fact book. 2nd edition. New York: Oxford University Press; 1992.
4. Peden M, Oyegbite K, Ozanne-Smith J, et al. World report on child injury prevention. Geneva (Switzerland): World Health Organization; 2008.
5. Jenkins R. Globalization, production, employment and poverty: debates and evidence. J Int Dev 2004;16:1–12.
6. McMichael AJ, Beaglehole R. The changing global context of public health. Lancet 2000;356(9228):495–9.
7. World Health Organization (WHO). WHO regional office. Available at: http://www.who.int/about/regions/en/. Accessed July 7, 2015.
8. World Bank. Country and lending groups. Washington, DC: World Bank; 2015. Available at: http://data.worldbank.org/about/country-and-lending-groups. Accessed July 7, 2015.
9. Haddon W. Options for the prevention of motor vehicle crash injury. Isr J Med 1980;16:45–65.
10. Ashagrei K. Statistics on working children and hazardous child labour in brief. Geneva (Switzerland): International Labour Organization; 1997. Available at: http://training.itcilo.it/actrav_cdrom2/en/osh/wc/child.htm. Accessed July 7, 2015.

11. Polanyi K. The great transformation. Boston: Beacon Press; 1944.
12. Labonte R, Schrecker T. Globalization and social determinants of health: introduction and methodological background (part 1 of 3). Global Health 2007;3:5.
13. Pappas G, Hyder AA, Akhter M. Globalization: toward a new framework for public health. Social Theor Health 2003;1:91–107.
14. Baumat Z. Globalization: the human consequences. New York: Columbia University Press; 1998.
15. Hanson G. The globalization of production. The National Bureau of Economic Research Reporter. 2001. Available at: http://www.nber.org/reporter/spring01/hanson.html. Accessed July 7, 2015.
16. McChesney R, Schiller D. The political economy of international communications: foundations for the emerging global debate about media ownership and regulation, technology, business and society programme paper No. 11. Geneva (Switzerland): Research Institute for Social Development; 2003.
17. Milberg W, Amengual M. Economic development and working conditions in export processing zones: a survey of trends. Geneva (Switzerland): International Labour Organization; 2008. Available at: www.oit.org/public/french/dialogue/download/wp3englishfinal.pdf. Accessed July 7, 2015.
18. Rogoff K, Wei SJ, Kose MA. Effects of financial globalization on developing countries: some empirical evidence, vol. 17. Washington, DC: International Monetary Fund; 2003. Available at: http://www.nber.org/~wei/data/prwk2003/prwk2003.pdf. Accessed July 7, 2015.
19. Global alliance of NGOs for road safety: about the alliance. Available at: http://www.roadsafetyngos.org/about-the-alliance/. Accessed July 31, 2015.
20. Khan UR, Sengoelge M, Zia N, et al. Country level economic disparities in child injury mortality. Arch Dis Child 2015;100:S29–33.
21. Coglianese C. Globalization and the design of international institutions. In: Nye JS Jr, Donahue JD, editors. Governance in a globalizing world. New York: Brookings Institution Press; 2000. p. 297–318.
22. Laflamme L, Hasselberg M, Burrows S. 20 years of research on socioeconomic inequality and children's—unintentional injuries understanding the cause-specific evidence at hand. Int J Pediatr 2010;2010. http://dx.doi.org/10.1155/2010/819687.
23. Ahmed FE. The rise of the Bangladesh garment industry: globalization, women workers, and voice. Natl Women's Stud Assoc (NWSA) J 2004;16(2):34–45.
24. Beneria L, Lind A. Global markets: threats to sustainable human development. In: Heyzer N, Kapoor S, Sandler J, editors. A commitment to the world's women: perspectives on development for Beijing and beyond. New York: UNIFEM; 1995.
25. MacKenzie D, Theoharides C, Yang D. Distortions in the international migrant labor market: evidence from Filipino migration and wage responses to destination country economic shocks. Discussion Paper No. 6498. Bonn (Germany): Institute for the Study of Labor; 2012.
26. McWilliams A, Siegel D. Corporate social responsibility: a theory of the firm perspective. Acad Manage Rev 2001;26:117–27.
27. Global Road Safety Partnership (GRSP) 2015. Available at: http://www.grsproadsafety.org/partners/current-partners. Accessed July 7, 2015.
28. Global Road Safety Partnership (GSRP). Press release: leading global businesses launch second phase of Global Road Safety Initiative, 2014. Available at: www.who.int/roadsafety/press_release_grsp.pdf. Accessed July 7, 2015.

29. The Guardian. Bangladesh textile factory fire leaves more than 100 dead. Reported by Jason Burke & Saad Hammadi. Available at: http://www.theguardian.com/world/2012/nov/25/bangladesh-textile-factory-fire. Accessed August 8, 2015.

30. The New York Times. Documents Indicate Walmart Blocked Safety Push in Bangladesh. Reported by Steven Greenhouse. Available at: http://www.nytimes.com/2012/12/06/world/asia/3-walmart-suppliers-made-goods-in-bangladeshi-factory-where-112-died-in-fire.html?_r=0. Accessed August 8, 2015.

31. The Guardian. Bangladesh garment factories still exploiting child labour for UK products. Reported by Miles Brignall & Sarah Butler. Available at: http://www.theguardian.com/world/2014/feb/06/bangladesh-garment-factories-child-labour-uk. Accessed August 8, 2015.

32. The New York Times. India Steadily increases its lead in road fatalities. Reported by Heather Timmons and Hari Kumar. Available at: http://www.nytimes.com/2010/06/08/world/asia/08iht-roads.html?_r=0. Accessed August 8, 2015.

33. British Broadcasting News. Health check: Bangladesh project to prevent toddlers drowning. Available at: http://www.bbc.com/news/health-31045033. Accessed August 8, 2015.

34. Hyder AH, Alonge O, He S, et al. Saving of children's lives from drowning in Bangladesh. Am J Prev Med 2014;47(6):842–5.

35. British Broadcasting News. World News Asia: swimming lessons in Bangladesh made law to stop drownings. Available at: http://www.bbc.com/news/world-asia-32239442. Accessed August 8, 2015.

# Adolescent Health Implications of New Age Technology

Cara Jacobson, Alexandra Bailin, Ruth Milanaik, DO,
Andrew Adesman, MD*

## KEYWORDS

- Adolescents • Internet addiction • Pornography • Cell phone • Cyberbullying
- Video games

## KEY POINTS

- New age technologies have become a prominent factor in the lives of adolescents, with the potential for a range of associated risks and serious consequences.
- Many studies have related the increased adolescent use of new age technology to adverse physical, emotional, and developmental effects.
- Texting while driving is one of the greatest risk behaviors related to new age technologies. Teens already constitute an at-risk population for motor vehicle accidents; technology-related distractions only further increase the likelihood of serious injury or loss of life.
- Pediatricians must educate adolescents and their parents about the potential risks associated with new age technology.
- Further research is needed to identify and delineate the impact of new age technologies on the health and development of adolescents.

## INTRODUCTION

Throughout the past decade, adolescent use of new age technology has increased dramatically. A 2009 survey found that on average, adolescents spend 11 hours of each day using technology.[1] However, heavy technology use is associated with poor academic performance, increased aggression, and low-quality relationships with parents and peers.[1–3] In general, increased new age technology use among adolescents has been related to poor mental and physical health. As youth exposure to

Disclosures: None.
Division of Developmental and Behavioral Pediatrics, Cohen Children's Medical Center of New York, Northwell Health, 1983 Marcus Avenue, Suite 130, Lake Success, NY 11042, USA
* Corresponding author.
E-mail address: aadesman@nshs.edu

new age technology continues to expand, it is vital that the health implications of Internet, cell phone, and video game use are noted and understood so that preventive measures can be taken to minimize their negative impact. This review examines the health implications of new age technology use among adolescents.

## INTERNET ADDICTION

Since its origin in the 1990s, use of the Internet has rapidly become a commonplace activity among adolescents.[4] According to a 2012 nationally representative phone survey of 812 teens aged 12 to 17 years, 80% have their own desktop or laptop computer, and of the 20% who do not, 67% have access to a computer they can use at home.[5,6] Given this dramatic increase in Internet use, many now view the Internet as potentially addictive.[7,8]

Internet addiction (IA) describes a loss of control over Internet use, which results in personal distress and symptoms of psychological dependence.[9] The proposed criteria for IA include the presentation of at least 5 of the 6 following criteria[10]:

- Spending an increasing amount of time online
- Failure to reduce use with concomitant feelings of restlessness and depression
- Staying online longer than originally intended
- Running the risk of losing a relationship or other opportunities due to Internet use
- Lying to conceal the extent of Internet use
- Using the Internet to escape negative feelings

Most studies suggest that male individuals have a higher frequency of IA,[7,11,12] which is likely due to their increased engagement in games, pornography, and gambling, all of which have been associated with IA.[13,14]

IA among adolescents has been found to be associated with depression, obsessive-compulsive disorder, attention-deficit hyperactivity disorder (ADHD), anxiety, stress, negative self-perception, and suicidal ideation.[11,12,15–17] Adolescents with IA are 2.5 times more likely to be depressed,[18] and 2 times more likely to engage in self-injurious behavior than typical adolescents.[19] Already-existing depression and hostility increase when adolescents become addicted to the Internet.[20] Furthermore, in a 2007 study of Korean adolescents, Ha and colleagues[16] found that a strong association between depression and IA existed even after controlling for differences in biogenetic temperament. These results suggest that adolescents with no history of mental health problems can develop depression due to excessive Internet use.

Adolescents with IA also tend to develop poor eating habits, including skipping meals, snacking, and loss of appetite. These adolescents do not consume enough of the recommended food groups; they also consume more than the recommended daily quantities of salt, fatty foods, fried foods, and foods high in simple sugars.[21] Unsurprisingly, studies have revealed an association between IA and a high body mass index (BMI).[22] The opposite is true as well; media plays a role in the development, maintenance, prevention, and treatment of eating disorders.[23] Time spent on the Internet is significantly related to body surveillance, internalization of the thin ideal, and drive for thinness.[24]

Last, IA is related to microstructural changes in adolescent brains, such as decreased gray matter volume.[25–27] Genetic polymorphisms, impairment of neurotransmitter systems, and anatomic and functional changes have been found in brains of individuals with IA.[28] However, these studies fail to determine the causality of this relationship and further longitudinal research should be conducted.

As it has been proven that IA leads to many health-related consequences among adolescents, it is essential that pediatricians and other health care professionals are aware of the implications of Internet addiction. Equipped with this knowledge, they can work toward the implementation of preventive, diagnostic, and treatment strategies. For example, there is evidence that promoting positive parent–adolescent interaction and attending to adolescent psychological needs should be included in preventive programs for future IA cases.[29] In addition, adolescents' own increased awareness and education regarding IA may prevent or at least mitigate the many negative consequences of such behavior.

## CYBERBULLYING

National studies have found that as many as 1 in 5 adolescents is involved in some type of bullying,[30] and bullying plays a large role in the high adolescent suicide rate. Unfortunately, the Internet serves as an additional medium through which adolescents can bully one another. The Youth Internet Safety Survey (YISS) defines online harassment, or cyberbullying, as "threats or other offensive behavior sent online to the youth or posted online about the youth for others to see."[31] Similar to traditional bullying, cyberbullying is usually composed of recurring behavior and a power imbalance between the bully and the victim.[32]

Cyberbullying has become increasingly pervasive in the lives of adolescents. In 2010, approximately 11% of adolescents were victims of cyberbullying, compared with 6% of adolescents in 2000. Cyberbullying has increased by 83% throughout the past decade.[33] According to the 2014 YISS, this increase in cyberbullying has been dramatic because "inhibitions that would otherwise restrain youth from engaging in harassment are reduced due to the anonymity and remoteness of online interactions."[33]

As technology is now being used as a vehicle for bullying, serious attention is warranted to investigate the extent and nature of this new form of aggression and the possible psychosocial effects it has on youth. For example, online harassment is significantly related to depression.[34] The study by Finkelhor and colleagues[34] surveyed 1501 youth ages 10 through 17, and found that 18% of the harassed youth reported 5 or more depressive symptoms, which was more than twice the rate (8%) for the overall sample.[34] Furthermore, similar to traditional bullying, cyberbullying is associated with suicidal ideation and suicidal behavior.[35,36] In a survey of 1973 middle school students, conducted by Hinduja and Patchin,[35] cyberbully victims were 1.9 times more likely to have attempted suicide, and cyberbully offenders were 1.5 times more likely to have attempted suicide than students who had not experienced online harassment.

Although there are several similarities between traditional bullying and cyberbullying, cyberbullying deserves to be addressed as its own unique risk factor. A 2014 meta-analysis determined that cyberbullying is more strongly related to suicidal ideation than is traditional bullying.[37] This study found that victims of traditional bullying had an increased risk for suicidal ideation by a factor of 2.16, whereas victims of cyberbullying had an increased risk by a factor of 3.12. Unlike traditional bully victims, cyberbully victims often feel that they have been degraded in front of a wider audience. Also, harmful material can be stored online, which can constantly remind victims of the incident.

In an Australian study conducted by Price and Dalgleish,[32] despite the serious impacts of cyberbullying, adolescents often did not seek support from others. The findings in this review stress the importance of instituting school-based programs aimed at reducing cyberbullying.[32] School antibullying policies often do not include prevention of cyberbullying, and in his study Bhat[38] suggests that cyberbullying prevention should be implemented in school antibullying policies. Interventions to prevent cyberbullying warrant much further attention and research.

## PORNOGRAPHY

The expansion of the Internet has enabled adolescents to access sexually explicit content easily. As adolescent accessibility to the Internet increases, more youth are exposed to online pornography.[31] According to a 2008 study conducted by Sabina and colleagues,[39] 72.8% of 563 college students surveyed (94% male students, 62% female students) had seen online pornography before turning 18. However, much of this adolescent exposure to pornography is involuntary. In YISS-2, approximately 1 in 3 youth said that they had experienced unwanted exposure to pornography, and 83% of youth were exposed when surfing the Web.[33] Female individuals have been found to report involuntary exposure more often than male individuals.[40] The YISS-2 attributes the increase in youth exposure to pornography to 3 factors: greater Internet accessibility, a change in technology, and more aggressive marketing strategies used by pornographic companies.[31]

Adolescent exposure to pornography has been found to have a variety of adverse health and social implications. For example, one study found that 59% of 15-year-olds to 24-year-olds agreed that exposure to pornography encourages adolescents to have sex before they are ready.[41] In addition, adolescent exposure to pornography has been associated with an increase in risky sexual behaviors. A study of 433 adolescents found that individuals who watched pornography were more likely to have engaged in anal sex, had sex with multiple partners, and used alcohol or drugs during sex.[42] In a 2001 study, 50% of youth surveyed thought that pornography encourages individuals to believe that unprotected sex is acceptable.[43] However, not all research has supported this association. For example, Luder and colleagues[44] found that among Swiss adolescents, risky sexual behaviors were not necessarily related to exposure to pornography.

Exposure to pornography, particularly violent pornography, may also be indicative of sexually aggressive behavior. In a 2006 study examining 10-year-old to 15-year-old adolescents surveyed nationally in the United States, intentional exposure to violent pornography was found to increase the odds of self-reported sexually aggressive behavior by nearly 6 times.[45] Another longitudinal study found that male adolescents who were exposed to pornography at an early age were more likely to engage in sexual harassment.[41] Adolescents who consume pornography were also found to be more likely to display forms of aggressive behaviors, such as theft, manipulation, and forced sexual intercourse.[46]

Pornography exposure may also affect adolescents' mental health. In a longitudinal analysis conducted by Mattebo,[47] frequent pornography use was largely associated with psychosomatic symptoms. Although frequent pornography use was less associated with depressive symptoms than psychosomatic symptoms at follow-up, female individuals who frequently used pornography at baseline were found to have depressive symptoms at follow-up. Additional research should be conducted to further understand the effects that pornography consumption has on adolescent mental health.

Many studies have addressed the impact of pornography consumption on adolescents' social development. Frequent pornography users were found to have weaker ties to social institutions and to have lower degrees of social integration.[14,48] In a 2010 study, Hunter and colleagues[49] found that early exposure to pornography is related to antisocial behavior. Furthermore, adolescents who use pornography frequently are significantly more likely to have abnormal conduct issues as well as addictive Internet use.[14]

As pornography appears to have a number of negative health effects on adolescents, it is important to educate them about these potential adverse consequences, especially regarding high-risk sexual behaviors. Given the popularity of the Internet, this may be the most influential sex educator for adolescents worldwide.

## TEXTING AND DRIVING

According to the National Center for Health Statistics, most adolescent deaths are the result of unintentional injuries.[50] Motor vehicle fatalities are responsible for 73% of these accidental deaths. In 2009, 3365 adolescents in the United States died in motor vehicle crashes[51,52] and in 2011, 2650 adolescents died in motor vehicle crashes; more than 292,000 suffered major injuries due to these accidents.[53] Although youth ages 15 to 24 represent only 14% of the US population, they represent 30% of the total costs of motor vehicle injuries among male individuals and 28% of the total costs of motor vehicle injuries among female individuals.

The National Highway Traffic Safety Administration found that distracted driving predominantly occurs in the adolescent age-group,[54] and cell phones play a significant role in adolescents' distracted driving. In a 2009 national survey conducted by the Allstate Foundation, 83% of 1000 teenagers reported using a cell phone while driving.[55] In a 2010 national survey of 1219 drivers, Wilson and Stimpson found that 43% of drivers ages 18 to 24 reported texting while driving.[56] Texting while driving is especially distracting and dangerous. A 2009 study revealed that texting was found to increase the risk of a car accident by 23 times.[57] In comparison, dialing a phone while driving increased the risk by 2.8 times and talking on or listening to the phone increased the risk by only 1.3 times.

Recently, new technology and education programs have been developed to prevent teens from texting while driving. For example, the Safe Texting Campaign developed an application that displays "Please Don't Text & Drive" on the home screen of cell phones when individuals are driving.[58] The application also replies to text messages when an individual is driving, letting the sender know that the individual is driving. Because of the severe danger of teen texting while driving, effective preventive measures, including advances in technology, revisions of high school health curricula, or the implementation of a zero-tolerance law for cell phone use while driving, should be further researched and promoted.

## TEXTING AND SLEEP

Although there have been limited studies on the topic, a link between texting and sleep problems has been suggested. In a 2011 study, White and colleagues[59] examined the effects of text messages on the sleep length and quality of 350 college students. Problematic cell phone use, addictive text messaging, problematic texting, and pathologic texting were significantly related to sleep quality, but not sleep length. In a study involving 84 first-year college undergraduates, Murdock[60] found that the amount of texting per day was directly associated with sleep problems. Furthermore, Fossum and colleagues[61] recently found that cell phone use was positively associated with insomnia.

In a survey of 346 US pediatricians, pediatricians chose the use of electronic devices and late-night texting/cell phone use as the predominant causes of sleep problems.[62] However, further longitudinal research should be conducted to better define this association.

## EXPOSURE TO RADIOFREQUENCIES

Because cell phones are a relatively new technology, scientists do not currently have long-term follow-up on their possible health effects.[63] However, because electric currents regulate physiologic functions of the human body, exposure to an electromagnetic field of sufficient strength can be expected to affect physiologic processes.[64] Due to the dramatic increase in cell phone use among children and adolescents, researchers have begun to investigate the potential negative effects that exposure to radiofrequency magnetic fields (RFEMF) have on health. Because of their developing nervous systems, smaller head sizes, higher conductivity of brain tissues, and increase in life exposure time, youth may have a greater susceptibility to RFEMF.[65,66] A 2013 Swedish study conducted by Davis and colleagues[67] revealed that brain tumor risk was significantly elevated for those who had used cell phones for at least a decade, but individuals who began using cell phones regularly before the age of 20 had a greater risk of ipsilateral glioma. It has been reported that exposure to radiation due to mobile phone use may alter the blood–brain barrier permeability.[68] If true, then this could possibly enable toxins in the bloodstream to cross the blood–brain barrier into brain cells.

Furthermore, in 2011, Mortazavi and colleagues[69] found that the amount of time that adolescents spent on cell phones was significantly related to the number of headaches, vertigo episodes, and sleeping problems experienced per month. However, conflicting findings on potential health risks tied to cell phone use have been published due to inconsistencies in research methods. For example, some studies have observed phone users for periods of time that are too short to show a significant association between cell phone use and an increased risk in brain cancer. It is clear that further large-scale, longitudinal research is necessary to comprehend the health effects of increased cell phone use.

## HEALTH IMPLICATIONS OF VIDEO GAME USE

As video games continue to rise in popularity among adolescents, concern regarding their health implications has also increased. Studies have found negative correlations between online game addiction and self-control.[70] Because of factors including violent scenes, hostile virtual reality, reinforcement of atrocities, symbolic enactment of cruelty, and replacement of aggression-inhibiting tendencies, violent computer games are believed to be more harmful than passive exposure to media.[70,71] Several studies have found that video game violence has a causal effect on aggressive behavior of adolescents. A 2010 meta-analysis revealed that in children and adolescents, violent video games are related to an increase in aggressive behavior and physiologic arousal, and a decrease in prosocial behavior.[72] No differences between male and female participants were found in the study.

Many studies have attempted to link video game use and obesity. However, according to the 2011 American Academy of Pediatrics (AAP) Policy Statement on "Children, Adolescents, Obesity, and the Media," researchers have found contradictory evidence.[73] For example, in 2004, Vandewater and colleagues[74] conducted a study in which children of higher percentile of BMI had only moderate usage of video games. The same study also found that some children of lower BMI percentile rank used electronic games more often. In addition, recent studies have observed that proactive video games are correlated with an increase in energy expenditure.[73] Therefore, video game use is not necessarily related to obesity.

The evidence regarding video game use and academic achievement is inconclusive. In 2009, Drummond and Sauer[75] analyzed data from more than 192,000 students in 22 countries and found that, contrary to the belief that video games have negative effects on academic achievement, video game use was found to have little impact on adolescent academic achievement in mathematics, science, and reading. Some researchers have proposed that video games actually promote problem-solving skills. In a 2013 study conducted by Adachi and Willoughby,[76] more strategic video game play was found to predict higher self-reported problem-solving skills over time than less strategic video game play. Empirical research regarding this relationship, however, is limited. The results also supported an indirect association between strategic video game play and academic grades. Strategic video game play predicted higher self-reported problem-solving skills, and higher self-reported problem-solving skills predicted higher academic grades. Due to a lack of consensus on many of the effects that video games have on adolescent health, further large-scale longitudinal research should be conducted.

## THE ROLE OF PEDIATRICIANS

Pediatricians play an important role in screening, counseling, and educating adolescents and parents regarding the risks associated with new age technology. According to the AAP, pediatricians should ask 2 questions to parents when seeing a patient: "How much time is the child spending with media?" and "Is there a television and/ or Internet-connected device in the child's bedroom?"[77] Pediatricians may advise parents to model positive "media diets," so that children learn to be selective and healthy when consuming technology. Parents should also be advised to establish technology-use restrictions, such as mealtime and bedtime curfews for devices.

When addressing cyberbullying, pediatricians should help parents and children in identifying people at school who can act as allies.[78] Furthermore, parents should be familiar with the signs of cyberbullying. Emotional signs include shy, moody, anxious, or aggressive behavior. Academic signs include a loss in interest in school and a drop in grades. The biggest red flag of cyberbullying is sudden withdrawal from technology.[79]

Parents should be encouraged to monitor technology use to prevent cyberbullying and exposure to inappropriate Web sites such as pornography. For example, parents may consider installing software that enables detailed tracking of sites that children have visited, or they can use filtering devices to control which Web sites children may visit. Parents may also consider keeping technological devices in common areas within the house, such as the living room or kitchen.[80]

Pediatricians should also collaborate with schools to promote education programs focused on positive technology use.[77] These programs may include implementation of technology that encourages student learning, or they may educate students on the dangers associated with technology use.

## SUMMARY

New age technologies, including the Internet, cell phones and video games, have become a permanent and increasingly prominent factor in the lives of adolescents. Given their immense and growing popularity, further research is needed to identify and delineate what impact these technologies may have on the health and development of adolescents. Realistically, although new age technologies have been truly transformative from a sociocultural standpoint, the challenge and mandate going forward is to be sure we fully recognize any adverse consequences they may have on children and adolescents and how these can best be mitigated.

## REFERENCES

1. Rideout VJ, Foehr UG, Roberts DF. Generation M2: media in the lives of 8–18 year olds. Menlo Park (CA): The Henry J. Kaiser Family Foundation; 2010.
2. David-Ferdon C, Hertz MF. Electronic media and youth violence: a CDC issue brief for researchers. Atlanta (GA): Centers for Disease Control and Prevention; 2009.
3. Richards R, McGee R, Williams SM, et al. Adolescent screen time and attachment to parents and peers. Arch Pediatr Adolesc Med 2010;166:258–62.
4. Borzekowski DL. Adolescents' use of the Internet: a controversial, coming-of-age resource. Adolesc Med Clin 2006;17:205–16.
5. Madden M, Lenhart A, Duggan M, et al. Teens and technology 2013. Washington, DC: PewResearch Internet Project; 2013. Available at: http://www.pewinternet.org/files/old-media//Files/Reports/2013/PIP_TeensandTechnology2013.pdf.
6. Lenhart A, Purcell K, Smith A, et al. Part 1: internet adoption and trends. Washington, DC: PewResearch Internet Project; 2010. Available at: http://www.pewinternet.org/2010/02/03/part-1-internet-adoption-and-trends/.
7. Pezoa-Jares RE, Espinoza-Luna IL, Vasquez-Medina JA. Internet addiction: a review. J Addict Res Ther 2012;S6:2.
8. National Highway Traffic Safety Administration. Distraction.gov: Official US government website for distracted driving. 2012. Available at: http://www.distraction.gov/content/get-the-facts/facts-and-statistics.html. Accessed July 13, 2015.
9. Brand M, Young K, Laier C. Prefrontal control and Internet addiction: a theoretical model and review of neuropsychological and neuroimaging findings. Front Hum Neurosci 2014;8:375.
10. Sadock BJ, Sadock VA. Kaplan & Sadock's comprehensive textbook of psychiatry. Vols. 1 and 2. 8th edition. Philadelphia: Lippincott Williams & Wilkins; 2004.
11. Şaşmaz T, Öner S, Kurt AÖ, et al. Prevalence and risk factors of Internet addiction in high school students. Eur J Public Health 2014;24:15–20.
12. Tsitsika A, Critselis E, Louizou A, et al. Determinants of Internet addiction among adolescents: a case-control study. Scientific World J 2011;11:876–85.
13. Morahan-Martin J, Schumacher P. Incidence and correlates of pathological Internet use among college students. Comput Human Behav 2000;16:13–29.
14. Tsitsika A, Critselis E, Kormas G, et al. Adolescent pornographic Internet site use: a multivariate regression analysis of the predictive factors of use and psychosocial implications. Cyberpsychol Behav Soc Netw 2009;12:545–50.
15. Yadav P, Banwari G, Parmar C, et al. Internet addiction and its correlates among high school students: a preliminary study from Ahmedabad, India. Asian J Psychiatr 2013;6:500–5.
16. Ha JH, Kim SY, Bae SC, et al. Depression and Internet addiction in adolescents. Psychopathology 2007;40:424–30.
17. Yen JY, Ko CH, Yen CF, et al. The comorbid psychiatric symptoms of Internet addiction: attention deficit and hyperactivity disorder (ADHD), depression, social phobia, and hostility (2007). J Adolesc Health 2007;41:94–9.
18. Lam LT, Peng ZW. Effect of pathological use of the Internet on adolescent mental health: a prospective study. Arch Pediatr Adolesc Med 2010;166:911–6.
19. LamL T, Peng Z, Mai J, et al. The association between Internet addiction and self-injurious behaviour among adolescents. Inj Prev 2009;15:403–8.

20. Ko C, Liu T, Wang P, et al. The exacerbation of depression, hostility, and social anxiety in the course of Internet addiction among adolescents: a prospective study. Compr Psychiatry 2014;55:1377–84.
21. Kim Y, Park JY, Kim SB, et al. The effects of Internet addiction on the lifestyle and dietary behavior of Korean adolescents. Nutr Res Pract 2010;4:51–7.
22. Canan F, Yildirim O, Ustunel TY, et al. The relationship between Internet addiction and body mass index in Turkish adolescents. Cyberpsychol Behav Soc Netw 2014;17:40–5.
23. Spettigue W, Henderson KA. Eating disorders and the role of the media. Can Child Adolesc Psychiatr Rev 2004;13:16–9.
24. Tiggemann M, Slater A. NetGirls: the Internet, Facebook, and body image concern in adolescent girls. Int J Eat Disord 2013;46:630–3.
25. Lin F, Zhou Y, Du Y, et al. Abnormal white matter integrity in adolescents with Internet addiction disorder: a tract-based spatial statistics study. PLoS One 2012;7:e30253.
26. Yuan K, Qin W, Wang G, et al. Microstructure abnormalities in adolescents with Internet addiction disorder. PLoS One 2011;6:e20708.
27. Zhou Y, Lin FC, Du YS, et al. Gray matter abnormalities in Internet addiction: a voxel-based morphometry study. Eur J Radiol 2011;80:93–6.
28. Pezoa-Jares RE, Espinoza-Luna IL. Neurobiological findings associated with Internet addiction: a literature review. Eur Psychiatry 2013;28:1.
29. Liu Q-X, Fang X-Y, Yan N, et al. Multi-family group therapy for adolescent Internet addiction: exploring the underlying mechanisms. Addict Behav 2014;42:1–8.
30. Teens and bullying. Pew Research Center; 2011. Available at: http://www.pewresearch.org/daily-number/teens-and-bullying/.
31. Mitchell K, Jones L, Finkelhor D, et al. Trends in unwanted online experiences and sexting: final report. Washington, DC: University of New Hampshire Scholars' Repository; 2014. p. 2–2014.
32. Price M, Dalgleish J. Cyberbullying: experiences, impacts and coping strategies as described by Australian young people. Youth Stud Aust 2010;29:51–9.
33. Sumter SR, Baumgartner SE, Valkenburg PM, et al. Developmental trajectories of peer victimization: offline and online experiences during adolescence. J Adolesc Health 2012;50:607–13.
34. Finkelhor D, Mitchell KJ, Wolak J. Online victimization: a report on the nation's youth. Alexandria (VA): National Center for Missing & Exploited Children; 2000.
35. Hinduja S, Patchin JW. Bullying, cyberbullying, and suicide. Arch Suicide Res 2010;14:206–21.
36. Fisher HL, Moffitt TE, Houts RM, et al. Bullying victimisation and risk of self harm in early adolescence: longitudinal cohort study. Br Med J 2012;344:e2684.
37. van Geel M, Vedder P, Tanilon J. Relationship between peer victimization, cyberbullying, and suicide in children and adolescents: a meta-analysis. JAMA Pediatr 2014;170:435–42.
38. Bhat CS. Cyber bullying: overview and strategies for school counsellors, guidance officers, and all school personnel. Aust J Guidance Counselling 2008;18:53–66.
39. Sabina C, Wolak J, Finkelhor D. The nature and dynamics of Internet pornography exposure for youth. Cyberpsychol Behav Soc Netw 2008;11:692–4.
40. Fergusson DM, Woodward LJ. Mental health, educational, and social role outcomes of adolescents with depression. Arch Gen Psychiatry 2002;59:225–31.

41. Brown JD, L'Engle KL. X-Rated: sexual attitudes and behaviors associated with US early adolescents' exposure to sexually explicit media. Comm Res 2009;36: 131–53.

42. Braun-Courville DK, Rojas M. Exposure to sexually explicit web sites and adolescent sexual attitudes and behaviors. J Adolesc Health 2009;45:158–64.

43. Rideout V. Generation Rx.com: how young people use the Internet for health information. Menlo Park (CA): The Henry J. Kaiser Family Foundation; 2001.

44. Luder MT, Pittet I, Berchtold A, et al. Associations between online pornography and sexual behavior among adolescents: myth or reality? Arch Sex Behav 2010;40:1037–45.

45. Ybarra ML, Mitchell KJ, Hamburger M, et al. X-rated material and perpetration of sexually aggressive behavior among children and adolescents: is there a link? Aggress Behav 2011;37:1–18.

46. Alexy EM, Burgess AW, Prentky RA. Pornography use as a risk marker for an aggressive pattern of behavior among sexually reactive children and adolescents. J Am Psychiatr Nurses Assoc 2009;14:442–53.

47. Mattebo M. Use of pornography and its associations with sexual experiences, lifestyles and health among adolescents. Digital comprehensive summaries of Uppsala dissertations from the faculty of medicine, 985. Uppsala (United Kingdom): Acta Universitatis Upsaliensis; 2014. p. 1–83.

48. Mesch GS. Social bonds and Internet pornographic exposure among adolescents. J Adolesc 2009;32:601–18.

49. Hunter JA, Figueredo AJ, Malamuth NM. Developmental pathways into social and sexual deviance. J Fam Viol 2010;25:143–50.

50. Miniño AM. Mortality among teenagers aged 12-19 years: United States, 1999-2006. NCHS data brief, no 37. Hyattsville (MD): National Center for Health Statistics; 2010.

51. Centers for Disease Control and Prevention (CDC), National Center for Injury Prevention and Control. Web-based injury statistics query and reporting system (WISQARS). 2010. Available at: www.cdc.gov/injury/wisqars/index.html. Accessed July 13, 2015.

52. National Highway Traffic Safety Administration (NHTSA). Fatality analysis reporting system (FARS), National Center for Statistics and Analysis. 2010. Available at: http://www-fars.nhtsa.dot.gov/People/PeopleAllVictims.aspx. Accessed July 13, 2015.

53. Centers for Disease Control and Prevention (CDC), National Center for Injury Prevention and Control. Web-based injury statistics query and reporting system (WISQARS). 2014. Available at: http://www.cdc.gov/motorvehiclesafety/teen_drivers/teendrivers_factsheet.html. Accessed July 13, 2015.

54. Ascone D, Lindsey T, Varghese C. An examination of driver distraction as recorded in NHT-SA databases. DOT HS 821 216. Washington, DC: National Highway Traffic Safety Administration; 2009. Available at: http://www-nrd.nhtsa.dot.gov/Pubs/821336.pdf.

55. Teen safe driving: shifting teen attitudes. Allstate Foundation; 2009. Available at: http://www.allstatefoundation.org/Shifting-Teen-Attitudes.

56. Wilson FA, Stimpson JP. Trends in fatalities from distracted driving in the United States, 1999 to 2008. American Journal of Public Health 2010;101:2213–9.

57. Box S. New data from Virginia Tech Transportation Institute provides insight into cell phone use and driving distraction. Blacksburg (VA): Virginia Tech News; 2009. Available at: http://www.vtnews.vt.edu/articles/2009/07/2009-571.html.

58. Preventing texting while driving through education and technology. Safe texting campaign. Available at: http://safetextingcampaign.com. Accessed July 13, 2015.
59. White AG, Buboltz W, Igou F. Mobile phone use and sleep quality and length in college students. Internat J Humanit Soc Sci 2011;1:5–58.
60. Murdock KK. Texting while stressed: implications for students' burnout, sleep, and well-being. Psychol Pop Media Cult 2013;2:207–21.
61. Fossum I, Nordnes L, Storemark S, et al. The association between use of electronic media in bed before going to sleep and insomnia symptoms, daytime sleepiness, morningness, and chronotype. Behav Sleep Med 2014;12(5):343–57.
62. Faruqui F, Khubchandani J, Price JH, et al. Sleep disorders in children: a national assessment of primary care pediatrician practices and perceptions. Pediatrics 2011;130:539–48.
63. Frumkin H, Jacobson A, Gansler T, et al. Cellular phones and risk of brain tumors. CA Cancer J Clin 2001;51:137–41.
64. Karinen A, Heinävaara S, Nylund R, et al. Mobile phone radiation might alter protein expression in human skin. BMC Genomics 2008;9:77.
65. Independent Expert Group on Mobile Phones. Report of the group (the Stewart Report). 2000. Available at: http://www.iegmp.org.uk/report/index.htm. fatalityfacts/teenagers/2009. Accessed July 13, 2015.
66. Kheifets L, Repacholi M, Saunders R, et al. The sensitivity of children to electromagnetic fields. Pediatrics 2005;118:e303–13.
67. Davis D, Kesari S, Soskolne C, et al. Swedish review strengthened grounds for concluding that radiation from cellular and cordless phones is a probable human carcinogen. Pathophysiology 2013;20:123–9.
68. Nittby H, Brun A, Eberhardt J, et al. Increased blood–brain barrier permeability in mammalian brain 7 days after exposure to the radiation from a GSM-910 mobile phone. Pathophysiology 2009;16:104–14.
69. Mortazavi SM, Atefi M, Kholghi F. The pattern of mobile phone use and prevalence of self-reported symptoms in elementary and junior high school students in Shiraz, Iran. Iran J Med Sci 2011;36:97–104.
70. Carnagey NL, Anderson CA. Violent video game exposure and aggression: a literature review. Minerva Psichiatr 2004;45:1–18.
71. Gentile DA, Anderson CA. Violent video games: the newest media violence hazard. Westport (CT): Media Violence and Children; 2003. p. 133–54.
72. Anderson CA, Shibuya A, Ihori N, et al. Violent video game effects on aggression, empathy, and prosocial behavior in eastern and western countries: a meta-analytic review. Psychol Bull 2010;138:153–73.
73. American Academy of Pediatrics. Policy statement: children, adolescents, obesity, and the media, 130. 2011. p. 201–8.
74. Vandewater EA, Shim M, Caplovitz AG. Linking obesity and activity level with children's television and video game use. J Adolesc 2004;27:71–86.
75. Drummond A, Sauer JD. Video-games do not negatively impact adolescent academic performance in science, mathematics or reading. PLoS One 2014;9: e88953.
76. Adachi P, Willoughby T. More than just fun and games: the longitudinal relationships between strategic video games, self-reported problem solving skills, and academic grades. J Youth Adolesc 2013;42:42–7.
77. American Academy of Pediatrics. Managing media: we need a plan. 2013. Available at: https://www.aap.org/en-us/about-the-aap/aap-press-room/pages/managing-media-we-need-a-plan.aspx. Accessed July 13, 2015.

78. American Academy of Pediatrics. Bullying and cyberbullying. Available at: https://www.aap.org/en-us/advocacy-and-policy/aap-health-initiatives/Medical-Home-for-Children-and-Adolescents-Exposed-to-Violence/Pages/Bullying-and-Cyberbullying.aspx. Accessed July 13, 2015.
79. National Crime Prevention Council. Cyberbullying: spotting the signs. 2010. Available at: http://www.ncpc.org/topics/cyberbullying/cyberbullying-tip-sheets/NCPC%20Tip%20Sheet%20-%20Spotting%20The%20Signs.pdf. Accessed July 13, 2015.
80. Broughton B. Keeping kids safe in cyberspace: pediatricians should talk to patients, parents about Internet dangers. AAP News; 2005. Available at: http://aapnews.aappublications.org/content/26/8/11.full.

# Ethical Issues in Pediatric Global Health

Lisa Adams, MD[a], Gautham K. Suresh, MD, DM, MS[b], Tim Lahey, MD, MMSc[a,c,*]

## KEYWORDS

• Ethics • Global health • Child welfare • Cultural competency • Poverty

## KEY POINTS

• Poverty and health disparities intensify the ethical challenges of pediatric health care.

• Ethical challenges in the pediatric global health context can arise at the individual and organizational levels.

• The individual ethical challenges in pediatric global health range from respect for aid recipient autonomy to balancing outreach work with other life priorities.

• The organizational ethical challenges in pediatric global health range from scarce resource allocation decisions to coping with corruption.

• Respectful and collaborative cross-cultural communications are key to the resolution of any ethical challenge in the pediatric global health context.

## INTRODUCTION

Children constitute a disadvantaged and vulnerable subset of the population, both as recipients of health care and as research subjects. Because children may not be able to speak or be heard about their wishes or interests in matters related to their health, their care depends on the reasoning and decisions made by adults: their parents, caregivers, and/or health care providers, a situation that can generate significant ethical challenges. Most adults care deeply for children, but may face difficult decisions that balance the child's immediate needs with other pressing interests, such as the needs of other dependents. These challenges are universal but exacerbated

Disclosures: None.
[a] Section of Infectious Diseases and International Health, Geisel School of Medicine at Dartmouth, 1 Rope Ferry Road, Hanover, NH 03755-1404, USA; [b] Department of Pediatric Medicine, Neonatology, The Newborn Center, Texas Children's Hospital, Baylor College of Medicine, 6621 Fannin, WT6104, Houston, TX 77030, USA; [c] Section of Infectious Diseases and International Health, Clinical Ethics Committee, Dartmouth-Hitchcock Medical Center, One Medical Center Drive, Lebanon, NH 03756, USA
* Corresponding author. Section of Infectious Diseases and International Health, Clinical Ethics Committee, Dartmouth-Hitchcock Medical Center, One Medical Center Drive, Lebanon, NH 03756.
E-mail address: Timothy.Lahey@Dartmouth.edu

Pediatr Clin N Am 63 (2016) 195–208
http://dx.doi.org/10.1016/j.pcl.2015.09.002
0031-3955/16/$ – see front matter © 2016 Elsevier Inc. All rights reserved.

by poverty, scarce health resources, and social inequities, the very essence of pediatric global health work.

Ethical issues affect many key areas of pediatric global health, including clinical care, medical education and training, health system improvement, and research. In this article, we discuss the complex ethical challenges that arise in the pediatric global health context at individual and organizational levels from the viewpoints of both low-income and middle-income countries (LMIC) and high-income countries (HIC). Decisions can range from issues pertinent to a single child's health, such as whether caregivers should solicit his or her assent to a surgical procedure, to issues that occur at a national level, such as whether receipt of age-appropriate vaccinations should be mandated for school entry. Collaborative and respectful communication can help resolve many of the ethical issues that arise in a pediatric global health context.

## SLOW PROGRESS IN CHILD HEALTH

Child health is historically neglected. More than 6 million children died in 2013, with more than half succumbing to preventable and/or treatable conditions.[1] Diarrheal diseases, pneumonia, and measles continue to be the leading causes of death in children despite the availability of vaccines, oral rehydration therapy, and antibiotics to prevent, treat, or cure these illnesses. In 1982, the executive director of the United Nations International Children's Emergency Fund (UNICEF), James P. Grant, called the high number of deaths in children a "silent emergency" to emphasize the global lack of awareness of this problem.[2] Despite considerable progress in reducing child mortality in the past decade, the total number of deaths in children younger than 5 years has gone from more than 8 million in 2005 to 6.6 million in 2012, the gains have not been evenly distributed.[3] A child born in a low-income country (LIC) is 30 times more likely to die before his or her fifth birthday than a child born in an HIC.[4] Such disparities are both unethical and unjust.

Drug development for childhood illnesses has lagged behind the development for diseases that primarily affect adults for several reasons, but certainly the lack of financial incentive for the pharmaceutical industry has been an important driver. Most of the world's children are dying in LICs from diseases associated with poor infrastructure. In these settings, there is little or no market incentive for companies to invest in drug discovery and development. Although an estimated 80,000 children who are negative for human immunodeficiency virus (HIV) die each year of the infectious disease tuberculosis (TB), one for which we have effective treatment, a lack of child-friendly formulations has made treating children with TB a challenge.[5] In at least one low-income setting, Tanzania, parents and caregivers report having to crush tablets, measure a specific fraction of the powder, and then mix it with food or drink to mask the bitter taste to administer each dose of medication to their child.[6] Despite having had effective medications for TB for more than 50 years, the first child-friendly formulations are expected to be available next year. Due to consistent advocacy, the history of unethical neglect of childhood morbidity and mortality is ending and child health issues are receiving greater attention and funding.

The exclusion of children from research trials for new drugs or diagnostics may have been motivated by the desire to protect children from potential harm, but has had the unintended consequence that interventions proven successful in adults were denied to children because of the lack of data in younger-age cohorts. Commenting on the dearth of data on TB in children as compared with adults, South African pediatrician Peter Donald remarked, "the time has come for the hidden epidemic of childhood

TB to emerge from the shadow of adult TB and be seen as a neglected child health problem of considerable proportions...."[7]

## THE HUMAN RIGHT TO HEALTH

In recognition of the heightened vulnerabilities of children to abuse and neglect, the United Nations (UN) codified the rights of children in 2 landmark documents. Its 1948 Universal Declaration of the Human Rights provided a broad framework for basic human rights, but it left significant gaps with regard to the unique needs of children. Consequently, in 1952, the UN adopted the Declaration of the Rights of the Child[8] and urged all of its member states to abide by these principles to protect and nurture its children. Concerned that the this general guidance needed specific actionable mandates, the UN General Assembly passed the UN Convention on the Rights of the Child in November 1989 and swiftly moved to implementation a few months later. Aimed at ensuring that governments, institutions, citizens, and families all act in a manner that promotes the best interests of the child, this was the first legally binding international document on protecting the rights of children.[9] These important foundational documents were followed years later by the creation of the UN Millennium Development Goals, which place significant emphasis on the health, education, and welfare of children.[10] Despite having high-level guidance regarding the treatment of children from a human rights perspective and admirable development targets designed to improve the welfare of the world's poorest children, ethical dilemmas involving children still occur.

## THE PERILS OF ACTING IN LOCO PARENTIS

Children are generally dependent on adults for their basic needs, such as food, shelter, and care. Generally, those adults will behave in accordance with the best interests of the child. When this is not the case, such as in cases of abuse or neglect, the child is best removed from that setting. Poverty complicates all of these dynamics.

The decision to remove the adult as a surrogate decision-maker is straightforward in extreme situations, it is unclear how to achieve the best interests of the child when the parent or caregiver is merely responding to complex incentives or when adults from different cultures, LMIC parents and HIC health care providers, for instance, perceive the best interests of the child differently.

Parents in many impoverished countries must choose between food for the family and education even when they know education is important to child well-being. Irregular attendance at clinic appointments or nonadherence to treatment recommendations can occur not from lack of commitment to a child's well-being but because competing demands such as work and care of other children preclude them.[11–16] We saw this dynamic frequently in our pediatric HIV clinic in Dar es Salaam, Tanzania, where children frequently missed appointments or doses of needed HIV medications not due to a failure to understand the importance of these interventions, but because their parents needed to provide care to another, acutely child in the family.

The Convention on the Rights of the Child, although an earnest attempt to establish the essential rights of children worldwide, does not resolve the complex background values, social structures, or provide a universally accepted approach to pediatric decision-making.[17] Except in the case of emancipated minors, parents or guardians have considerable latitude in making decisions for their child. Local religious, social, and legal frameworks across countries generally support this practice. Health care providers have a duty to act in the best interests of their patients. Ethical conflicts can arise when medical recommendations are at odds with the decisions parents or guardians are making for their child.

In the context of a global health partnership, individuals from LMICs can come into loose collaboration with individuals from HICs, such as the United States. As those individuals may not share cultural assumptions, and thus see the prioritization of various aspects of child health differently, ethical issues can arise. As an example, an HIC provider may perceive a child as neglected because he or she is doing manual labor instead of attending school, whereas a parent from an LMIC may prioritize obtaining adequate resources to feed the family over child education. In such cross-cultural interactions, ethical issues can arise that may have different resolutions depending on the resources available and locally prevalent cultural assumptions.

The complexity of such decision-making requires respectful and culturally humble interactions between individuals from different areas of the world.

### Ethical Issues That Arise for Individual Providers

Major ethical issues that arise at a provider level in the pediatric global health context include respect for the autonomy of aid recipients, scope of professional duties in LMICs, and balancing outreach work with other life priorities (**Box 1**).

#### Respect for the autonomy of aid recipients

What moral responsibility, if any, do HICs have to assist LMICs in the care of their pediatric population? Many types of assistance are provided through bilateral funding, direct health care service delivery, technical assistance, training, and donations of materials and supplies. In some instances, this assistance can range from beneficial to neutral to harmful.[18] Much of the assistance HICs have provided to LMICs has been paternalistic, with wealthy countries deciding what poorer countries must need, or should have. One notable example is the frequency with which inappropriate drug

---

**Box 1**
**Ethical issues in pediatric global health pertinent to individual providers and organizations**

*General issues*

- Lack of adequate consultation regarding issues pertaining to LMIC site
- Unequal burdens and benefits of partnerships
- Inadequate identification and evaluation of benefits to LMIC
- Funding differentials

*Individual providers*

- Respect for autonomy of aid recipients
- Assent, consent, and disclosure
- Scope of professional duties in LMICs
- Balancing global health work with other priorities

*Organizations*

- Allocation of scarce resources
- Conflicts of interests
- Corruption and kickbacks

*Abbreviation:* LMIC, low-and middle-income countries.

donations have been made to LICs, particularly in postdisaster or crisis situations.[19,20] These donations are frequently not appropriate for the needs of the population, are misused, and can interfere with local pharmaceutical policies and production. Thus, the legacy of colonialism can continue through the practices of humanitarian assistance long after colonized countries achieve their independence. Such paternalistic actions are not only unhelpful, they disrespect the recipient country's autonomy, and worse, burden the country with the challenge and cost of disposing of inappropriate or expired medications. These ill-conceived programs violate the precept of nonmaleficence in medical bioethics, and also the important medical axiom "primum non nocere" or "first, do no harm."[21]

Fortunately, today more global health initiatives are being led by recipient countries, thereby ensuring that they are responsive to their actual needs. For example, the Rwandan Human Resources for Health program is fully led by the Rwandan Ministry of Health (MOH). In addition, the Rwandan MOH contracts directly with US medical schools for their faculty time rather than having a US-based entity as the intermediary.[22] Additionally, adding the voices of high-income activists and policy-makers to those of our low-income partners has been effective in advocating that resources and research be directed to the previously neglected childhood diseases that result in the disproportionate number of deaths of poor children. Organizations such as the Global Alliance for TB Drug Development, based in New York, or Drugs for Neglected Diseases initiative (DNDi), based in Geneva, are 2 such examples of groups that advocate and support drug development and distribution for otherwise neglected diseases among vulnerable patient populations, including children. This can help ensure that pediatric global health engagement is focused primarily on the true needs of the host countries and not on the ego gratification that can come to people from HICs who choose to work in LMICs.

Engaging in support and assistance of others from a culture different from one's own is fraught with ethical challenges. Although the goal may be to benefit the pediatric population in that country or community, well-intentioned outsiders wanting to act benevolently but who do not understand the cultural context can do a significant amount of damage. Too often, we try to impose our cultural and social priorities onto those we are trying to assist, disrespecting their autonomy and acting in an offensive (at best) or dangerous (at worst) manner. Attempts to provide aid or care to others without a deep sense of the cultural complexities or social dynamics of the recipient community or an understanding of its priorities are generally doomed to failure.

One of the most difficult ethical challenges in pediatric global health has been how to approach the practice of female genital mutilation or cutting (FGM) in many countries in sub-Saharan Africa. Most Westerners find this practice abhorrent and unethical. This raises the distinction of moral universalism, the stance that some ethical dictums are absolute regardless of cultural, religious, or other belief systems, and moral relativism, which holds that standards of what is right or wrong will vary by culture. For the moral relativists, to indicate there is a universal moral code is akin to moral imperialism. For moral universalists, FGM is simply wrong in any setting. However, showing respect for another's culture and traditions need not require that one agree with its beliefs. The World Health Organization and human rights groups consider FGM a violation of the human rights of girls and women.[23] What, then, is the ethical responsibility of health care providers in this situation? It is important to understand that parents who subject their daughters to the FGM typically do so because they love their daughters.[24] Recognizing the power and importance of local traditions should guide how physicians approach this culturally bound practice. However, the health risks and detrimental consequences associated with FGM are significant, and physicians have a duty to inform parents of these if considering FGM for their daughters.[25] Some pediatricians have found that a respectful dialogue, held in a neutral, nonjudgmental manner, allows parents to speak openly about this practice. In the countries in which FGM is still practiced, broad community mobilization efforts focused on improving health literacy and education about human rights have been shown to be effective and have been successfully replicated.[26]

Other issues related to sexual health can also present an ethical quagmire for health care providers. Discussions of sexual debut, contraception, and prevention of sexually transmitted disease including HIV can be a source of potential tension in the provider-parent-patient (child) triad. The question of gradual gaining of independence and when agency is fully conferred to the child will vary by community and can even differ at the level of the family or individual. Determining a family's views in an open and nonjudgmental manner will again be an important guide for health care providers, but the ethical challenges arise when parental beliefs differ from what the medical and social science evidence indicates. In cases in which there is disagreement between the parent and provider, does the provider's duty to the patient (child) supersede the parental authority for deciding what health information the child receives?

Similar to sharing sexual health information, the issue of when to disclose HIV status to an infected child can lead to ideological standoffs between parents and providers. At our pediatric HIV clinic in Tanzania, our first foray with this challenge occurred when a grandparent (a respected physician in the community) told providers that his 13-year-old grandson was too young to be informed of his HIV status. (Fortunately, this situation was eventually resolved via tactful negotiation with local physicians.) When the provider or organization is an outsider to the community, this tension is often further exacerbated. Examples abound of situations in which local families or communities have been angered by what they construe as foreign providers or international organizations promoting a Western ideology that is in direct conflict with their culture and social belief system. One such program that we have been affiliated with uses soccer coaches to educate youth about HIV prevention through promoting personal efficacy. Despite its foundation in social learning theory and youth mental health development, this program initially faced criticism for importing a presumed Western approach to more traditional cultures in Southern Africa. Engaging in an ongoing respectful dialogue with parents and/or community leadership and allied community-based groups is essential to resolving such ideological clashes. The health care provider should, however, uphold his or her ethical obligation to provide sound, evidence-based health information that will promote the health of the patient.[27] Doing this against a backdrop of open inquiry and honest conversation with respect for individual and local beliefs will be the most effective approach for reaching a mutually agreeable resolution.

### Assent, consent, and disclosure

Perhaps the most prevalent ethical challenge that arises in the care of children worldwide revolves around the balance of paternalism with respect for patient autonomy. The youngest children cannot give true informed consent, yet respect for child autonomy mandates that adults involved in their care attempt to engage their autonomy in an age-appropriate fashion. The term for a child's approval of an intervention for which they cannot give full informed consent is "assent."[28]

The age threshold above which providers should seek not just assent but full consent varies according to local custom and also according to the intellectual and decision-making capacity of individual children.[29] The treatment of infectious diseases exemplifies this dynamic. An infant with a severe ear infection is treated with antibiotics without asking permission, whereas clinicians providing intravenous antibiotics to an 8-year-old boy hospitalized with pneumonia would ask the boy's assent before inserting the intravenous catheter. By contrast, an adolescent with a sexually transmitted disease might be treated without parental notification should the adolescent request it.

In a global health context, judgments about the age of assent versus the age of consent, and which health issues can be handled privately may vary by country and may be informed by cultural factors about which a provider may be only partially aware. As a result, a provider from an HIC who is comfortable providing treatment for an adolescent with a sexually transmitted disease without consulting the parents may face staunch parental opposition when practicing in a country in which the prevalent culture prioritizes parental authority over child privacy, in contrast to the provider's home country.

There is no single correct approach to the resolution of the ethical conflicts that arise as a result of such different base assumptions. Ultimately the HIC provider may provide the same level of care to the adolescent with a sexually transmitted disease in an LMIC context as would be done in an HIC setting, but perhaps put more emphasis on encouraging parental consultation in the LMIC context out of respect for the locally prevalent practices. To shape defensible ethical decision-making, ideally the HIC provider should consult with host country providers and community leaders regarding local cultural assumptions that might influence general pediatric health care so that when sensitive individual situations arise, the response can be respectful of such host country cultural preferences.[30]

### Scope of professional duties in low-income and middle-income settings

Resource scarcity is a daily challenge for individuals working in pediatric global health. In many ways, scarcity can conflict with provider professional obligations. Health care workers can feel unable to execute on the mandate to provide the best care possible for patients, for instance, if resources are too scarce to allow for the provision of standard medicines and surgical procedures. Simple acceptance of what is possible given local resource limitations can be expedient, and may even be seen as culturally competent, but may perpetuate local resource limitations by representing a failure to fight those limitations. Yet, pragmatically, health care providers working in LMICs need to care for children with the resources available to them. They must, therefore, make transparent decisions about what kind of care they can provide responsibly within those locally specific limitations, and which kinds of care are simply precluded until pitched efforts to improve funding succeed. Health care workers, both local and foreign, can, and should, advocate for improved conditions and better resources for their patients in such settings.

A key component of the satisfaction of professional obligations to provide the best care possible within the limits of the local context is a commitment to working within the scope of one's professional practice. It is common for students and other early-career providers to be asked to provide a level of service that would be deemed outside the scope of their professional practice in an HIC. For instance, we have mentored medical students asked to perform unsupervised delivery of babies in Africa and another who performed unsupervised cranial burr hole procedures in adolescents with intracranial bleeding after traumatic brain injuries while volunteering in a South American jungle clinic. In both cases, students were told that without their help the patients would die. Situations like these pose a difficult ethical challenge: pediatric global health providers may feel obligated to choose between denial of services or the provision of services they would never attempt in their host country.

There is no simple solution to this conundrum. LMIC medical systems have shown that nonphysician providers can be trained to render high-quality care to children. For example, in areas with low numbers of physicians, nurses and other nonphysician providers (eg, community health workers or peer-counselors) can deliver high-quality antiretroviral therapy (ART) to children with HIV.[31] This is a good reminder that the system of health care provision in HICs like the United States can be wasteful and inefficient and likely benefit from adopting innovative community-based approaches proven effective in LMICs. Yet it is important for providers from HICs not to enforce inadequate access to appropriate quality services in LMICs by allowing or encouraging trainees to practice outside of their scope for the purposes of their own education, by engaging in such practices themselves, or by accepting ad hoc medical services by inadequately trained providers who seem to address a pressing medical need but in fact do not do so sufficiently. One way of discriminating between innovation and unprofessional provision of substandard of care is to measure outcomes and engage in quality improvement work to improve them when needed.

### Balancing global health work with other life priorities

Health care providers who care for children in a global health context are often highly committed people who want the best for children. Given the enormity of the obstacles to optimal child health in such settings, providers can be impelled to work demanding schedules that conflict with other life priorities, such as giving attention to their own families and/or provision for personal health and well-being. Although potentially appropriate in short-term crises, an excessive engagement with the work of pediatric global health to the exclusion of other personally meaningful life priorities is usually not sustainable and may in the long term undermine the efficacy and durability of pediatric global health work through the development of burnout.[32] As a result, there is an ethical argument to be made that the ideal approach to pediatric global health work is a balanced engagement that promotes long-term commitment and is not ultimately undermined by neglect of other major life obligations and enjoyment. Not only can trumpeting this concept help protect sustained global health work, but it can improve recruitment to the work if potential candidates recognize pediatric global health work can be balanced with other life goals.

### Ethical Issues That Arise at an Organizational Level

Individual health care providers working in pediatric global health face formidable ethical challenges that are complementary to but somewhat different from those faced by people leading organizational or governmental pediatric global health efforts. These ethical issues include scarce resource allocation decision-making, the potential conflicts of interest that can arise with pediatric global health interventions, and even corruption. We address each of these issues in the following sections.

### Allocation of scarce resources

Health care providers working in LMICs all face challenging decisions about the allocation of scarce resources. Children are usually unable to advocate for resources themselves, so their health needs are frequently prioritized lower in disbursements from governmental and other aid agencies. This problem is particularly acute in the sphere of pediatric global health. This can bring core health needs of children into conflict, for instance when funding for preventive measures like vaccines or nutritional interventions is seen as diverting support from efforts directed at acute and lethal illnesses, such as the treatment of diarrheal diseases and malaria.

Choices between competing health needs of children can be made all the more challenging by the balkanization of aid efforts in pediatric global health. If one agency supports vaccine development and another distributes oral rehydration solution for pediatric diarrheal disease, then health programs may feel obligated to choose between them or divide resources in ways that do not capitalize on potential synergies (eg, separate and distinct trainings for each rather than one on comprehensive child health). One way of eluding this trap of dichotomous thinking is for aid efforts to move from vertical to horizontal approaches to health care, such as has been promoted through the integrated community case management of childhood illness.[33] This strategy still places emphasis on childhood illness assessment and treatment rather than the marrying of illness assessment with disease prevention and health promotion, but has certainly been a step in the right direction.

The identification of synergies between potentially competing priorities in pediatric global health, and thus the trap of categorizing child health in distinct disease silos, helps, yet amid inadequate resources some challenges are unavoidable. From there, the optimal approach involves both a pragmatic response to the limits of funding and vigorous resistance of those selfsame limitations. In addition, respect for the autonomy of children in global health settings mandates partnership with host country decision-makers so that allocation decisions reflect local priorities and not solely those imposed by HIC providers. Further, an iterative collaborative process of reassessment of the wisdom of resource distribution decisions, and an alignment of the next wave of decisions to evolving health needs, is critical. This can avoid inadvertent misallocation of resources, such as can occur if the most effective organizations target pediatric health needs that are less urgent than those prioritized by less effective organizations. The proper allocation to prioritized health issues is a key role of host country governments, which can help align the distribution of nongovernmental organizations to national pediatric health priorities.

### Conflicts of interest that can arise when pediatric global health interventions are motivated by commercial, religious, political, or research agendas

Pediatric global health interventions can be implemented or affected by commercial, religious, and political agendas. These can be promulgated by service agencies themselves, such as when pediatric formula companies offer free or cut-rate access to substandard nutritional options or medications to mothers in LMICs. An internationally decried research example is the unregulated experimental provision by Pfizer of the nonstandard antibiotic trovofloxacin to pediatric patients with meningitis in Nigeria in 1996.[34] Another example, this time involving a government-supported organization, comes from the President's Emergency Plan for AIDS Relief (PEPFAR). In its early days of program implementation, PEPFAR disbursed funds only to organizations that abided by its pledge against sex work and abstinence-only education programming even though the former could endanger adolescent sex workers,[35–37] and the latter was demonstrably less effective than other prevention measures in keeping youth safe.[38]

### Corruption and kickbacks

Corruption occurs worldwide, but by virtue of their dependent status, children are especially vulnerable to it. It is thus unsurprising that child mortality rates are associated with corruption.[39] Corrupt individuals, and organizations, can cadge funds from both governmental and nongovernmental organizations in HICs and LMICs alike. Corruption may be widespread in particular countries like Nigeria, in which it has been described as part of the fabric of certain segments of the local culture,[40] but it is particularly distressing when it depletes funds meant for children in need. Outrage is appropriate, as is a systematic avoidance of corrupt individuals and organizations.[41] These natural and ultimately productive inclinations, however, should be modulated by the recognition that definitions of corruption can vary from culture to culture, and even when a particular activity is universally understood as corrupt, it may appear more egregious when perceived across a gradient of cultural difference. This sensibility should lead to collaboration with local leaders who can help health care providers working in a pediatric global health context to identify collaborative guidelines for the definition and response to corruption.

### The Crucial Need for Global Health Ethics Education for Trainees and Faculty

In recent years, there has been rapid development of global health programs at US universities, with faculty and trainees actively engaged in service, education, and research missions.[42] Given the complex ethical issues this engagement will engender,[43] academic institutions and departments engaged in pediatric global health programs should implement competency-based curriculum in global pediatric health for trainees and faculty.[44,45] The Consortium of Universities of Global Health Education Committee recently published a broad, interprofessional global health competency framework, which may lead to further curricula development, implementation, and evaluation.[46] It is crucial to have meaningful and ethical experiences for trainees and other health care providers engaged in short-term global health research or service projects, protect communities from potential harm, and foster sustainable partnerships to improve global health and reduce disparities.[47] A Working Group on Ethics Guidelines for Global Health Training (WEIGHT) has developed best practice guidelines.[48] An innovative, 10-case online curriculum "Ethical Challenges in Short-term Global Health Training" (freely available at http://ethicsandglobalhealth.org) has been developed by Johns Hopkins Berman Institute of Bioethics in collaboration with Stanford University Center for Innovation in Global Health.[49] This and other freely available online curricula related to short-term global health ethics education are depicted in **Box 2**. Given the wide array of ethical, social, and cultural issues in global health research conducted in LMICs, there is a growing interest in the development of Consultation Services in Research Ethics (CSRE) to complement the traditional institutional review board ethics review.[50] The role of CSRE may be particularly useful to implement global health research projects funded and implemented by organizations and researchers in HICs. The conduct and design of pediatric global health research should comply with current international research regulations and conform to high ethical standards to protect the rights and

---

**Box 2**
**Free online curricula for short-term global health ethics education**

- Stanford Center for Innovation in Global Health and Johns Hopkins Berman Institute of Bioethics, "Ethical Challenges in Short-term Global Health Training" http://ethicsandglobal health.org

- Unite for Site Volunteer Ethics and Online Professionalism Course http://www.uniteforsight. org/international-volunteering/

- University of British Columbia, "Ethics of International Engagement and Service-Learning Project" http://ethicsofisl.ubc.ca/

*Data from* DeCamp M, Rodriguez J, Hecht S, et al. An ethics curriculum for short-term global health trainees. Global Health 2013;9:5.

safety of research participants. The ethical issues related to child health research in LMICs are shown in **Box 3**.[51]

### Importance of Cultural Humility and Collaboration

We have discussed the myriad ethical issues that arise in a pediatric global health context either at an individual or organizational level. Each can bring LMIC and HIC individuals into collaboration, and potentially conflict, and thus effective skills in cross-cultural communication are necessary regardless of the situational particulars.

A key consideration in all such circumstances is a true partnership between LMIC and HIC players in which local LMIC prioritization of health needs strongly shapes the pediatric global health interventions funded in large part by HIC donors. One critical component of this collaboration is the gradual transfer of economic or programmatic autonomy to LMIC partners as capacity on the ground allows it. Put another way, the best pediatric global health programs plan for the eventual obsolescence of the HIC donors and shift the LMIC and HIC collaborations into truly equitable partnerships based on common research and educational interests.

### SUMMARY

To meet the health needs of vulnerable children in a global health context, adults from LMICs and HICs must collaborate across cultural differences and amid resource constraints. This work is an ethical minefield (see **Box 1**). At an individual level, the ethical issues that inevitably arise include navigating pediatric assent and consent to defining professional role boundaries in resource-limited settings. No less challenging are the ethical issues that arise at an organizational level, from difficult decisions regarding the allocation of scarce resources to balancing the complicated mixture of commercial, religious, and political agendas that can motivate pediatric global health outreach work. This complicated skill set is summarized in **Fig. 1**. Although each issue has its individual challenges and approaches to resolution, in every case the establishment of respectful cross-cultural, multidisciplinary, and interprofessional partnerships between LMIC and HIC providers is indispensable.

---

**Box 3**
**Ethical issues in pediatric global health research**

- Promote equity in child health
- Identify local research needs
- Develop culturally sensitive research methods
- Adherence to universal ethical standards of care
- Commitment to distributive justice
- Establish a valid informed consent/assent process
- Capacity building of local ethical review to protect research subjects
- Impact of research on child health within the community
- Community engagement
- Benefit sharing and what should happen after research completion

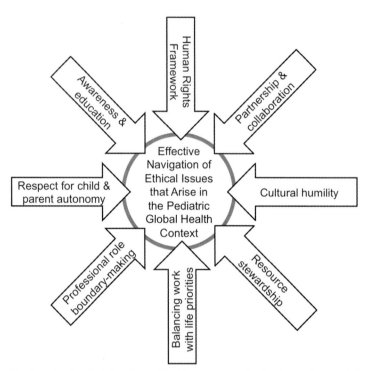

**Fig. 1.** Critical methods of addressing ethical issues that arise in the pediatric global health context.

## REFERENCES

1. World Health Organization. Children: reducing mortality. 2014. Available at: http://www.who.int/mediacentre/factsheets/fs178/en/. Accessed May 28, 2015.
2. Grant JP. Children in dark times: a year of silent emergency. Draper Fund Rep 1982;(11):1–4.
3. United Nations Children's Fund. Every child counts: revealing disparities, advancing children's rights. New York: United Nations Children's Fund; 2014. Available at: http://www.unicef.org/gambia/SOWC_report_2014.pdf. Accessed June 9, 2015.
4. Jones G, Steketee RW, Black RE, et al, Bellagio child survival study Group. How many child deaths can we prevent this year? Lancet 2003;362(9377):65–71.
5. World Health Organization. Global tuberculosis report 2014. 2015. Available at: http://apps.who.int/iris/bitstream/10665/137094/1/9789241564809_eng.pdf?ua=1. Accessed September 29, 2015.
6. Adams LV, Craig SR, Mmbaga EJ, et al. Children's medicines in Tanzania: a national survey of administration practices and preferences. PLos One 2013;8(3): e58303.
7. Donald PR. Childhood tuberculosis: the hidden epidemic. Int J Tuberc Lung Dis 2004;8(5):627–9.
8. United Nations. Geneva declaration of the rights of the child. 1924. Available at: http://www.un-documents.net/gdrc1924.htm. Accessed May 28, 2015.
9. Oberg CN. Embracing international children's rights: from principles to practice. Clin Pediatr 2012;51(7):619–24.

10. United Nations. We can end poverty: millennium development goals and beyond 2015. 2015. Available at: http://www.un.org/millenniumgoals/. Accessed June 9, 2015.

11. Kalyango JN, Hall M, Karamagi C. Appointment keeping for medical review among patients with selected chronic diseases in an urban area of Uganda. Pan Afr Med J 2014;19:229.

12. Samuels RC, Ward VL, Melvin P, et al. Missed appointments: factors contributing to high no-show rates in an urban pediatrics primary care clinic. Clin Pediatr 2015;54(10):976–82.

13. Pesata V, Pallija G, Webb AA. A descriptive study of missed appointments: families' perceptions of barriers to care. J Pediatr Health Care 1999;13(4):178–82.

14. Bigna JJ, Noubiap JJ, Plottel CS, et al. Factors associated with non-adherence to scheduled medical follow-up appointments among Cameroonian children requiring HIV care: a case-control analysis of the usual-care group in the MORE CARE trial. Infect Dis Poverty 2014;3(1):44.

15. Tweya H, Gugsa S, Hosseinipour M, et al. Understanding factors, outcomes and reasons for loss to follow-up among women in Option B+ PMTCT programme in Lilongwe, Malawi. Trop Med Int Health 2014;19(11):1360–6.

16. Weigel R, Makwiza I, Nyirenda J, et al. Supporting children to adhere to antiretroviral therapy in urban Malawi: multi method insights. BMC Pediatr 2009;9:45.

17. Engelhardt HT Jr. Beyond the best interests of children: four views of the family and of foundational disagreements regarding pediatric decision making. J Med Philos 2010;35(5):499–517.

18. Van Tilburg C. Controversies in medical aid to developing countries: balancing help and harm. Int Health 2015;7(3):147–8.

19. van Dijk DP, Dinant G, Jacobs JA. Inappropriate drug donations: what has happened since the 1999 WHO guidelines? Educ Health (Abingdon) 2011; 24(2):462.

20. Bero L, Carson B, Moller H, et al. To give is better than to receive: compliance with WHO guidelines for drug donations during 2000-2008. Bull World Health Organ 2010;88(12):922–9.

21. Smith CM. Origin and uses of primum non nocere–above all, do no harm! J Clin Pharmacol 2005;45(4):371–7.

22. Binagwaho A, Kyamanywa P, Farmer PE, et al. The human resources for health program in Rwanda–new partnership. N Engl J Med 2013;369(21):2054–9.

23. World Health Organization. Female genital mutilation. 2014. Available at: http://www.who.int/mediacentre/factsheets/fs241/en/. Accessed May 28, 2015.

24. Jaeger F, Caflisch M, Hohlfeld P. Female genital mutilation and its prevention: a challenge for paediatricians. Eur J Pediatr 2009;168(1):27–33.

25. Hearst AA, Molnar AM. Female genital cutting: an evidence-based approach to clinical management for the primary care physician. Mayo Clin Proc 2013; 88(6):618–29.

26. Ellsberg M, Arango DJ, Morton M, et al. Prevention of violence against women and girls: what does the evidence say? Lancet 2015;385(9977):1555–66.

27. Lieberman LD, Fagen MC, Neiger BL. Evaluating programs that address ideological issues: ethical and practical considerations for practitioners and evaluators. Health Prom Pract 2014;15(2):161–7.

28. De Lourdes Levy M, Larcher V, Kurz R. Ethics Working Group of the Confederation of European Specialists in Pediatrics. Informed consent/assent in children. Statement of the Ethics Working Group of the Confederation of European Specialists in Paediatrics (CESP). Eur J Pediatr 2003;162(9):629–33.

29. Informed consent, parental permission, and assent in pediatric practice. Committee on Bioethics, American Academy of Pediatrics. Pediatrics 1995;95(2):314–7.

30. Prainsack B, Buyx A. Solidarity in contemporary bioethics–towards a new approach. Bioethics 2012;26(7):343–50.

31. Kredo T, Adeniyi FB, Bateganya M, et al. Task shifting from doctors to non-doctors for initiation and maintenance of antiretroviral therapy. Cochrane Database Syst Rev 2014;(7):CD007331.

32. Raviola G, Machoki M, Mwaikambo E, et al. HIV, disease plague, demoralization and "burnout": resident experience of the medical profession in Nairobi, Kenya. Cult Med Psychiatry 2002;26(1):55–86.

33. Young M, Wolfheim C, Marsh DR, et al. World Health Organization/United Nations Children's Fund joint statement on integrated community case management: an equity-focused strategy to improve access to essential treatment services for children. Am J Trop Med Hyg 2012;87(5 Suppl):6–10.

34. Malakoff D. Human research. Nigerian families sue Pfizer, testing the reach of US law. Science 2001;293(5536):1742.

35. Silverman JG. Adolescent female sex workers: invisibility, violence and HIV. Arch Dis Child 2011;96(5):478–81.

36. Masenior NF, Beyrer C. The US anti-prostitution pledge: first amendment challenges and public health priorities. PLoS Med 2007;4(7):e207.

37. Ditmore MH, Allman D. An analysis of the implementation of PEPFAR's anti-prostitution pledge and its implications for successful HIV prevention among organizations working with sex workers. J Internat AIDS Soc 2013;16:17354.

38. Santelli JS, Speizer IS, Edelstein ZR. Abstinence promotion under PEPFAR: the shifting focus of HIV prevention for youth. Glob Public Health 2013;8(1):1–12.

39. Hanf M, Van-Melle A, Fraisse F, et al. Corruption kills: estimating the global impact of corruption on children deaths. PLoS One 2011;6(11):e26990.

40. Smith DJ. Corruption, NGOs, and development in Nigeria. Third World Q 2010;31(2).

41. Eaton L. Global Fund toughens stance against corruption. BMJ 2005;331(7519):718.

42. Merson MH. University engagement in global health. N Engl J Med 2014;370(18): 1676–8.

43. Provenzano AM, Graber LK, Elansary M, et al. Short-term global health research projects by US medical students: ethical challenges for partnerships. Am J Trop Med Hyg 2010;83(2):211–4.

44. Howard CR, Gladding SP, Kiguli S, et al. Development of a competency-based curriculum in global child health. Acad Med 2011;86(4):521–8.

45. Tzel R, Kurbasic M, Staton D, et al. Academic Pediatric Association, Global Health Task Force. Faculty competencies for global health. Pediatrics 2015;135(6):e1535.

46. Jogerst K, Callender B, Adams V, et al. Identifying interprofessional global health competencies for 21st-century health professionals. Ann Glob Health 2015;81(2):239–47.

47. Pinto AD, Upshur RE. Global health ethics for students. Dev World Bioeth 2009; 9(1):1–10.

48. Crump JA, Sugarman J, Working Group on Ethics Guidelines for Global Health Training (WEIGHT). Ethics and best practice guidelines for training experiences in global health. Am J Trop Med Hyg 2010;83(6):1178–82.

49. DeCamp M, Rodriguez J, Hecht S, et al. An ethics curriculum for short-term global health trainees. Glob Health 2013;9:5.

50. Lavery JV, Green SK, Bandewar SV, et al. Addressing ethical, social, and cultural issues in global health research. PLoS Negl Trop Dis 2013;7(8):e2227.

51. Roth D. An ethics-based approach to global child health research. Paediatr Child Health 2003;8(2):67–71.

# Index

*Note:* Page numbers of article titles are in **boldface** type.

## A

Pediatr Clin N Am 63 (2016) 209–220
http://dx.doi.org/10.1016/S0031-3955(15)00188-1
0031-3955/16/$ – see front matter © 2016 Elsevier Inc. All rights reserved.

**pediatric.theclinics.com**

# Moving?

## Make sure your subscription moves with you!

To notify us of your new address, find your **Clinics Account Number** (located on your mailing label above your name), and contact customer service at:

**Email: journalscustomerservice-usa@elsevier.com**

**800-654-2452** (subscribers in the U.S. & Canada)
**314-447-8871** (subscribers outside of the U.S. & Canada)

Fax number: 314-447-8029

**Elsevier Health Sciences Division**
**Subscription Customer Service**
**3251 Riverport Lane**
**Maryland Heights, MO 63043**

*To ensure uninterrupted delivery of your subscription, please notify us at least 4 weeks in advance of move.

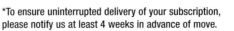

ELSEVIER